Cervical Cancer

Jaime G. de la Garza-Salazar
Flavia Morales-Vásquez
Abelardo Meneses-Garcia
Editors

Cervical Cancer

Springer

Editors
Jaime G. de la Garza-Salazar
Instituto Nacional de Cancerología
Mexico City
Mexico

Abelardo Meneses-Garcia
Instituto Nacional de Cancerología
Mexico City
Mexico

Flavia Morales-Vásquez
Instituto Nacional de Cancerología
Mexico City
Mexico

ISBN 978-3-319-45230-2 ISBN 978-3-319-45231-9 (eBook)
DOI 10.1007/978-3-319-45231-9

Library of Congress Control Number: 2017941082

Printed on acid-free paper

This Springer imprint is published by Springer Nature
The registered company is Springer International Publishing AG
The registered company address is: Gewerbestrasse 11, 6330 Cham, Switzerland

There are few books in relation of cervical cancer, but a good number of articles reporting the prevention programs and management of the surgical, radiotherapy and the Systemic treatments. Our interest is to give you in this book information about the history of the cervical cytology and the most recent epidemiology and the State of the Art in all aspects of prevention, diagnosis and the different treatments. Statistics Reports in 2012 were registered more than 14 millions new cases and 8.2 millions deaths in women and men, Cervical cancer is the third most common malignancy among women, with approximately half a million newly diagnosed cases and over 200,000 deaths annually, 85% of women dying from cervical cancer reside in developing countries
We dedícate this book to all women that have had cervical cancer and also to all women that they are able to detect the early disease, also to gynecologist and oncologist as well the general physicians that are in charge in the management of these patients. Hoping that some day in the future we can erradícate this disease with more aggressive preventive programs and the development of new vaccines.
Jaime G. de la Garza-Salazar

Preface

Cervical cancer is the third most common malignancy among women, with approximately half a million newly diagnosed cases and over 200,000 deaths annually. Although most cases of cervical cancer can be prevented by routine screening and treatment of precancerous lesions, cervical cancer is the leading cause of cancer mortality among women in developing countries.

Every year in our institution treat hundreds of patients with this neoplasia, and we want to improve the results. Dr. Jaime G. de la Garza-Salazar, Medical Oncologist, has promoted for decades the fight against cancer in Mexico and Latin America, with medical education, investigation and diffusion. Dr. Jaime G. de la Garza-Salazar thought of this book as an opportunity to drive the best results in diagnosis, treatment, palliation and research available to all doctors in the world who face this type of cancer.

With the support of Dr. Meneses and Springer this effort sees the light.

The aim of the present book is to present a general view of the Cervical Cancer and improve the prognosis of patients with this disease.

Virtually all cases of invasive cervical cancer are associated with infection by high-risk strains of human papilloma virus (VPH). Effective primary and secondary prevention programs, as well as effective treatment for early-stage invasive cancer have dramatically reduced the burden of cervical cancer in high-income countries; 85% of the mortality from cervical cancer now occurs in low- and middle-income countries.

Despite the fact that the HPV vaccine protects against high-risk HPV and has been available since 2006, only 33.4% of girls age 13–17 have completed the 3 dose vaccine.

The treatment of cervical cancer is stage-specific. While early stage disease can be cured with radiotherapy or surgery, the most effective treatment for locally advanced stage patients is concurrent chemotherapy and pelvic irradiation. Typically, once weekly cisplatin is administered intravenously while a combination of external beam radiation and brachytherapy is used to treat the pelvic tumor.

Recent findings from large scale genomic sequencing of human cervical tumors has suggested that targeted therapies may present a better option. Of note, it was recently shown that addition of angiogenesis inhibitor, bevacizumab, to combination chemotherapy in patients with recurrent, persistent, or metastatic cervical cancer improved median overall survival. Despites advances in treatment, patients with metastatic cancers and those with recurrent or persistent disease have limited treatment options.

In this work, we discuss the literature supporting novel drug delivery strategies for cervical cancer treatment and highlight some of the current advancements in local and systemic treatments, for early and advanced disease.

We have special focus in persistent and recurrent cervical cancer, the Palliative Care constitutes an option oriented toward improving the life quality and symptom management of these patients and that of their relatives. The early and integral incorporation onto the handling is important for the symptomatology, physical, psychological and spiritual relief of these patients.

Mexico City, Mexico Flavia Morales-Vásquez

Acknowledgments

This book was partially supported by the Consejo Nacional de Ciencia y Tecnología, grant number 271928, Red Temática, Colegio Mexicano para la Investigación del Cáncer.

We would like to acknowledge the following persons: Luis Herrera Alonso (English translation and style correction), Sandra Garnica (secretarial work), Edmundo Alvarez (computer systems advisor), and Abha Krishnan (Project Coordinator for Springer Nature).

About the Editors

Dr. Jaime G. de la Garza-Salazar born in Monterrey, N.L., Mexico, December 12, 1934. Studies: Medical Doctor, Universidad Autónoma de Nuevo León, Mexico, 1952–1958; Postgraduate in Internal Medicine and Medical Oncology, South Texas Medicine School, San Antonio, Texas, USA, 1959–1964; Mayo Clinic, Rochester, Minnesota, 1965–1966. Doctor Honoris Causa, granted by Universidad Autónoma de Puebla, and Doctor in Medicine-Honoris Causa, granted by Universidad Autónoma de Nuevo León, Mexico; 11th Cino del Duca Award; Achievement in Cancer Research, 14th International Congress on Anti-Cancer Treatment, February 4, 2003 (Paris, France). Former general director of "Instituto Nacional de Cancerología-Mexico" (1993–2003). Distinguished Achievement Award, American Society of Clinical Oncology (ASCO) Chicago, Illinois. Author: *Inflammatory Breast Cancer*, Springer, October 2012, and *Benign Disease of the Breast*, Nova Publishers.

Dr. Flavia Morales is a medical oncologist who developed her career as a physician at Instituto Nacional de Cancerología (INCan) in Mexico. Dr. Morales is professor of oncology at the Embryology Department, School of Medicine, at Universidad Nacional Autonoma de Mexico (UNAM) and assistant professor of medical oncology at the Oncology Department in Instituto Nacional de Cancerología-UNAM. She graduated at "Universidad Veracruzana" as medical surgeon. She completed her residency in internal medicine in 1997 and then continued her residency in medical oncology. Dr. Morales has completed a master's degree in medical sciences. She attended as an oncology observer (2004–2005) at MD Anderson Cancer Center in the Breast Cancer Department "Nellie B. Connally." Her main research interests include breast and gynecologic cancers and fertility and pregnancy in patients with cancer. She has been particularly involved in the development of oncology clinical research in Mexico.

Dr. Abelardo Meneses born in Puebla, México. Studies: Medical Doctor, Universidad Autónoma de Puebla, Mexico; Ph.D., Medical School, Instituto Nacional Politécnico; Postgraduate in General Pathology and Oncological Pathology; he had a Master´s degree in Molecular Oncology. Centro de Investigación Biomédica,

Spain. He is member of Academia Mexicana de Cirugía, member of Academia Nacional de Medicina, member of Sistema Nacional de Investigadores, and general director of "Instituto Nacional de Cancerología-Mexico" (2013–2018). Co-author: *Inflammatory Breast Cancer*, Springer, October 2012, and *Benign Disease of the Breast*, Nova Publishers. Member of the Southwest Oncology Group. He has written more than 140 articles with more than 1484 citations in the Citation Index.

Contents

Contributors

José Luis Aguilar-Ponce Internal Medicine Subdirection, Instituto Nacional de Cancerología-México, Mexico City, Mexico

Francisco Javier Alcalá-Prieto Department Surgical Oncology, Instituto Nacional de Cancerología-México, Mexico City, Mexico

Roberto Alejandro Cruz-Morales Department of Radiology, Instituto Nacional de Cancerología-México, Mexico City, Mexico

Silvia Allende-Pérez Head of Palliative Care Service, Instituto Nacional de Cancerología-México, Mexico City, Mexico

Oscar Arrieta-Rodríguez Department of Medical Oncology, Instituto Nacional de Cancerología-México, Mexico City, Mexico

Horacio Astudillo-de la Vega Laboratory of Traslational Investigation and Celular Therapy, Hospital de Oncología, Centro Médico Nacional "Siglo XXI", IMSS, México City, Mexico

Salim Abraham Barquet-Muñoz Gynecologic Tumors Deparment, Instituto Nacional de Cancerología-México, Mexico City, Mexico

Department of Radiation Oncology, Centro Médico ABC, Mexico City, Mexico

Department of Gynecologic Oncology, Instituto Nacional de Cancerología-México, Mexico City, Mexico

Luis Benitez-Bribiesca Deparment of Investigation at Instituto Mexicano del Seguro Social (IMSS), Instituto Nacional de Cancerología, Mexico City, Mexico

Monika Blake-Cerda Department of Radiation Oncology, Instituto Nacional de Cancerología-México, Mexico City, Mexico

Claudia Cano-Blanco Department of Medical Oncology, Instituto Nacional de Cancerología-México, Mexico City, Mexico

David F. Cantú-de-León Division of Research, Instituto Nacional de Cancerología-México, Mexico City, Mexico

Lucely Cetina-Pérez Clinical Research Department, Instituto Nacional de Cancerología-México, Mexico City, Mexico

José G. Chanona-Vilchis Department of Pathology, Instituto Nacional de Cancerología-México, Mexico City, Mexico

Clinical Research Department, Instituto Nacional de Cancerología-México, Mexico City, Mexico

Cristian Yaoska Corea-Urbina Gynecologic Tumors Deparment, Instituto Nacional de Cancerología-México, Mexico City, Mexico

Jaime Alberto Coronel-Martínez Clinical Research Department, Instituto Nacional de Cancerología-México, Mexico City, Mexico

Jaime G. de la Garza-Salazar Department of Clinical Investigation, Instituto Nacional de Cancerología-México, Mexico City, Mexico

Georgina Domínguez-Ocadio Palliative Care Service, Instituto Nacional de Cancerología-México, Mexico City, Mexico

E. Erica Ruiz-Garcia Laboratory of Traslational Investigation, Instituto Nacional de Cancerología-México, Mexico City, Mexico

Jorge Fernández-Retana Facultad de estudios superiores Iztacala, Universidad Nacional Autónoma de México, Mexico City, Mexico

Laboratory of Funtional Genomics, Unidad de Biomedicina, FES-IZTACALA, UNAM, Tlalnepantla, Mexico

Frank D. Ferris Research and Education at OhioHealth in Columbus, Columbus, OH, USA

Carlos Galindo-Sarco Department of Radiology, Instituto Nacional de Cancerología-México, Mexico City, Mexico

Dolores Gallardo-Rincón Department of Medical Oncology, Instituto Nacional de Cancerología-México, Mexico City, Mexico

Francisco Osvaldo García-Pérez Department of Radiology, Instituto Nacional de Cancerología-México, Mexico City, Mexico

Aarón González-Enciso Gynecologic Tumors Deparment, Instituto Nacional de Cancerología-México, Mexico City, Mexico

Roque Alberto Guadarrama-Fleites Department of Radiation Oncology, Instituto Nacional de Cancerología-México, Mexico City, Mexico

Mauricio Hernández-Ávila Instituto Nacional de Salud Pública, México City, Mexico

Angel Herrera-Gómez Department Surgical Oncology, Instituto Nacional de Cancerología-México, Mexico City, Mexico

David Isla-Ortiz Department of Gynecologic Oncology, Instituto Nacional de Cancerología-México, Mexico City, Mexico

Paula Juarez-Sánchez Department of Pathology, Instituto Nacional de Cancerología-México, Mexico City, Mexico

Eduardo Lazcano-Ponce Instituto Nacional de Salud Pública, México City, Mexico

Leith León-Maldonado Instituto Nacional de Salud Pública, México City, Mexico

Alhely López-Arias Clinical Research. Instituto Nacional de Cancerología-México, Mexico City, Mexico

Horacio N. López-Basave Department Surgical Oncology, Instituto Nacional de Cancerología-México, Mexico City, Mexico

C. Lopez-Camarillo Universidad Autonoma de la Ciudad de Mexico, Mexico City, Mexico

Guinevere V. López-Tecamachaltzi Department of Radiology, Instituto Nacional de Cancerología-México, Mexico City, Mexico

Juan P. Marquez-Manriquez Tumor Vaccine Group, University of Washington, Seattle, WA, USA

Jorge Martínez-Tlahuel Department of Medical Oncology, Instituto Nacional de Cancerología-México, Mexico City, Mexico

Unit of Biomedical Research in Cancer, Instituto de Investigaciones Biomédicas, Universidad Nacional Autónoma de México, Mexico City, Mexico

Abelardo Meneses-García Department of General Direction, Instituto Nacional de Cancerología-México, Mexico City, Mexico

Alejandro Mohar-Betancourt Unit of Epidemiology, Instituto Nacional de Cancerología-México, Mexico City, Mexico

Gonzalo Montalvo-Esquivel Department Surgical Oncology, Instituto Nacional de Cancerología-México, Mexico City, Mexico

Flavia Morales-Vásquez Department of Medical Oncology, Instituto Nacional de Cancerología-México, Mexico City, Mexico

Aida Mota-García Department of Radiation Oncology, Instituto Nacional de Cancerología-México, Mexico City, Mexico

Irlanda Pacheco-Bravo Department of radiology, Instituto Nacional de Cancerología-México, Mexico City, Mexico

Adriana Peña-Nieves Unit of Epidemiology, Instituto Nacional de Cancerología-México, Mexico City, Mexico

Dana A Pérez-Camargo Palliative Care Service, Instituto Nacional de Cancerología-México, Mexico City, Mexico

Carlos Pérez-Plasencia Department of Investigation Genomics Laboratory, Instituto Nacional de Cancerología-México, Mexico City, Mexico

Milagros Pérez-Quintanilla Gynecologic Tumors Deparment, Instituto Nacional de Cancerología-México, Mexico City, D.F, Mexico

Bonifacio Ramón-Ortega Department of Radiation Oncology, Instituto Nacional de Cancerología-México, Mexico City, Mexico

Erik Ramos Tumor Vaccine Group, University of Washington, Seattle, WA, USA

Juan Armando Reyes-Pérez Department of Radiology, Instituto Nacional de Cancerología-México, Mexico City, Mexico

Nancy Reynoso-Noveron Unit of Epidemiology, Instituto Nacional de Cancerología-México, Mexico City, Mexico

Maryori Ortiz Rodríguez Unit of Epidemiology, Instituto Nacional de Cancerología-México, Mexico City, Mexico

Laboratory of Funtional Genomics, Unidad de Biomedicina, FES-IZTACALA, UNAM, Tlalnepantla, Mexico

Jorge Salmerón Instituto Nacional de Salud Pública, México City, Mexico

Mónica Lizzette Serrano-Arévalo Department of Cytopathology, Instituto Nacional de Cancerología-México, Mexico City, Mexico

Guadalupe Elizabeth Trejo-Durán Department of Radiation Oncology, Instituto Nacional de Cancerología-México, Mexico City, Mexico

Ana María Cano Valdez Department of Pathology, Instituto Nacional de Cancerología-México, Mexico City, Mexico

Julio César Velasco-Rodríguez Department of Medical Oncology, Hospital Español de México, Mexico City, Mexico

Emma Verástegui-Avilés Palliative Care Service, Instituto Nacional de Cancerología-México, Mexico City, Mexico

Lidia Faridi Villegas-González Department of Cytopathology, Instituto Nacional de Cancerología-México, Mexico City, Mexico

Chapter 1
Introduction

Jaime G. de la Garza-Salazar, Abelardo Meneses-García, Oscar Arrieta-Rodríguez, José Luis Aguilar-Ponce, and Paula Juarez-Sánchez

Abstract Cervix epidermoid carcinoma (CxCa) is the most frequent neoplasia of the feminine genital tract among the so-called third world countries. In countries referred to as first world countries early detection and treatment has given positive long-term results in women with CxCa. In Western Europe, Australia and New Zealand, for every 100,000 women diagnosed at least two will die from this disease. According to the WHO, in eastern Africa the amount of deaths among 30-year-old women is much higher (27.6%).

Although most cases of cervical cancer can be prevented by routine screening and treatment of precancerous lesions, cervical cancer is the leading cause of cancer mortality among women in developing countries.

The aim of the present chapter is to present a general view about the history of the Cervical Cancer, we think this knowledge improve today the results in the management of these patients.

Keywords Cervical cancer • Papanicolaou • Chemotherapy • Radiotherapy • Metastasis • Neoplasias

J.G. de la Garza-Salazar, MD
Department of Clinical Investigation, Instituto Nacional de Cancerología-México, Mexico City, Mexico

A. Meneses-García, MD, PhD
Department of General Direction, Instituto Nacional de Cancerología-México, Mexico City, Mexico

O. Arrieta-Rodríguez, MD
Department of Medical Oncology, Instituto Nacional de Cancerología-México, Mexico City, Mexico

J.L. Aguilar Ponce, MD
Internal Medicine Subdirection, Instituto Nacional de Cancerología-México, Mexico City, Mexico

P. Juarez-Sánchez, MD (✉)
Department of Pathology, Instituto Nacional de Cancerología-México, Av. San Fernando No 22, Col. Sección XVI, Mexico City 14080, Mexico
e-mail: cendifarma2006@yahoo.com.mx

J.G. de la Garza-Salazar et al. (eds.), *Cervical Cancer*,
DOI 10.1007/978-3-319-45231-9_1

Cervix epidermoid carcinoma (CxCa) is the most frequent neoplasia of the female genital tract among the so-called third world countries. In countries referred to as first world countries early detection and treatment has given positive long-term results in women with CxCa. In Western Europe, Australia and New Zealand, for every 100,000 women diagnosed at least two will die from this disease. According to the WHO, in eastern Africa the amount of deaths among 30-year-old women is much higher (27.6%). In detection campaigns, the most useful technique so far has been the Papanicolaou procedure, however it has some weak points, including "false positives" results that lead to unnecessary and repetitive biopsies; even worse is the report of "false negative" results, where the changes go unnoticed. This facts together with the socio-cultural problems of countries such as Africa, set back even more the successful detection and standard treatment of the disease [1]. Race, ethnic group and immigration status contribute to the high prevalence of CxCa in the US by making pelvic exploration and Papanicolaou sampling a forbidden practice because of cultural and language barriers [2].

The statistic reports of 2012 registered more than14 million new cases and 8.2 million deaths [3]. In that same year, more than 83,000 women were diagnosed with CxCa [3] and almost 36,000 of them died from this disease in America. If current trends are not changed, the number of deaths in Latin America will raise 45% by the year 2030.Death rates are three times higher in Latin America and the Caribbean than in North America, which evidences their enormous health disparities. Approximately 85% of the women dying from CxCa reside in developing countries. In the US, the early clinical stages of the disease have reported a substantial increase in women under 26 year's old [3, 4].

1.1 History of the Vaginal Cytology

There is an interesting story behind Vaginal Cytology, the most effective method for the early detection of CxCa and it's a story not known by most of gynecologists nor oncologists. Is the eponym of the vaginal exfoliative cytology an exam designed by Papanicolaou, by Felix-Archimede Pouchet (Fig. 1.1), by Eliseo Ramírez, by Aurel

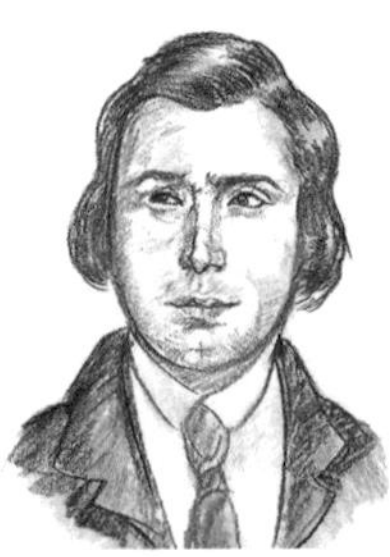

Fig. 1.1 Felix-Archimede Pouchet

Babeş-Constantin Daniel or by both Charles Stockard and Giorgio Papanicolaou [5–7] (Fig. 1.2). Actually, it seems that the gynecological study was initiated in Paris by the naturalist Felix-Archimede Pouchet (1847), who studied the morphological changes associated with the normal menstrual cycle [5].

It has long been discussed whether the vaginal exfoliative cytology exam should be called "Papanicolaou test". Mexicans say that the founder of such an exam, who was even credited for it by the Greek Papanicolaou, was the Mexican Eliseo Ramírez-Ulloa (Fig. 1.3). Meanwhile, the Romanians will say that the test was designed by Aurel Babes and Constantin Daniel; for this reason the bibliography should be revised to clarify any doubts regarding this matter.

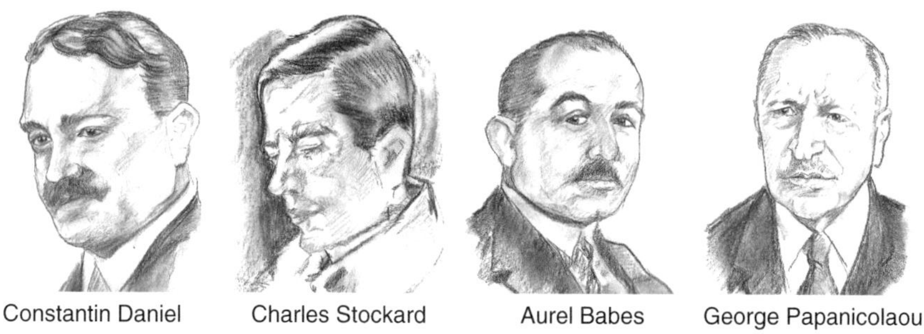

Fig. 1.2 Constantin Daniel, Charles Stockard, Aurel Babes and George Papanicolaou

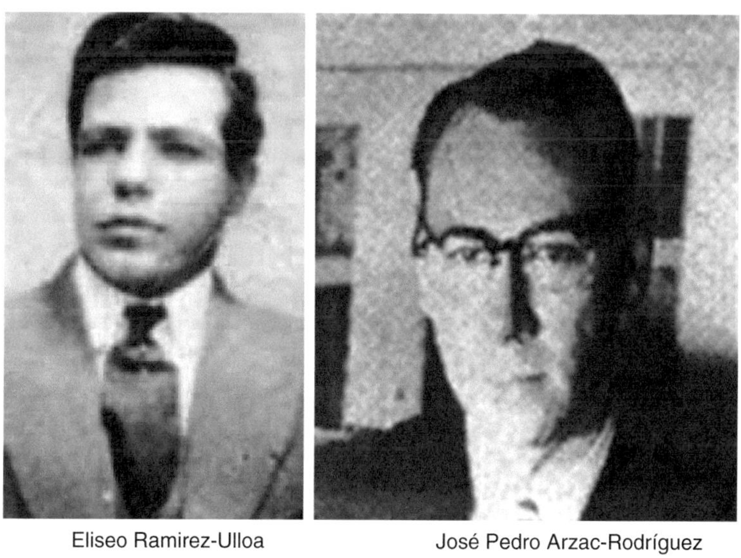

Fig. 1.3 Eliseo Ramirez-Ulloa and José Pedro Arzac-Rodríguez

George Papanicolaou mention in a publication on the Am. J. Anat. on 1933 as follows:

> "A Mexican gynecologist, Ramírez published, in 1928, a study of the human vaginal smear cycle. He recognized five provisional types of cells: I) Cells with a large and round nucleus clearly outlined, finely reticulated, and taking a violet-reddish color with Leischmann's stain; cytoplasm reticulated, pale-blue, with or without inclusions. II) Cells with a large round or oval nucleus having a thick reticulum, granular or semigranular; cytoplasm spongy, bluish, with inclusions and vacuoles. III) Cells with a much smaller nucleus having a thick reticulum or forming granules, irregularly outlined, taking a blue-violet color; cytoplasm condensed, bluish, vacuolated with inclusions. IV) Cells with a small, pyknotic granular or simply structureless nucleus of bluish or wine shade; cytoplasm spongio-granular with abundant inclusions and with or without large vacuoles. V) Anucleate cells and cells with only a trace of a nucleus. The nucleus appears as a mass of granules, which seem to be dispersed in the granular cytoplasm. All the granulations, nuclear or cytoplasmic, display the same bluish color". "Ramirez found that during menstruation the prevailing cellular type is: I (49 per cent), II (27 per cent), III (20 percent), IV (4 per cent), and V (0); leucocytes, scarce at first, increase toward the end. During the post menstrual period (2–3 days after menstruation), the cell percentages were as follows: I (1 per cent), II (9 per cent), III (24 per cent), IV (60 per cent), V (6 per cent); many polynuclear neutrophilic leucocytes. During the early interval (4–8 days after menstruation): I (0), II (15 per cent), III (25 per cent), IV (52 per cent), and V (8 per cent). During the interval (8 days after menstruation): I (0), II (1 per cent), III (42 per cent), IV (45 per cent), and V (12 per cent); leucocytes exceptional" "Ramirez found the leucocytes scarce in the beginning and increasing in numbers toward the end of menstruation. Shortly after menstruation, there were many polymorph nuclear neutrophilic leucocytes. With the end of menstruation, epithelial cells showing small pyknotic nuclei exceeded gradually in number those with larger nuclei. Cells encumbered with leucocytes, as observed by us especially toward the end of the menstrual phase, have been occasionally seen by Moser, though not in relation to any definite stage".

1.2 History of the Vaginal Cytology in Mexico

Patricia Alonso de Ruiz [7] says:

> The cytological studies on our country date from many years ago, in the twenties from last century; Dr. Eliseo Ramirez Ulloa performed some morphological studies, evaluating the cellular characteristics of the material peeled during the menstrual phase and it points out some interesting morphological data, this descriptions can be found on both the recompilation of his works and on the no-longer-published Mexican Journal of Biology. Afterwards, during the forties, Dr. José Pedro Arzac managed to get the staining reactives after reading some of the work of Dr Papanicolaou and traveling to the US to meet with him. After evaluating a considerable amount of cases at the Sanatorio Español, Dr. Arzac published his findings in the Mexican Journal of Gynecology and Obstetrics [7], where he clearly mentions the advantages of using cytology to identify malignant cells [7].

Jesús Kumate-Rodríguez [7] says:

> Eliseo Ramírez (1888–1940), a self-learning investigator, made the most important and original contribution of this century to medical sciences: he discovered the morphological changes of the vaginal cytology that take place during the menstrual cycle and was 6 months ahead of the discoveries of Dr. Papanicolaou. However, his findings went largely unnoticed

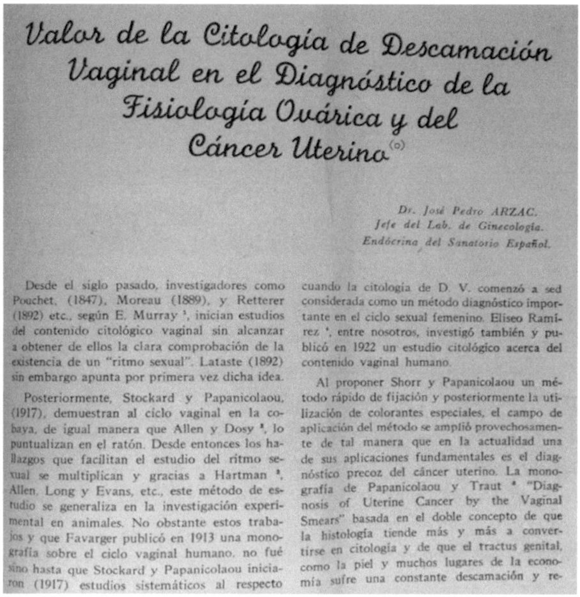

Valor de la Citología de Descamación Vaginal en el Diagnóstico de la Fisiología Ovárica y del Cáncer Uterino(o)

Dr. José Pedro ARZAC.
Jefe del Lab. de Ginecología.
Endócrina del Sanatorio Español.

Desde el siglo pasado, investigadores como Pouchet, (1847), Moreau (1889), y Retterer (1892) etc., según E. Murray [1], inician estudios del contenido citológico vaginal sin alcanzar a obtener de ellos la clara comprobación de la existencia de un "ritmo sexual". Lataste (1892) sin embargo apunta por primera vez dicha idea.

Posteriormente, Stockard y Papanicolaou, (1917), demuestran al ciclo vaginal en la cobaya, de igual manera que Allen y Dosy [2], lo puntualizan en el ratón. Desde entonces los hallazgos que facilitan el estudio del ritmo sexual se multiplican y gracias a Hartman [3], Allen, Long y Evans, etc., este método de estudio se generaliza en la investigación experimental en animales. No obstante estos trabajos y que Favarger publicó en 1913 una monografía sobre el ciclo vaginal humano, no fué sino hasta que Stockard y Papanicolaou iniciaron (1917) estudios sistemáticos al respecto cuando la citologia de D. V. comenzó a sed considerada como un método diagnóstico importante en el ciclo sexual femenino. Eliseo Ramírez [4], entre nosotros, investigó también y publicó en 1922 un estudio citológico acerca del contenido vaginal humano.

Al proponer Shorr y Papanicolaou un método rápido de fijación y posteriormente la utilización de colorantes especiales, el campo de aplicación del método se amplió provechosamente de tal manera que en la actualidad una de sus aplicaciones fundamentales es el diagnóstico precoz del cáncer uterino. La monografía de Papanicolaou y Traut [5] "Diagnosis of Uterine Cancer by the Vaginal Smears" basada en el doble concepto de que la histología tiende más y más a convertirse en citología y de que el tractus genital, como la piel y muchos lugares de la economía sufre una constante descamación y re-

Fig. 1.4 Dr. José Pedro Arzaćs publication

> because of factors such as Dr. Ramírez publishing in mexican journals of local distribution, having written in spanish and the absence of receptive media that would have given rise to critics, stimulus, and more projection of his discovery… [7].

On the same paper mentioned above, Fernando Quijano-Pitman says:

> A very important contribution of that decade was the one accomplished by Eliseo Ramírez, with the vaginal cytology test to study the menstrual cycle; this lead to the establishment of the cytological diagnosis of cervix cancer, which was later on expanded to the cytological diagnosis of other regions and organs. This technique is now called Papanicolau test. This author, acknowledged in several occasions with all due honorability and integrity, the priority of Eliseo Ramirez, who should be considered as the father and initiator of cytological diagnosis [7].

On 1945, the Mexican researcher José Pedro Arzac (Fig. 1.3) published an article (Fig. 1.4) referring to the works that he carried out together with Dr. Ramírez [7].

1.3 The Work Submitted to the Mexican Association of Gynecology and Obstetrics (1945), the References Uses Obsolete Parameters

Traditional we know that CxCa is a multifactorial disease that is consistently influenced by the age at which sexual activity started, the number of sexual partners, a low socio-economic and cultural status, the number of births and tobacco

consumption. The finding of some of the carcinogens of tobacco in cervix mucous has led to the supposition of their association and participation in the carcinogenesis of the latter. The association between CxCa and the use of the contraconceptives mentioned by some authors is still a matter of discussion [8]. A pending issue to be solved is that of women with CxCa who are also seropositive for Human Immunodeficiency Virus (HIV); in these patients the cervical dysplasia is multifocal, of rapid progression and highly recurrent (although it is possible that they pass away earlier because of the immunodeficiency).

Up until now, the treatment for HIV+/HPV+ women that present cervical intraepithelial neoplasia (CIN) is not so effective, and often the standard treatment for VIH/AIDS can reduce the symptoms of early lesions. Women with advanced CxCa and VIH/AIDS generally receive the same treatment than women without VIH/AIDS [9].

In Mexico, during the last years the frequency and late diagnosis of CxCa has importantly diminished and is now preceded by the primary carcinoma of the mammary gland, which is first in frequency and death rate; this has been because of the early detection programs for both diseases initiated on 1995 with the "National Program for the Prevention and Control of Cervical and Breast Cancer". CxCa incidence, the way it is presented and it's relation with HPV-16, 18 will be subject to a broad analysis and literature revisions in the matter of rate of prevalence, biogenetics and treatment [10–12] according to the accepted standards of diagnosis and treatment (WHO, Society of Gynecologist Pathologists – SPG, FIGO).

The Human Papilloma Virus (HPV) has been marked as responsible for the malignant transformation of the cervical epithelium and recently other molecular alterations have been identified such as the over-expression of HER-2neu and c-myc or the mutation of H-ras, K-ras or c-myc, which evidences the presence of other factors (although these changes could be secondarily attributed to HPV). The investigations point at VPH genes E6 and E7, which might be involved in the etiopathogeny of CxCa, given that these genes stimulate cell proliferation by suppressing the regulatory functions of Retinoblastoma protein (Rb) and that of p53 [13]. Other factors associated with a bad prognosis are DNA ploidy, $p27^{Kip1}$ expression, p53, c-erbB-2 and COX2 [14].

Independent of the discoveries implicated in the etiology of CxCa, the HPV type identified in the tumor seems to have an importance in the prognosis, reason for which it has been proposed to analyze these groups as a complimentary part of the cytological test. HPV 18, for instance, is associated to a particularly adverse prognosis and it is not uncommon to find it in tumors with a low rate of survival. It is possible that the new variations found on the L1 gene of this virus can be used in the design of diagnosis reactives and an HPV vaccine [14, 15]. Recently two anti-HPV vaccines have been commercialized (HPV4 and HPV2) [16] based on non-infectious particles that are similar to the virus and are obtained via DNA recombination techniques. Both vaccines are equally safe and it has been proven that they give almost full protection against pre-cancerous lesions. HPV vaccine for girls and young adolescents (9–12 years old) can prevent up to 70% of the new CxCa cases [17].

The recommended dose of these vaccines for these particular groups is three doses via intramuscular injection in a period of 6 months. The second and third doses are applied two and 6 months after the first dose respectively. The vaccine brand can be substituted for another during the three dose series. HPV vaccine may be administered simultaneously to the vaccines [16]. The amount of doses required from this vaccine is currently a matter of analysis; it has not yet been established if booster doses are necessary. Some studies have shown that two doses are as effective as the three recommended doses [17].

Independent of the screening problems identified by the National Program for the Prevention and Control of Cervical Cancer (PNDCU, according to its original name in Spanish) such as coverage and quality [18], and in spite of the failure registered in programs based on vaginal cytology the Pap test continues to be the best resource to reduce the CxCa mortality, and most likely can be improved with the strategically use of the resources available (including scientific, economic and screening resources) in each of the 32 states of the Mexican Republic in order to create and apply a surveillance system that not only allows early detection but also guaranties timely treatment.

We know that the death rate of this neoplasia is three times higher in Latin America and the Caribbean than in the rest of North America. This fact evidenced the enormous differences that exist in health and the roll of sociocultural factors, for which it has been estimated that the treatment of these groups followed by the treatment of the identified pre-cancerous lesions, is a cost-effective prevention strategy of great value. In 2004 the Mexican Health Secretary created the Popular Insurance, which cover 100% of the expenses for the integral treatment of women with early or advanced lesions in the cervix (including diagnose, surgery, radiotherapy and chemotherapy). Thanks to this insurance early diagnose and integral treatment have considerably increased the healing of this disease and prolonged the survival of patients with CxCa [19].

In our experience and in accordance with the recommendations of the American Joint Committee (AJCC) and those of FIGO established to determine the TNM Classification (Tumor, Nodes and Metastases) and the clinical stage (Table 1.1), we consider as fundamental elements the history and clinical exploration (abdominal and pelvic) associated with other laboratory studies and/or studies such as X rays, (thorax and urography), computerized tomography, magnetic resonance using the emission of ultra-fine particles of iron oxide (USPIO), positron emission tomography (PET), whose sensibility and specificity is between 99 and 100%. The study of the sentinel lymph node seems to be a good option to define a pelvic lymphadenectomy [20].

Once the CxCa has been established, the treatment is, in general terms, multidisciplinary (surgery, radiotherapy, chemotherapy and target therapy) and must be fundamental in the clinical and laboratory findings. The cone biopsy, cryotherapy and/or surgical electro-incision are procedures recommended for EC0 to 1A1 and invasion of the endocervix have been discarded. Clinical stage and histology are both invaluable information to define the therapeutic conduct (adenocarcinoma has lower survival rates than epidermoid carcinoma when compared stage by stage)

Table 1.1 TNM and FIGO classification for Cérvix Carcinoma

(T) Primary tumor, (N) Lymph nodes, (M) Metastasis		
TNM system	**FIGO**	**Surgical-pathological Characteristics**
TX		**Primary tumor cannot be evaluated**
T0		**There is no evidence of the primary tumor**
Tis		**Carcinoma in situ (pre-invasive carcinoma)**
T1	I	Cervix-confined carcinoma (with no dispersion to the uterus)
T1a	IA	Invasive carcinoma, microscopically diagnosed, maximum stroma invasion with no more than 5 mm from the epithelial-base and horizontal extension of 7 mm or less. Invasion of vascular space (venous or lymphatic) does not affect classification
T1a1	IA1	Invasion of the stroma with a depth ≤3.0 mm and horizontal extension ≤7.0 mm
T1a2	IA2	Invasion of the stroma with a depth >3.0 mm and horizontal extension ≤5.0
T1b	IB	Clinically visible, cervix- confined lesion or microscopic lesion with characteristics of T1a/IA2
T1b1	IB1	Clinically visible lesion with ≤4.0 cm as its maximum size
T1b2	IB2	Clinically visible lesion with >4.0 cm as its maximum size
T2	II	Carcinoma that invades the lower portion of the uterus but not the pelvic wall or that invades on its lower portion a third of the vagina
T2a	IIA	Tumor without parametrial invasion
T2a1	IIA1	Clinically visible lesion with ≤4.0 cm on its greater diameter
T2a2	IIA2	Clinically visible lesion with >4.0 cm on its greater diameter
T2b	IIB	Tumor with parametrial invasion
T3	III	The tumor extends to the pelvic wall and/or includes on its lower portion a third of the vagina and/or causes hydronephrosis or obstructs renal function
T3a	IIIA	The tumor invades on its lower portion a third of the vagina without extending to the pelvic wall
T3b	IIIB	The tumor extends to the pelvic wall ad causes hydronephrosis (renal insufficiency)
T4	IV	The tumor invades the mucous tissue of the bladder or that of the rectum and/or extends below to the true pelvis (bullous edema is not enough to classify the tumor as T4)
T4a	IVA	The tumor invades the mucous tissue of the bladder or that of the rectum (bullous edema is not enough to classify the tumor as T4)
T4b	IVB	The tumor extends beyond the true pelvis
Regional lymph nodes (N)		
NX	Regional lymph nodes cannot be evaluated	
N0	Without metastasis to regional lymph nodes	
N1	With metastasis to regional lymph nodes	
Distant metastasis (M)		
M0	Without distant metastasis	
M1	With distant metastasis (including peritoneal dissemination; compromising of the lymph nodes from the supra-ventricular, mediastinum or para-aortic regions; lungs, liver or bones)	

Cervical Cancer Staging: Cecelia H Boardman, MD; Chief Editor: from Memorial Sloan-Kettering – Yukio Sonoda, MD

besides, analysis of surgical margins allows to evaluate for additional treatments. Radical trachelectomy (for EC, IA2 and IB), originally described on 1986 by the French gynecologist Daniel Dargent, allows young women to retain their reproductive function. Lymphadenectomy is performed afterwards.

Simple hysterectomy (abdominal or robot-assisted laparoscopic) and radical hysterectomy are prescribed in case of EC, IA2, IB and least frequent in young women with EC IIA. Pelvic exenteration is used to treat a recurrent CxCa. This technique removes: the bladder, vagina, rectum, might also include part of the colon depending on the extension of the neoplasia. Reconstruction includes nel-bladder with urostomy and colostomy. Vaginal reconstruction is possible and will be referenced broadly on the designated chapter.

Pelvic lymphadenectomy is usually carried out during simple or radical hysterectomy or during trachelectomy [21]. The patients that are primarily treated with surgery, with positive margins, lymphovascular space invasion and lymphatic metastasis must receive concomitant chemo-radiation.

External radiotherapy (for EC IB1) plus 3D based MRI brachytherapy seems to improve the local control of the disease. Complementary hysterectomy after the radiotherapy evaluated by the RTGO group in a randomized trial did not show survival differences between both arms and only showed a potential benefit for women with persistent disease. Another option is combined radio-surgery.

EC IB2 standard treatment is chemo-radiotherapy. The most frequently used scheme for chemotherapy is Cisplatin (40 mg/m [2]) in a weekly scheme. Acute gastro-intestinal and hematologic toxicity are frequent. The usefulness of adjuvant therapy post-chemo-radiation has not yet been defined nor extensively studied, however a randomized study with cisplatin and gentamicin proved to be useful. Complementary surgery can be an option for patients with persistent disease.

In Mexico, we began the chemotherapy for patients with advanced CxCa with good results over 42 years ago (de la Garza et al. 1973) (Fig. 1.5). We studied 25 patients of the Oncological Hospital of the Mexican Institute, IMSS, (according to its original name in spanish) who presented advanced CxCa (15 with pelvic activity, six with lung metastasis and five with hepatic metastasis). We used 5-fluorouracil (5-FU), cyclophosphamide, vincristine, and methotrexate. In those years, it was hard to convince oncologists (surgeons and radiotherapists) of the potential benefit of the treatment. One patient's lung metastasis disappeared completely, demonstrating in Mexico that CxCa was sensitive to chemotherapy treatment [22].

1.4 Chemotherapy and Concomitant Radiotherapy for Cervical Cancer

In 1999, Rose P.G. et al. performed an innovative, randomized trial using radiotherapy and three regimes of concurrent chemotherapy, in representation of the Gynecological Oncology Group, in patients with advanced CxCa. On the first group, they used only cisplatin (40 mg/m [2] for 6 weeks). The second group received

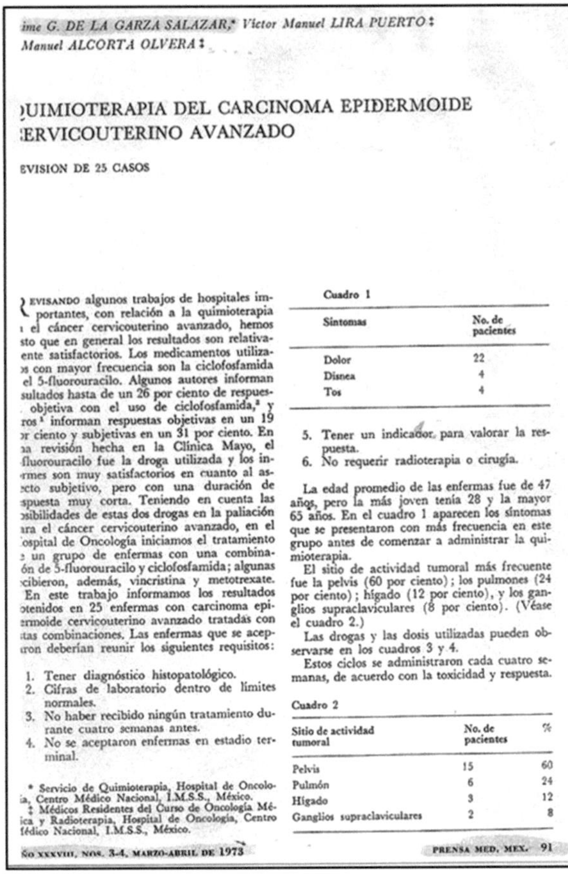

ime G. DE LA GARZA SALAZAR,* Victor Manuel LIRA PUERTO ‡
Manuel ALCORTA OLVERA ‡

)UIMIOTERAPIA DEL CARCINOMA EPIDERMOIDE
:ERVICOUTERINO AVANZADO

EVISION DE 25 CASOS

EVISANDO algunos trabajos de hospitales importantes, con relación a la quimioterapia 1 el cáncer cervicouterino avanzado, hemos sto que en general los resultados son relativaente satisfactorios. Los medicamentos utiliza)s con mayor frecuencia son la ciclofosfamida el 5-fluorouracilo. Algunos autores informan sultados hasta de un 26 por ciento de respues. objetiva con el uso de ciclofosfamida,[2] y ros[3] informan respuestas objetivas en un 19)r ciento y subjetivas en un 31 por ciento. En 1a revisión hecha en la Clínica Mayo, el fluorouracilo fue la droga utilizada y los in·rmes son muy satisfactorios en cuanto al as:cto subjetivo, pero con una duración de :spuesta muy corta. Teniendo en cuenta las)sibilidades de estas dos drogas en la paliación ıra el cáncer cervicouterino avanzado, en el :ospital de Oncología iniciamos el tratamiento : un grupo de enfermas con una combinaón de 5-fluorouracilo y ciclofosfamida; algunas :cibieron, además, vincristina y metotrexate. En este trabajo informamos los resultados)tenidos en 25 enfermas con carcinoma epi:rmoide cervicouterino avanzado tratadas con :tas combinaciones. Las enfermas que se aceparon deberían reunir los siguientes requisitos:

1. Tener diagnóstico histopatológico.
2. Cifras de laboratorio dentro de límites normales.
3. No haber recibido ningún tratamiento durante cuatro semanas antes.
4. No se aceptaron enfermas en estadio terminal.

* Servicio de Quimioterapia, Hospital de Oncoloía, Centro Médico Nacional, I.M.S.S., México.
‡ Médicos Residentes del Curso de Oncología Méica y Radioterapia, Hospital de Oncología, Centro Iédico Nacional, I.M.S.S., México.

Cuadro 1

Síntomas	No. de pacientes
Dolor	22
Disnea	4
Tos	4

5. Tener un indicador para valorar la respuesta.
6. No requerir radioterapia o cirugía.

La edad promedio de las enfermas fue de 47 años, pero la más joven tenía 28 y la mayor 65 años. En el cuadro 1 aparecen los síntomas que se presentaron con más frecuencia en este grupo antes de comenzar a administrar la quimioterapia.

El sitio de actividad tumoral más frecuente fue la pelvis (60 por ciento); los pulmones (24 por ciento); hígado (12 por ciento), y los ganglios supraclaviculares (8 por ciento). (Véase el cuadro 2.)

Las drogas y las dosis utilizadas pueden observarse en los cuadros 3 y 4.

Estos ciclos se administraron cada cuatro semanas, de acuerdo con la toxicidad y respuesta.

Cuadro 2

Sitio de actividad tumoral	No. de pacientes	%
Pelvis	15	60
Pulmón	6	24
Hígado	3	12
Ganglios supraclaviculares	2	8

ÑO XXXVIII, NOS. 3-4, MARZO-ABRIL DE 1973 PRENSA MED. MEX. 91

Fig. 1.5 The Mexican publication: Prensa Médica de México. Marzo-Abril 1973

cisplatin (50 mg/m [2] on days 1 and 29) followed by 5 FU in 96 h days 1 and 29 (4 g/m [2]) and orally administered hydroxyurea (2 g/m [2], twice a week). The third group received only orally hydroxyurea (3 g/m [2]). The women included had epidermoid carcinoma, adenosquamous carcinoma and adenocarcinoma in stages IIB, III o IVA without compromised lymph nodes. The group concluded that the radiotherapy and chemotherapy regimens that included cisplatin improved the survival rate and progression-free survival among the women with locally advanced CxCa.

> "Based on significant improvement in both progression-free survival and overall survival when cisplatin-based chemotherapy was administered during radiation for various stages of cervical cancer. Led The National Cancer Institute to issue an alert: released a clinical alert to practicing oncologists on February 23, 1999 [23]"

On 2002 Rose PG and Bundy BN analyzed and compared six clinical trials (GOG: Gynecologic Oncology Group; SWOG Southwest Oncology Group; RTOG Radiotherapy Oncology Group y del NCIC National Cancer Institute of Canada) [24] and noted:

> "This clinical alert outlined the findings of the five clinical trials that had been completed and recommended ". . . strong consideration should be given to the incorporation of concurrent cisplatin-based chemotherapy with radiation therapy in women who require radiation therapy for treatment of cervical cancer." These five randomized trials, involving approximately 1,800 women, demonstrated a 30% to 50% improvement in survival when cisplatin-based chemotherapy was administered concurrently with radiation therapy, in this issue".

On the other hand, Rose PG said [25]:

> "Based on the results of these five randomized trials, the National Cancer Institute (NCI) released a Clinical Announcement stating that cisplatin-based chemotherapy, as used in these trials (i.e. concurrently with radiation therapy), as the new standard of therapy for cervical cancer"
>
> Pearcey et al [26], "reported in a National Cancer Institute of Canada (NCIC)–sponsored trial comparing cisplatin-based chemotherapy given concurrently with radiation versus radiation alone for patients with locally advanced cervical cancer. This represents the sixth randomized trial that uses cisplatin-based chemotherapy administered concurrently during radiation therapy for cervical cancer. The authors, who conclude . . . the balance of evidence favors the use of combined-modality treatment for the types of patients studied in this trial."

In another study carried out in Mexico in which neo-adjuvant chemotherapy (NAC) was used on patients with CxCa EC IB and IIA and that was published on 2000, Dueñas et al. [27] reported that besides giving an elevated rate of response, the combination of cisplatin, vincristine and bleomycin (PVB) seems to reduce the risk factors for recurrence (Fig. 1.6). NAC is still a matter of polemics on an internationally level and is currently under investigation by the EORTC (55994). A systematic revision with meta-analysis of individual patient data has proven the superiority of NAC followed by surgery, in terms of global survival. In spite of the results NAC is not consider standard treatment for two reasons: the inferiority of the control arm (radiotherapy only) compared with the current standard, and the second reason: the results of the GOG 141. The combined chemotherapy on EC IVB based on cisplatin and topotecan has a potential benefit on the average total survival, on the period free

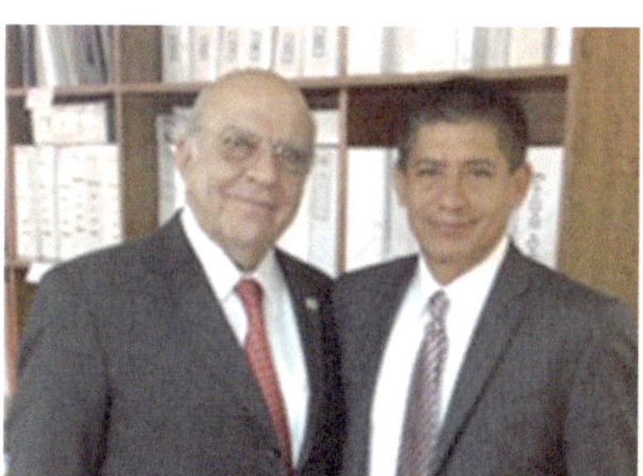

Jaime de la Garza   Alfonso Dueñas

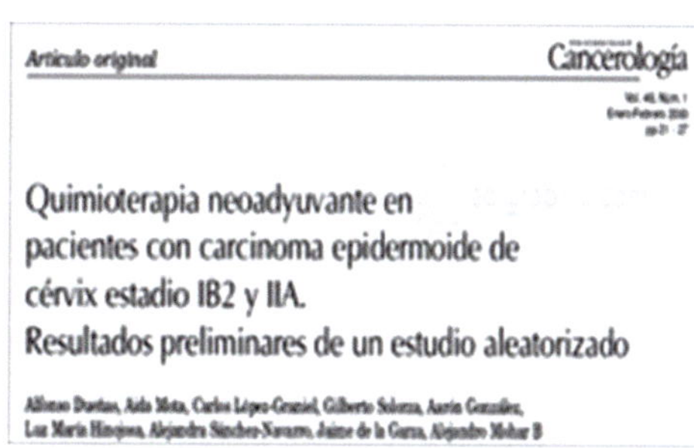
Artículo original

Cancerología

Quimioterapia neoadyuvante en pacientes con carcinoma epidermoide de cérvix estadio IB2 y IIA. Resultados preliminares de un estudio aleatorizado

Fig. 1.6 Jaime de la Garza and Alfonso Dueñas — The Mexican publication: Cancerología

of disease and in the number of responses. A study of the GOG compared four doublets of cisplatin and showed no superiority against the scheme that uses cisplatin plus paclitaxel.

For many patients with locally recurrent disease and/or metastasis palliative chemotherapy can be an option. In some cases with central pelvic recurrence, pelvic surgery is recommended and radiotherapy might result useful [24] in patients who have not been previously radiated.

Usually, in patients with CxCa in early clinical stages local treatment is enough; this does not apply for patients with an advanced disease because in many women there is relapse to the initial treatment due more to chemo-resistance rather than to the tumors extension; this has made it necessary to focus on investigating new therapeutic strategies such as molecular ones. Now days, only 15–20% of the patients respond to chemotherapy. Cisplatin is the most used drug perhaps because it induces a response in 20–40%, nonetheless relapses are not rare. Recently, many combinations have been tried with modest results; only the combination of cisplatin with topotecan seems to be more effective.

Molecular CxCa studies on CaSki and SiHa cell lines have analyzed the problem of chemo-resistance (both cell lines include an integrated form of HPV16) and have found that both types of cell respond differently to the *treatment* with cell-death inducing agents (epirubicin). CaSki cells are more sensible to these treatments than SiHa cells, which suggests that the levels of p53 and/or pro-caspase 8 could be involved. Chemo-resistance is a multifactorial process in which the differences in neoplasic reproduction [28] could be involved, or the differences in angiogenic capacity, which could complicate the distribution of anti-neoplasia medication (bioavailability).

The follow-up of treated patients with CxCa includes gynecological exploration, Pap test every 3 months during the first two years, every 6 months during the next 3 years and annual basis from the on. PET/CT is usefully in the early detection of local recurrence and/or metastasis.

1.5 The Sexuality of CxCa Patients

The appearance or confirmation of the disease undoubtedly generates fears, anguish and survival expectations that deteriorate the personality. This topic is poorly treated and not known even though it constitutes a real and current concern. Whether it is as a direct consequence of the disease, or because of the treatments, or because of the combined impact some couple pre-existing problems might arise or become exacerbated. Some problems are directly related to the disease (dispauremia, anemia and anorexia). However, sexuality (proximity and physics contact) remains present even in the terminal patient. There is no doubt that the specialists must carefully evaluate this problem and the physician, with the sole propose of providing the cancer patient with a satisfying life quality [29].

1.6 Other Primary Tumors of the Cervix

1.6.1 Epithelial Lineage Tumors

There are other metaplastic changes that occur in the cervical epithelium (glandular or stromal) that represent different stages of a morphological continuum (from increasing stage dysplasia, to in situ carcinoma and invasive cancer). In this regard, glandular atypical dysplasia has become a matter of recent discussion [30]. It was initially described in pregnant women with a history of use of oral contraceptives, inflammatory diseases or in irradiated patients; for this reasons its relevance as a pre-malignant lesion is not widely accepted [31]. According to some informs the percentage of cases like the former associated with a cervical or endometrial malignant tumor is high. Nine percent to thirty-eight percent of women with CIN level 2 or 3 present in situ adenocarcinoma and 3–17% have invading carcinomas [32, 33]. Malignant adenomioma can be associated to the Peutz-Jeghers syndrome has mutations of the STK11 gene (a tumor suppressor gene responsible for the syndrome localized in 19p13.3) [34, 35].

The endocervical carcinoma has a different prognosis and treatment than those used for the epidermoid carcinoma. This neoplasia constitutes only a fraction of the malignant cervical neoplasias (15–20%), its cytological diagnose is less effective than with the epidermoid variant [36]. It affects young women and, apart from the smoking habit, it shares similar risk factors to the epidermoid variety (especially the infection with the oncogenic variants of HPV). In advance stages they are difficult to treat (are more resistant to radiotherapy, have shorter periods of tumor-free survival and its prognosis is less favorable). Adenosquamous variants seem to be associated to the use of oral contraceptives and like the papillary or villoglandular variants they share as triggering factor the HPV infection.

The WHO recognizes and classifies this tumors (Table 1.1 and 1.2) [37, 38]. Other tumors that do not fit in the described categories are:

- Adenosquamous carcinoma
- Carcinoma of polished-glass cell

Table 1.2 WHO, infiltrating adenocarcinomas

I. Mucinous Adenocarcinoma
II. Endometrioid Adenocarcinoma
Endocervical
Intestinal (enteroid)
Signet ring cells
Minimum deviation
Villoglandular
III. Clear-cell Adenocarcinoma
IV. Serous Adenocarcinoma
V. Adenocarcinoma Mesonephric

- Adenoid-cystic carcinoma
- Adenoid-basal carcinoma
- Neuro-endocrine carcinomas
- Carcinoid
- Typical carcinoid
- Small cell carcinoma
- Big cell carcinoma
- Undifferentiated Carcinoma

Polished-glass cell carcinoma constitutes 1–2% of cervical carcinomas. It presents itself in young women, its growth is fast and there is usually early distant metastasis; has a poor response to radiotherapy but the results with chemotherapy are promising. This tumor lacks on hormone receptors (to estrogen or progesterone). The density of eosinophil infiltrate as part of the immune-inflammatory response in the tumor should be a study subject. The adenoid-cystic carcinoma presents itself in black women <60 years old. It is an aggressive recurrent tumor with metastasic tendencies.

1.6.2 Neuro-endocrine Tumors

It was originally recognized in the cervix by Albores-Saavedra on 1972 [39]. The small cell variant constitutes merely 5% of all the primary carcinomas of the cervix and the variant of big cells represents 0.087–0.6% of cervical carcinomas; it has been reported that both subtypes are associated to HPV 16, 28, 31 and 33 [40], they are characterized by their highly aggressive behavior and its tendency to give rise to early metastasis. In these cases the rate of 5-year survival s 54.8–31.5%. Because of its rareness, there is no consensus on the treatment of these neoplasias [41, 42]. Mixed histopathological presentation is less frequent and, Aely Riu et al. have recently reported it in a 26-year-old patient, association with HPV 18 and 16 was proven, which leads to the supposition that anti-HPV vaccine could be of use.

1.6.3 Mesenchymatous-Origin Tumors

Primary leiomyoma of the cervix are rare. The malignant variant is also rare. Polypoid lesions of fibrous-connective and glandular component (adenomyoma and adenofibroma) are usually benign and their cervical location is not frequent. Müllerian mixed tumor is also not frequent in cervix compared with it counterpart in the uterus. More frequent in post-menopausal women and is usually a polypoid mass. Müllerian adenosarcoma shows malignant changes in the mesenchyma.

1.7 Metastatic Tumors on to the Cervix

The rarity of metastasis of an extra-genital carcinoma to the cervix has been attributed to high fibrous content, centrifugal lymphatic drainage, reduced blood flow, the small anatomical size and finally the lack of systematic studies of the cervix looking for the lesion and the tendency to only consider the existence of primary carcinomas in the cervix.

Metastasis to the cervix do occur and mainly in breast stomach and colorectal carcinomas [43–47].

References

1. German academics tackle cervical cancer in Africa with SAP HANA. www.eticcs.org/german-academics-tackle-cervical-cancer-in-africa-with-sap-hana. 20 Nov 2015.
2. Segnan N. Socioeconomic status and cancer screening. In: Kogevinas M, Pearce N, Susser M, Boffetta P, editors. Social inequalities and cancer. Lyon: International Agency for Research on Cancer; 1997. p. 369–76.
3. Cervical cancer. www.paho.org/hq/index.php?option=com_topics&view=article&id=348&Itemid=40936&lang=en, 2012.
4. Cancer en cifras, www.infocancer.org.mx/globocan-2012-con776i0.html, 2012.
5. Diamantis, A, Androutsos G. Highlights from the history of hormonal cytology. Hormones Athens Grecia. 2002;7(2):184–6. ISSN 1109-3099. PMID 18477558.
6. Papanicolaou GN. The sexual cycle in the human female as revealed by Vaginal Smears. Am J Anat. 1933;52: 519–637? Amer J Anat. 1933;52:519.
7. Alonso P, Kumate RJ, Quijano FP, Aréchiga H, Somolinos J. Sociedad Latinoamericana de Citopatología (SLAC). Contribuciones mexicanas al conocimiento médico. México: Fondo de Cultura Económica; 1993. p. 96–7. Arzoz JP. Work presented before the Asociacion Mexicana de Ginecología y Obstetricia. 1945.
8. Beral V, Hannaford P, Kay C. Oral contraceptive use and malignancies of the genital tract results from the Royal College of general practitioners' oral contraception study. Lancet. 1988;2:1331–5.
9. HIV and AIDS-Related Cancer: treatment options. Approved by the Cancer.Net Editorial Board; 2014.
10. Berumen J, Casas L, Segura E, Amezcua JL, Garcia-Carranca A. Genome amplification of human papillomavirus types 16 and 18 in cervical carcinomas is related to the retention of E1/E2 genes. Int J Cancer. 1994;56:640–5.
11. Lizano M, Berumen J, Guido MC, Casas L, Garcia-Carranca A. Association between human papillomavirus type 18 variants and histopathology of cervical cancer. J Natl Cancer Inst. 1997;89:1227–31.
12. Jaime B, Rosa M. O, Eduardo L, et al. Asian-American variants of human papillomavirus 16 and risk for cervical cancer: a case–control study. J Natl Cancer Inst. 2001;93(17):1321330. doi:10.1093/jnci/93.17.1325.
13. Lombard I, Vincent-Solomon A, Validire P, et al. Human papillomavirus genotye as a major determinant of the course of cervical cancer. J Clin Oncol. 1998;16:2613–9.
14. Berumen J, Rosa M. O, Eduardo L, et al. Asian-American variants of human papillomavirus 16 and risk for cervical cancer: a case–control study. JNCI J Natl Cancer Inst. 2001;93(17): 132–3. doi:10.1093/jnci/93.17.1325.

15. Shen M, Ding X, Li T, Chen G, Zhou X. Sequence variation analysis of HPV-18 isolates in southwest China. P Los One. 2013;8(2):e56614. doi:10.137/journal. Pone. 0056614. Epub 25 Feb 2013.
16. American College of Obstetricians and Gynecologists. Committee opinion no. 588: human papillomavirus vaccination. Obstet Gynecol. 2014;123(3):712–8.
17. Kreimer AR, et al. Proof-of-principle evaluation of the efficacy of fewer than three doses of a bivalent HPV 16/18 vaccine. J Natl Cancer Inst. 2011;103(19):1444–51. doi:10.1093/jnci/djr319. Epub 2011 Sep 9.
18. OPS and PAHO. 2013. www.paho.org/cancer.
19. Torres-Poveda KJ, Cruz-Valdéz A, Madrid-Mariana V. Epidemiologia del Cáncer cervicouterino. Gaceta Mexicana de Oncología (Sociedad Mexicana de Oncología). 2014;13(Suppl4):4–17.
20. Janicek MF, Averette HE. Cervical cancer: prevention, diagnosis, and therapeutics. CA a Canc J Clin. 2001;51(2):92–114.
21. Surgery for cervical cáncer. American Cancer Society. 2015. 26 Feb. www.cancer.org ›... › Detailed Guide.
22. de la Garza JG. et al. Quimioterapia del Carcinoma Epidermoide cervicouterino avanzado, Prensa Med. Mex. Año XXXVIII, mzo, de 1973. Nos 3–4.
23. Rose PG, Bundy BN, Watkins EB, et al. Concurrent cisplatin-based radiotherapy and chemotherapy for locally advanced cervical cancer. N Engl J Med. 1999;340:1144–53. doi:10.1056/NEJM199904153401502.
24. Rose PG, Bundy BN. Chemoradiation for locally advanced cervical cancer: does it help? J Clin Oncol. 2002;20(4):891–3.
25. Rose PG. Chemoradiotherapy for cervical cáncer. Eur J Canc. 2002;38(2):270–8.
26. Pearcey R, Brundage M, Drouin P, et al. Phase III trial comparing radical radiotherapy with and without cisplatin chemotherapy in patients with advanced squamous cell cancer of the cervix. J Clin Oncol. 2002;Vl 20(4):966–72. American Society for Clinical Oncology.
27. Dueñas A, Mota A, López-Garniel C, et al. Quimioterapia neoadyuvante en pacientes con carcinoma epidermoide de cérvix, estadio IB2 y IIA. Resultados preliminares de un estudio aleatorizado. Cancerologia. 2000;46(1):21–7.
28. Filippova M, Filippov V, Williams VM, et al. Research article: cellular levels of oxidative stress affect the response of cervical cancer cells to chemotherapeutic agents. BioMed Res Inter. 2014;2014(574659):14. http://dx.doi.org/10.1155/2014/574659.
29. Grau Abalo JA, del Llantá Abreu MC, Roger MC, González GF. La sexualidad en pacientes con cáncer: algunas consideraciones sobre su evaluación y tratamiento. Rev Cubana Oncol. 1999;15(1):49–65.
30. Brown LJ, Wells M. Cervical glandular atypia associated with squamous intraepithelial neoplasia: a premalignant lesion? J Clin Pathol. 1986;39:22–8.
31. Gloor E, Hurlimann J. Cervical intraepithelial neoplasia (adenocarcinoma in situ and glandular dysplasia): a correlative study of 23 cases with histologic grading, histochemical analysis of mucins, and immunohistochemical determination of the affinity of four lectins. Cancer. 1986;58:1272–80.
32. Cervical cancer statistics, www.cancer.ca/en/cancer-information/cancer-type/cervical/statistics/?region=ab, 2016.
33. de Marques JPH, Costa LB, de Sosa AP et al. Atypical glandular cells and cervical cancer. Sistematic Rev Rev Assoc Med Bras. 57:2. Sao Paulo Abr. ISSN 0104–4230.
34. Cosme A, Ojeda E, San Vicente MT et al. Sindrome de Peutz Jeghers asociado a múltiples tumores epiteliales. Rev Gastroenterol y Hepatol Dic. 2001;24(10):495–499.
35. Francis JMA, Torres EP, Sahagun FB, Sindrome de Peutz Jeghers. Articulo de Revisión. Rev. Hospital General de México, SS. Abril. 2006;68(2):99–105.
36. Jiménez-Ayala M, Portillo BJ-A. Citopatología glandular del endocérvix. Diagnóstico diferencial. Rev Española de Patologia. 2003;36(1):11–20.
37. Tavassoli FA, Devilee P, editors. World Health Organization classification of tumors. Pathology and genetics of tumors of the breast and female genital organs. Lyon: IARC Press; 2003.

38. Hardison D. Hernández: Carcinoma de cérvix, tipos histológicos y factores pronóstico. Patología Quirúrgica. X Congreso Virtual Hispano-americano de Anatomía Patológica. 1–30 noviembre 2009 #2090. ISBN 978.84–692-76778.
39. Albores-Saavedra J. Primary carcinoid of the uterine cérvix. Pathologia. 1972;19:185–93.
40. Horn L-C, Lindner K, Szepankiewicz G et al. p16, p14, p53, and cyclin D1 expression and HPV analysis in small cell carcinomas of the uterine cervix. Inter J Gynecol Pathol. 25:182 Y186. Lippincott Williams & Wilkins, Baltimore O 2006 International Society of Gynecological Pathologists. 182. doi:10.1097/01.pgp.0000185406.85685.df.
41. Kumar S, Nair S, Alexander M. Carcinomatous meningitis occurring prior to a diagnosis of large cell neuroendocrine carcinoma of the uterine cérvix. J Postgrad Med. 2004;50:311–2.
42. Wang KL, Yang YC, Wang TY, Chen JR, Chen TC, Chen HS, et al. Neuroendocrine carcinoma of the uterine cervix: a clinicopathologic retrospective study of 31 cases with prognostic implications. J Chemother. 2006;18:209–16.
43. Berhili S, El Khannoussi B, Kadiri S, et al. Case report, uterine cervix metastasis from a sigmoid adenocarcinoma: a rare presentation of an uncommon tumor. Gynecolo Oncol Res Pract. 2014;1:6. doi:10.1186/2053-6844-1-6.
44. Chereau E, Ballester M, Gonin J, Leusieur B, Darai E. Cervical metastases from colorectal cancer. World J Oncol. 2011;2(2):83–4.
45. Sozen I, Small L, Kowalski M, Mayo SW, Hurwitz CA. Adenocarcinoma of the cervix metastatic from a colon primary and diagnosed from a routine pap smear in a 17-year-old woman: a case report. J Reprod Med. 2005;50:793–5.
46. Zulfiqar M, Liu S, Shi D, Madan S, Jacques S, King L, Shidham V, Giorgadze T. Metastatic colorectal adenocarcinoma in cervico-vaginal cytology specimens confirmed by immunocytochemical stains on liquid base specimens: two study cases with review of the literature. Cytojournal. 2013;10:9. doi:10.4103/1742-6413.112297.
47. Francisco Mucientes H, Pamela Villalobos H, Vanessa Klaassen H, et al. Casos Clínicos Metástasis de carcinoma de células en anillo de sello al cuello uterino. Rev chil obstet ginecol. 2013;78(3):229–235 230.

Chapter 2
Cervical Cancer Epidemiology

Nancy Reynoso-Noverón, Adriana Peña-Nieves, Maryori Ortiz Rodríguez, and Alejandro Mohar-Betancourt

Abstract Cervical cancer is a worldwide public health problem. In 2012, cervical cancer was the fourth most common disease in women and the seventh around the world, representing approximately 9 of every 10 deaths in less developed regions (87%). In Mexico, its relevance is also considerable; it is the neoplasia with the second highest incidence rates and the second leading cause of death among women of all ages. The most affected age groups are from 50–59 and 30–49 years old. Persistent infection with human papilloma virus (HPV) is a necessary factor for its development. There are certain risk factors that have been associated with cervical cancer, such as tobacco consumption, sexually transmitted diseases (STDs), oral contraceptive use and age at onset of sexual activity. In federal states such as Morelos or Chiapas, this disease has a greater impact on mortality partly because of social differences among the population. Although the strengthening of detection procedures, treatment and timely diagnosis have contributed to an important decrease in the mortality attributed to this cause in our country, there is still a need to keep improving the areas of prevention and promotion.

Keywords Neoplasia • Cervix • Mexico • Epidemiology • Detection • Prevention

N. Reynoso-Noverón, MD, PhD (✉) • A. Peña-Nieves, MSc • M.O. Rodríguez, MSc
Unit of Epidemiology, Instituto Nacional de Cancerología-México,
Av. San Fernando No 22, Col. Sección XVI, Mexico City 14080, Mexico
e-mail: nrn231002@yahoo.com.mx

A. Mohar-Betancourt, MD, PhD
Unit of Epidemiology, Instituto Nacional de Cancerología-México,
Av. San Fernando No 22, Col. Sección XVI, Mexico City 14080, Mexico

Unit of Biomedical Research in Cancer, Instituto de Investigaciones Biomédicas, Universidad Nacional Autónoma de México, Mexico City, Mexico

J.G. de la Garza-Salazar et al. (eds.), *Cervical Cancer*,
DOI 10.1007/978-3-319-45231-9_2

2.1 Impact of Cervical Cancer (CC)

2.1.1 In the World

In spite of being preventable, cervical cancer (CxCa) is the fourth most common type of cancer among women and the seventh among the general population. In 2012, 528,000 new cases were reported, accounting for an age-adjusted incidence rate of 14.0 per 100,000 women (Fig. 2.1). High-risk regions (with estimated age-standardized incidence rates of >30 per 100,000 women) include eastern Africa (42.7), Melanesia (33.3) and southern and middle Africa (31.5 and 30.6,

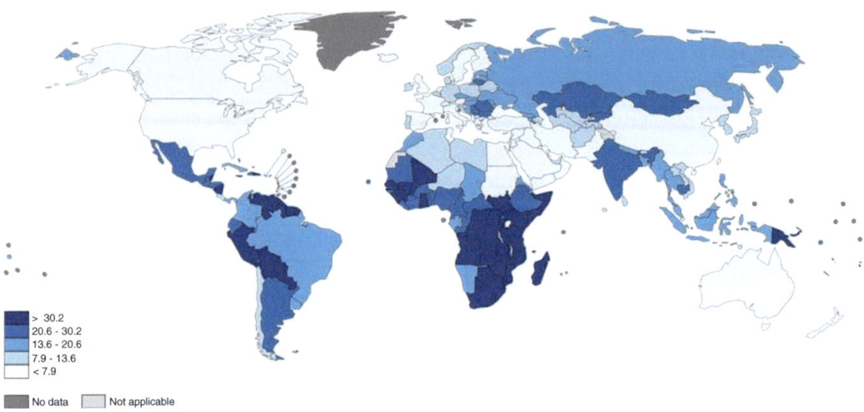

Fig. 2.1 Worldwide estimated incidence of cervical cancer in 2012* (Source: GLOBOCAN, 2012. Map production: IARC. World Health Organization http://globocan.iarc.fr/Pages/fact_sheets_cancer.aspx). *Estimated age-standardized rates per 100,000 women

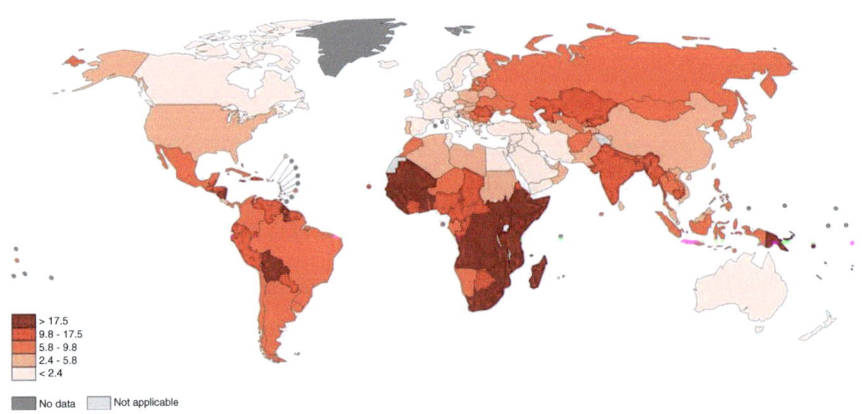

Fig. 2.2 Worldwide estimated mortality of cervical cancer in 2012*. GLOBOCAN, 2012. Map production: IARC. World Health Organization http://globocan.iarc.fr/Pages/fact_sheets_cancer.aspx. *Estimated age-standardized rates per 100,000 women

respectively). The lowest rates were present in Australia/New Zealand (5.5) and western Africa (4.4). In 2012, approximately 266,000 deaths were estimated around the world, which represents 7.5% of all female deaths attributed to cancer and an age-standardized mortality rate of 6.8 per 100,000 women (Fig. 2.2) [1].

Of the World Health Organization (WHO) regions, Africa and southeastern Asia have the highest mortality around the world (21.5 and 11.3 deaths per 100,000, respectively). Notably, approximately 9 of 10 deaths due to this malignant tumor occur in less developed regions [1]. A large majority of the global burden (approximately 85%) occurs in the less developed regions, where it accounts for 12% of almost all cancer cases in women. This disease affects primarily young women of low socio-economic status during their reproductive age, which also impacts their families. Thus, this type of cancer demonstrates the lack of equality in health status that exists [2].

2.1.2 Latin America and the Caribbean

According to GLOBOCAN, in 2012 in Latin America and the Caribbean, cervical cancer had an age-standardized rate of incidence of 21.2 per 100,000 women and a mortality rate of 8.7 per 100,000 women, which represents approximately 69,000 new cases and approximately 29,000 deaths. It is the second most common malignant tumor only after breast cancer, which is responsible for more new cases (27% and 12.2%, respectively) and deaths (14.9% and 9.9%, respectively) in these regions.

The countries with the highest estimated mortality rates are Guyana, Nicaragua, Paraguay, Surinam, Belize and Haiti, and those with the highest age-standardized incidence rates are Guyana, Surinam, French Guiana, Nicaragua and Paraguay (Table. 2.1). The estimated 1-year prevalence rate for this disease in the adult population is of 54,508 cases, but it is expected that the prevalence rates are four times higher (227,273 cases) (Fig. 2.3) [3].

Regarding the mortality rates in the year 2012, 28,565 deaths were reported in this region, with an age-standardized rate of 8.7 per 100,000 women. This rate corresponds to 10.7% of all deaths around the globe [3].

Currently, in the Americas, it is estimated that deaths due to CxCa are responsible for a great amount of years of potential life lost. As reported by the Pan-American Health Organization (PAHO), 74,855 women of 13 different countries of Latin America died because of cervical cancer between 1996 and 2001, of which 50,032 were from 25 to 64 years old. This finding indicates that more than 1.56 million years of potential life were lost because of the premature death of these women. When the morbidity burden is calculated in disability-adjusted life-years (which is equivalent to losing 1 year of healthy life), the WHO estimations suggest that in Latin America, this disease is responsible for 471,000 disability-adjusted life-years, which implies a much higher burden in comparison to any other type of cancer in women [4].

Table 2.1 Incidence and mortality rates of malignant cervical neoplasia in the Americas in 2012

País	New Cases	Deaths	Incidence rate[a]	Mortality rate[a]
Argentina	4956	2127	8.2	8.4
Bahamas	44	15	20.6	7.0
Barbados	44	15	25.4	7.2
Belice	43	17	32.7	14.9
Brasil	18,503	8414	16.3	7.3
Chile	1441	734	12.8	6.0
Colombia	4661	1986	18.7	8.0
Costa Rica	297	116	11.4	4.4
Cuba	1287	569	17.1	6.7
Ecuador	2094	1026	29.0	14.0
El Salvador	823	388	24.8	11.9
Guatemala	1393	672	22.3	12.2
Guayana Francesa	35	12	36.6	13.1
Guyana	161	71	46.9	21.9
Haití	1048	575	24.9	14.6
Jamaica	392	185	26.3	11.9
México	13,960	4769	23.3	8.1
Nicaragua	934	424	36.2	18.3
Panamá	351	134	18.7	7.1
Paraguay	1022	439	34.2	15.7
Perú	4636	1715	32.7	12.0
Puerto Rico	259	84	11.4	2.8
República Dominicana	1507	600	30.7	12.3
Surinam	107	44	38.0	15.7
Trinidad y Tobago	209	105	24.5	12.0
Uruguay	402	175	19.0	7.1
Venezuela	4973	1789	32.8	12.3

Source: GLOBOCAN 2012 (IARC). Consulted: 29/01/2016
[a]Incidence and Mortality Rates were age-standardized for 100,000 women

In agreement with the PAHO data, in the Americas, 83,000 women were diagnosed with cervical cancer in 2012, and 36,000 of them died because of this disease. If this tendency continues, the number of deaths will increase by 45% by 2030. The death rates for Latin America and the Caribbean continue to be three times higher than in North America, which serves as a testimony for the considerable inequalities in health status that exist [5].

Regarding the number of deaths due to this cause, among all the other neoplasias, ten countries stand out in the Latin America and Caribbean region, with proportions higher than 11%. These same countries can be sub-classified into two groups, the first sub-group, where ≥18% of the total deaths are due to malignant neoplasias (Guyana, 21.3%; Paraguay, 18.7%; Haiti, 18.3%; and Suriname, 17.7%), and the

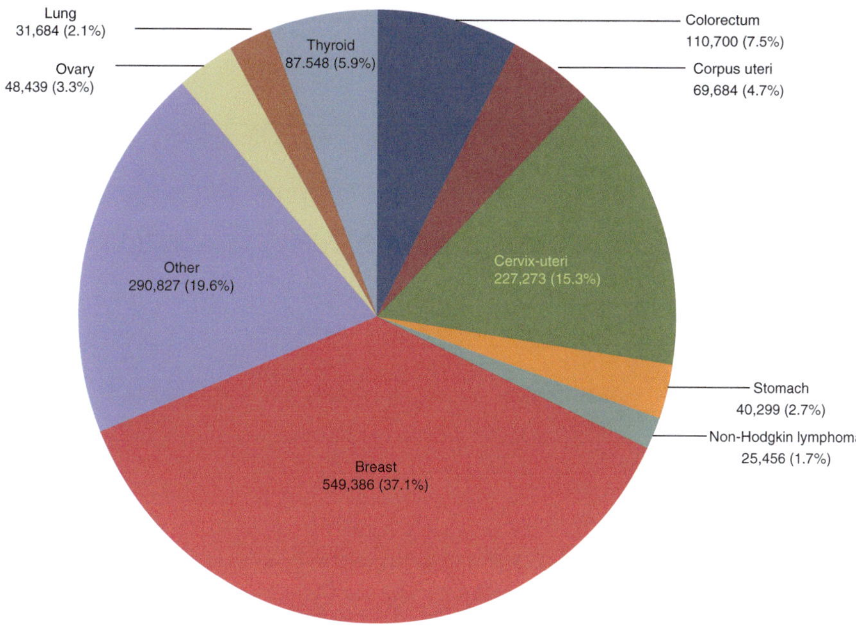

Fig. 2.3 Five-year estimated prevalence of cancer cases in women of Latin America and the Caribbean in 2012. Total population: 1,481,296 women (Source: GLOBOCAN 2012 (IARC). Consulted: 17/11/2015). Población total: 1,481,296 mujeres. Fuente: GLOBOCAN 2012 (IARC). Consultado el 17 de noviembre de 2015

second sub-group, where the ratio is slightly lower (Venezuela, Dominican Republic, Trinidad and Tobago, Jamaica, Mexico and El Salvador) (Table 2.2) [3].

2.1.3 In Mexico

Both the incidence and mortality of this malignant neoplasia are associated with demographic transition because there is a direct relationship between population aging and the appearance of new cases. However, lifestyle and the response capacity of the health departments limit the regional picture of this situation.

In México, cervical cancer is considered a public health problem, and this cancer is the second most common cause of malignant tumors in women ≥25 years old. Cervical cancer made up 9% (529,800) of all new cancer cases and 8% (275,100) of the total of female deaths due to cancer in 2008. Unfortunately, this type of cancer predominantly affects women in their reproductive years who find themselves in a vulnerable economic and social state, which implies a considerable impact both economically and socially and is currently the second cause of death by neoplasias in women in their reproductive years (40–59 years old) as well as in older women (55–59 years old) [6].

Table 2.2 Ratio of malignant neoplasia-caused deaths due to cervical cancer in women of the Americas in 2012

Country	Total deaths by malignan tumors[a]	Death by cervical cancer	Share of total (%)
Argentina	31,260	2127	6.8
Barbados	244	15	6.1
Brasil	103,606	8414	8.1
Canadá	35,230	503	1.4
Chile	12,063	734	6.1
Colombia	19,052	1986	10.4
Costa Rica	2005	116	5.8
Cuba	10,351	569	5.5
El salvador	3379	388	11.5
Estados Unidos	293,353	6605	2.3
Guyana	333	71	21.3
Haití	3146	575	18.3
Jamaica	1442	185	12.8
México	40,053	4769	11.9
Panamá	1353	134	9.9
Paraguay	2345	439	18.7
República Dominicana	4044	600	14.8
Surinam	248	44	17.7
Trinidad y Tobago	811	105	12.9
Uruguay	3756	175	4.7
Venezuela	11,280	1789	15.9

Source: GLOBOCAN, 2012
[a]All cancer types excluding non-melanoma skin cancer

2.1.3.1 Morbidity

The General Direction of Epidemiology of Mexico gathers information regarding the incidence rates and number of new cases in their annual reports. These data show that 3063 new cases were reported in Mexico in 2014 (incidence rate of 6.1 cases for every 100,000 women older than 10 years), whereas in 1992, the number of cases reported was 4378; this represents a decrease of 30% in the total number of cases presented in Mexico in the last 22 years. Considering the different age groups, the highest incidence rate is present in women older than 45 years, specifically in those between 60–64 years of age (incidence rate of 15.5), followed by those between 45 and 49 years of age (incidence rate of 12.6), and last, but close to the former, the group of women between 50 and 59 years old (incidence rate of 12.4; in all three cases, the rates are calculated for every 100,000 women more than 10 years of age).

The CxCa case distribution was heterogeneous across the different federal states of the republic in 2014 (Fig. 2.4), with the highest incidence rates were reported in the states of Colima, Campeche and Aguascalientes (43.4, 18.6 and 15.6 per 100,000

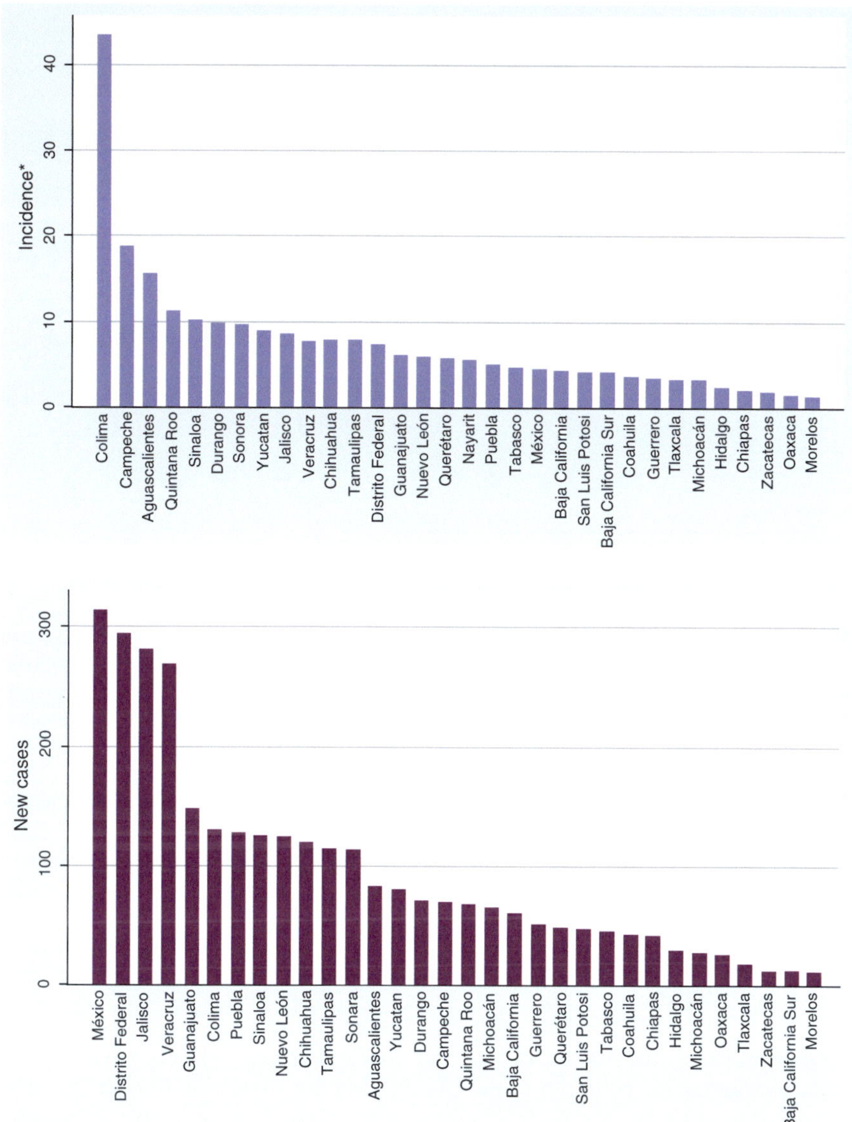

Fig. 2.4 Number of new cervical cancer cases and incidence rates* by federal state. *Rates were calculated per 100,000 women more than 10 years of age (Source: SUIVE/DGE/Secretariat of Health/United States of Mexico)

women more than 10 years of age, respectively), and the lowest incidence rates were reported in the states of Zacatecas, Oaxaca and Morelos (1.8, 1.5, and 1.3 for every 100,000 women more than 10 years of age, respectively).

Of the total cervical cancer cases registered in 2014, the majority were reported by the Mexican Social Security Institute (IMSS), followed by the Secretariat of

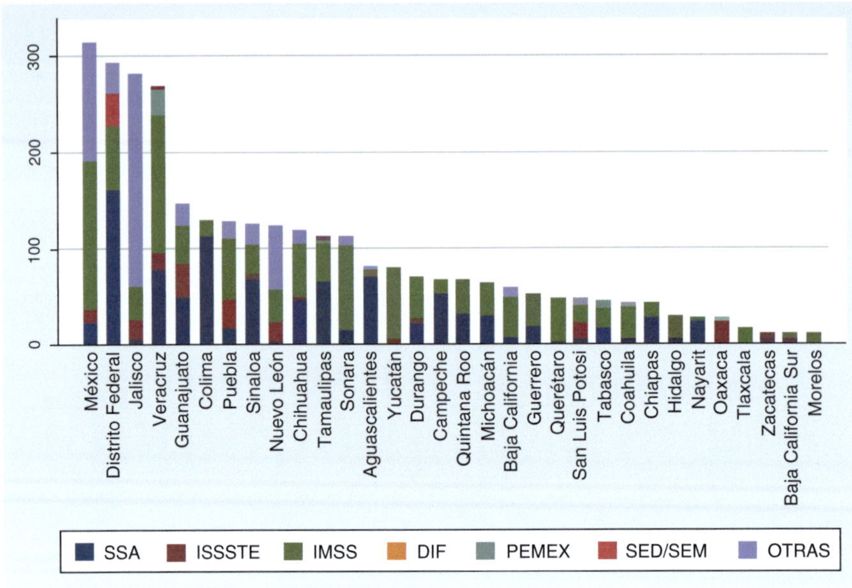

Fig. 2.5 New cases per federal state and notifying institution in Mexico in 2014. IMSS: also includes PROSPERA, and SED/SEM includes information from the Secretariat of National Defense and the Secretariat of the Navy (SEDENA and SEMAR, respectively, according to their original names in Spanish) (Source: SUIVE/DGE/Secretariat of Health/United States of Mexico)

Health and other institutions. In federal states where the Secretariat of Health is not the main reporting institution, such as Jalisco, Nuevo León, Yucatán and Baja California, its role is replaced by the IMSS or the Insurance and Social Security Institute for State Workers (ISSSTE) (Fig. 2.5).

2.1.3.2 Mortality

Cervical cancer is the second cause of death due to cancer among women since 2006, and among the countries of the Organization for Economic Cooperation and Development (OECD), Mexico is the country with the highest mortality rate because of cervical cancer.

A total of 3784 female deaths were registered in Mexico in 2013, with a raw rate of 7.0 deaths per 100,000 women. Specifically, in the group of women 25 years and older, 3776 deaths were recorded, with a raw rate of 11.3 deaths per 100,000 women and an average age of death of 59 years old [5]. A total of 67,277 deaths were registered between 1998–2013, and the most affected age groups were from 50 to 69 years old, followed by the group of 30–49 years of age, while the least affected group was that of the youngest women (between 10 and 29 years old) (Fig. 2.6).

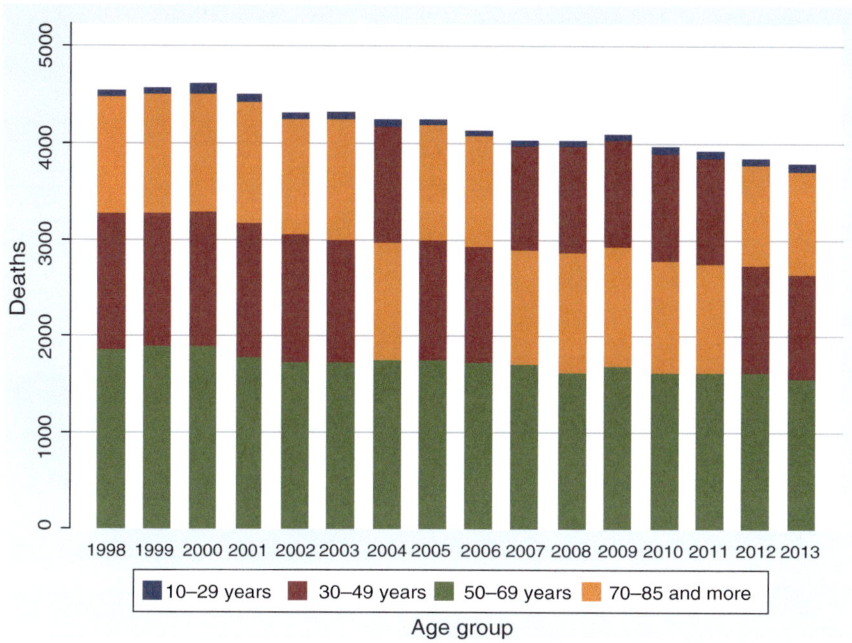

Fig. 2.6 Mortality due to cervical cancer by age group in Mexico in 1998–2013 (Source: General Directorate of Information of the Secretariat of Health of Mexico. INEGI to elaborate the leading causes of death with the Mexican list)

Between 2000 and 2013, the raw mortality rates fell from 18.9 to 11.3 deaths per 100,000 women above 25 years old, which represents a decrease of 40.2% in 13 years. If the federal states are considered during the last year (Fig. 2.7), there are different impact levels of this neoplasia; note the mortality rates between 12.7 and 18.6 deaths per 100,000 women ≥25 years old in the states of Morelos, Chiapas, Veracruz and Sonora (18.6, 17.2, 16.4 and 15.9, respectively) and the states with 8.1 or less deaths per 100,000 women ≥25 years old, which are Aguascalientes, Baja California Sur and Mexico City [7].

2.2 Risk Factors

Studies indicate that persistent infection with human papilloma virus (HPV) is a necessary requirement for the development of cervical cancer [8, 9]. It is transmitted by sexual contact, affecting 8 of every 10 persons (men and women) at some point of their life. Only one woman of every 10 that acquire this infection will develop cancer [10]. Certain factors that were formerly believed to be associated with an increased risk of developing cervical cancer are now known to be risk factors for HPV infection. Some of these risk factors are as follows [11–17]:

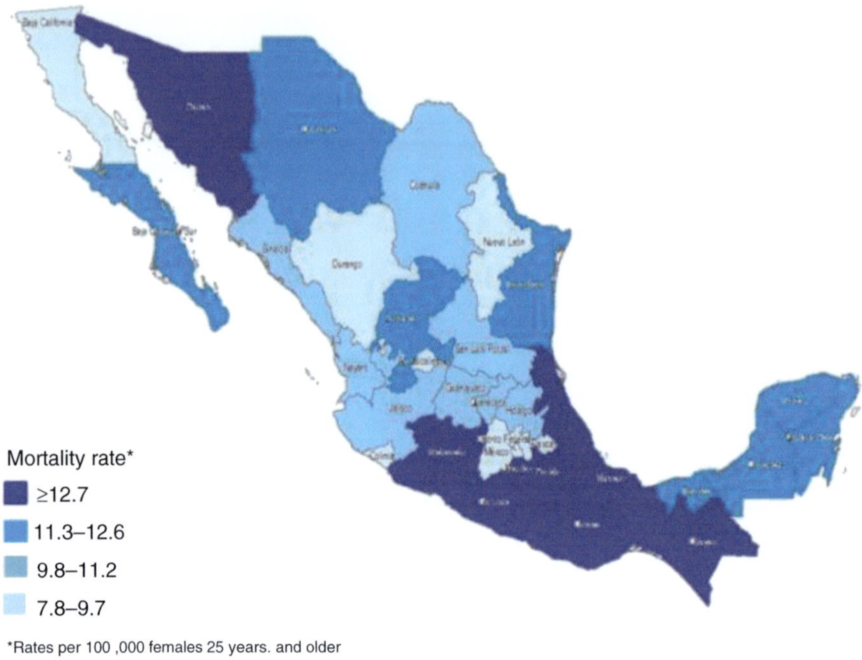

Fig. 2.7 Cervical cancer mortality rate in Mexico in 2013

- Tobacco consumption
- STDs (herpes and chlamydia)
- Use of oral hormones
- Nutritional deficiencies
- Age of onset of sexual activity and absence of protection during adolescence
- High-risk sexual behavior throughout lifetime (multiple sexual partners)

This neoplasia is 100% preventable with measures such as vaccinating against HPV, using condoms, and avoiding tobacco consumption, as well as early detection and treatment of pre-cancerous lesions.

In Mexico, the HPV type prevalence distribution is not known; recent studies have reported the prevalence and genotype distribution of HPV in Mexico in women with cervical cancer, with low- and high-grade squamous intra-epithelial lesions and with normal cytology. Of 8706 samples of tissues from Mexican females, which were stratified according to diagnosis (499, cervical cancer; 364, high-grade lesions; 1425, low-grade lesions; and 6418, normal cytology); the most frequent genotypes were as follows [18]:

- HPV 16 (63.1%), HPV 18 (8.6%) HPV 58 and HPV 31 (5%) for CxCa
- HPV 16 (28.3%), HPV 58 (12.6%), HPV 18 (7.4%) and HPV 33 (6.5%) for high-grade lesions

- HPV 16 (13.1%), HPV 33 (7.4%), HPV 18 (4.2%), HPV 18 (4.2%) and HPV 58 (2.6%) for low-grade lesions
- HPV 16 (3.4%), HPV 33 (2.1%), HPV 18 and HPV 58 (1.2% for normal cytology)

Additionally, a study conducted in heterosexual couples reported that the prevalence of HPV infection is 13.7% for women. The most frequently detected high-risk types were HPVs 59, 16, 31, 52 and 58, and the low-risk types detected were HPV 62, 71, 81 and 54 among women [19].

2.3 Evolution of the Cervical Cancer Program in Mexico

In the last decade, the reduction in mortality may be attributed to a low incidence caused by the combination of prevention activities implemented in health services together with diagnosis opportunity, treatment delivery and improvements in health care service quality and access [20, 21].

In Mexico, actions have been taken to address public health matters in the last 10 years, which has increased the current understanding of this neoplasia. One such example is Mexico's National Institute of Cancerology, a public assistance institution created on November 25th, 1946, that specializes in providing treatment for different types of cancer, together with the public health measures designed, including national campaigns against cancer. In 1974, the first National Cervical Cancer Early Detection Program was created, and it used the Pap test or cytology as the means of detection because it had been established for decades, it was the reference test for cervical cancer screening around the world, and it had reduced the mortality of this disease in developed countries with plenty of resources [22].

In 1996, the health care system of Mexico had only enough resources and infrastructure to carry out about three million Pap tests per year for a population of more than 16 million women between 25 and 65 years old. In that same year, the official Mexican standards dictated that Pap test were recommended on a yearly basis for women with an active sexual lifestyle, without delimiting an age limit, and women with a colposcopy diagnosis of HPV and even presenting slight dysplasia were attended at the colposcopy clinic with cryosurgery, electro-surgery or laser in accordance with the technical protocol of the country. At that same time, the National Cervical Cancer Early Detection Program did not consider epidemiological surveillance an important factor, which could have guaranteed the follow-up and treatment of the anomalies detected in women in which a Pap test had been carried out [23].

In 1997, steps were taken to improve the early detection and surveillance of patients, namely, the National Committee for the Prevention and Control of Cervical and Breast Cancer was created. Then, in 1998, the Secretariat of Health created the General Direction of the Prevention and Control of Cervical Cancer [24]. Additionally, since 2004, the Popular Insurance Program began including cervical

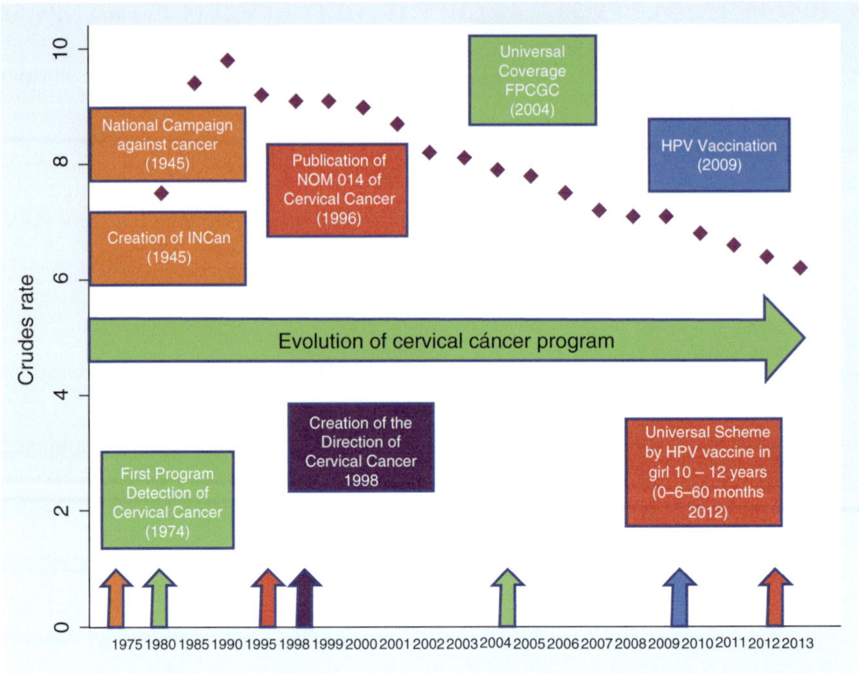

Fig. 2.8 History of the actions implemented in the country to counteract CxCa (Source: Adapted from the Secretary of Health. National Center for Gender Equality and Reproductive Health)

cancer with support from the Fund for the Protection of Catastrophic Expenses, which means that any woman, no matter her economic situation or her geographical location, could be attended free of charge in the accredited hospitals of the Popular Insurance Program [25]. The recent implementations in the health care system, such as programmed vaccination in an extended dose scheme, with two doses at 0–2 months or 0–6 months and a third dose after 60 months in girls between 9 and 11 years old (Fig. 2.8), are worth mentioning [26].

Finally, there is evidence that socioeconomic improvement and the implementation of early detection programs have significantly influenced the slowing and reduction of the mortality rates due to cervical cancer. In Mexico, this reduction is a priority, and according to the results of the ENSANUT 2012, 44.3% of women between 25 and 65 years of age had a Pap test performed in the year prior to this survey, while 37.1 and 29.4% had their tests performed 1 year before the ENSANUT 2006 and ENSA 2000 surveys. In addition, in 2012, women were also administered tests for the detection of HPV (10% of women between 35 and 50 years old) (Fig. 2.9) [27].

However, despite the benefit of preventative care, there is still a tendency to allocate a strong majority of healthcare expenditures for curative measures while neglecting preventative efforts. Healthy eating habits, an increase in physical activity, controlled alcohol consumption, and the promotion of safe sex and vaccination for

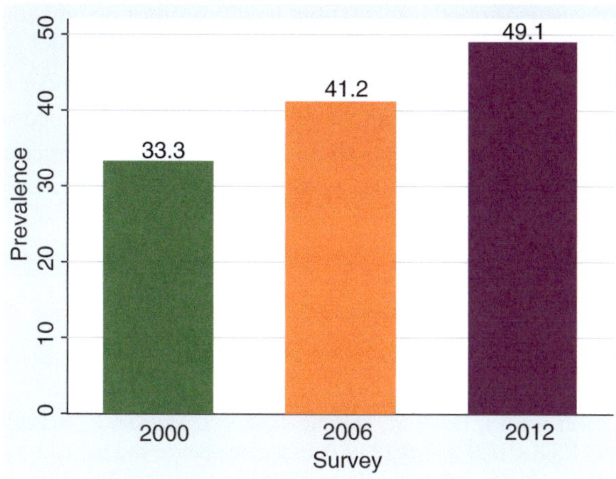

Fig. 2.9 Prevalence of the use of the Pap test during the last 12 months in women between 25 and 64 years old. Mexico ENSA, ENSANUT 2006 and 2012 (Source: ENSANUT 2012)

the prevention of the main serotypes of HPV associated with this type of cancer can reduce its incidence [10].

2.4 The Role of the Health Care System in Mexico to Prevent Mortality and Morbidity Due to Cervical Cancer: Conclusions

In spite of the difficulties, the health care system has managed to partially reduce the mortality rate due to cervical cancer through a cervical cancer prevention program, although not at the same pace at which it has been reduced in more developed countries. Thus, it is necessary to perform constant monitoring of the mortality rates due to cervical cancer with the purpose of evaluating the advances made by these programs and determining the need for interventions. It is also necessary to implement cancer archives based on the population to be able to evaluate the real impact of the implemented interventions in the future and simultaneously design and carry out interventions that allow us to develop prevention-focused policies that are more cost-effective for the healthcare system [21].

It is also necessary to continue the improvement process. Integral programs that include education, HPV vaccination, screening, treatment and palliative care, together with a monitoring and evaluation component for the prevention and control of cervical cancer, are key elements to reduce the impact of this disease.

Cervical cancer is the result of a persistent infection by certain types of HPV and develops over the course of many years, offering various windows of opportunity for its prevention, including vaccination, screening and treatment of pre-cancerous lesions.

Given the above-mentioned information, health promotion and education should have the main objective of providing women, their families and the population with the information that allows them to understand that cervical cancer is preventable; therefore, it is necessary for women to receive the screening services that the health service offers. Furthermore, women should be encouraged to receive appropriate treatment when required and provided with better access to diagnostic services and adequate and timely treatment.

References

1. Ferlay J, Soerjomataram I, Ervik M, Dikshit R, Eser S, Mathers C, Rebelo M, Parkin DM, Forman D, Bray F. GLOBOCAN 2012 v1.0, cancer incidence and mortality worldwide: IARC CancerBase No. 11 [Internet]. Lyon: International Agency for Research on Cancer; 2013. Available from: http://globocan.iarc.fr, accessed on 11/12/2015.
2. Almonte M, Murillo R, Sánchez GI, Jerónimo J, Salmerón J, Ferreccio C, Lazcano-Ponce E, Herrero R. New paradigms and challenges in cervical cancer prevention and control in Latin America. Salud Publica Mex 2010;52:544–59.
3. International Agency for Research on Cancer. Incidence and mortality rates of cervical cancer in the Americas 2012. GLOBOCAN 2012. Consulted: 11/17/2015.
4. Lewis MJ. Análisis de la situación de cáncer cervicouterino en América Latina y el Caribe. Washington, D.C. Organización Panamericana de la Salud / Organización Mundial de la Salud (OPS/OMS); 2004. p. 40.
5. Organización Panamericana de la Salud & Organización Mundial de la Salud. Nota informativa. Consulted: 01/26/2016; available at: http://www.paho.org/hq/index.php?option=com_topics&view=article&id=348&Itemid=40936&lang=es.
6. Torres-Poveda KJ, Cruz-Valdez A, Madrid-Marina V. Epidemiología del Cáncer Cérvico Uterino. Gaceta Mexicana de Oncología. 2014;13(4):4–17.
7. Secretaría de Salud. Centro Nacional de Equidad de Género y Salud Reproductiva. Información estadística. Available at: http://cnegsr.salud.gob.mx/contenidos/Programas_de_Accion/CancerdelaMujer/InfEstad.html. Consulted on: 11/13/2015.
8. Bosch FX, Lörincz A, Muñoz N, Meijer CJ, Shah KV. The causal relation between human papillomavirus and cervical cancer. J Clin Pathol. 2002;55:244–65.
9. Muñoz N, Bosch FX, de Sanjose S, et al. Epidemiologic classification of human papillomavirus types associated with cervical cancer. N Engl J Med. 2003;348:518–27.
10. Secretaría de Salud. Programa de Acción Específico. Prevención y control del cáncer de la mujer 2013-2018. 98 pages. Disponible en: http://www.spps.gob.mx/programas-accion2013-2018.html.
11. Collins SI, Mazloomzadeh S, Winter H, et al. Proximity of first intercourse to menarche and the risk of human papillomavirus infection: a longitudinal study. Int J Cancer. 2005;114:498–500.
12. Ho GY, Bierman R, Beardsley L, Chang CJ, Burk RD. Natural history of cervicovaginal papillomavirus infection in young women. N Engl J Med. 1998;338:423–8.
13. Herrero R, Castle PE, Schiffman M, et al. Epidemiologic profile of type-specific human papillomavirus infection and cervical neoplasia in Guanacaste, Costa Rica. J Infect Dis. 2005;191:1796–807.
14. Hernández-Giron C, Smith JS, Lörincz A, Lazcano E, Hernandez-Avila M, Salmerón J. High-risk human papillomavirus detection and related risk factors among pregnant and nonpregnant women in Mexico. Sex Transm Dis. 2005;32:613–8.
15. Smith JS, Green J, Berrington de González A, et al. Cervical cancer and use of hormonal contraceptives: a systematic review. Lancet. 2003;361:1159–67.

16. Plummer M, Herrero R, Franceschi S, et al. Smoking and cervical cancer: pooled analysis of the IARC multi-centric case–control study. Cancer Causes Control. 2003;14:805–14.
17. International Collaboration of Epidemiological Studies of Cervical Cancer. Carcinoma of the cervix and tobacco smoking: Collaborative reanalysis of individual data on 13,541 women with carcinoma of the cervix and 23,017 women without carcinoma of the cervix from 23 epidemiological studies. Int J Cancer. 2006;118:1481–95. doi:10.1002/ijc.21493.
18. Peralta R et al. Prevalence of human papillomavirus in the cervical epithelium of Mexican women: meta-analysis. Infect Agent Cancer. 2012;7:34.
19. Parada R, Morales R, Giuliano AR, et al. Prevalence, concordance and determinants of human papillomavirus infection among heterosexual partners in a rural region of central Mexico. BMC Infect Dis. 2010;10:223.
20. Lazcano-Ponce E, Palacio-Mejía LS, Allen-Leigh B, Yunes-Diaz E, Alonso P, Schiavon R. Decreasing cervical cancer mortality in México: effect of Papanicolaou coverage, birth rate, and the importance of diagnostic validity of cytology. Cancer Epidemiol Biomark Prev. 2008;17:2808–17.
21. Torres-Sánchez LE, Rojas-Martínez R, Escamilla-Núñez C, de la Vara-Salazar E, Lazcano-Ponce E. Cancer mortality trends in Mexico, 1980–2011. Salud Publica Mex 2014;56: 473–91.
22. Organización Mundial de la Salud & Organización Panamericana de la Salud. El cáncer cérvicouterino en las Américas 2014. Available at: http://190.34.154.93/rncp/sites/all/files/OPS-Nota-Informativa-Cancer-Cervicouterino-2014.pdf.
23. Lazcano-Ponce E, Sue Moss s, Alonso P, Salmerón J y Hernández M. Cáncer Cérvicouterino, diagnostico, prevención y control. Programa de detección oportuna de cáncer de cuello uterino en países en vías de desarrollo. El caso de México. Chapter 14. Mexico, D.F: Editorial Médica Panamericana; 2000. 254 pp.
24. Instituto nacional de las mujeres INMUJERES. El enfoque de género en la producción de las estadísticas sobre salud en México. Guía para el uso y una referencia para la producción de información. Available at: http://cedoc.inmujeres.gob.mx/documentos_download/100665.pdf.
25. Aracena-Genao B, González-Robledo M, González-Robledo L, Palacio-Mejía L, Nigenda-López G. El fondo de protección contra gastos catastróficos: tendencia, evolución y operación. Salud Publica Mex. 2011;53:s407–15.
26. Lazcano-Ponce E, Aranda Flores C, Aguado-Pérez A, Cruz-Valdez y Bojalil R. Vacunas para proteger de la infección por virus de papiloma humano. Gaceta Mexicana de Oncología. 2014;13(Suppl 4):39–47.
27. Gutiérrez JP, Rivera-Dommarco J, Shamah-Levy T, Villalpando-Hernández S, Franco A, Cuevas-Nasu L, Romero-Martínez M, Hernández-Ávila M. Encuesta Nacional de Salud y Nutrición 2012. Resultados Nacionales. Cuernavaca. México: Instituto Nacional de Salud Pública (MX); 2012.

Chapter 3
Malignant Transforming Mechanisms of Human Papillomavirus

H. Astudillo-de la Vega, E. Ruiz-Garcia, C. Lopez-Camarillo, Jaime G. de la Garza-Salazar, A. Meneses-Garcia, and L. Benitez-Bribiesca

Abstract HPVs transforming activities represent the viral replication strategy that is driven to replicate viral genomes and to establish long-term maintenance in a tissue. High-risk-HPV-infected cells and carcinogenesis progression are terminal events, since cancer cells contain integrated HPV genomes and do produce viral progeny. High-risk HPV (HR-HPV) genome integration indeed represents a consequence of HPV E6/E7- induced genomic instability. HR-HPV E6 and E7 proteins critically contribute to viral life cycle and transforming activity. HR-HPV E7 proteins bind to pRB and decreased efficiency. HR-HPV E6 proteins efficiently interact with TP53 and promote for TP53 degradation. High-risk HPVs can frequently persist for decades in an infected host cell at a low number of copies. One of the events of HPV-induced carcinogenesis is the HPV genome integration into a host chromosome, and it is probably a failed viral mechanism. High Risk-HPV E6 proteins and E7 contribute to immortalization of primary human epithelial cells by induction of telomerase activity. Data evidences suggest that microbial dysbiosis is associated with malignant

H. Astudillo-de la Vega, MD MSc PhD (✉)
Laboratorio de Investigación Traslacional y Terapia Celular, Hospital de Oncología, Centro Médico Nacional "Siglo XXI", IMSS, Av. Cuauhtemoc 330, Col. Doctores, CP 06720 México DF, Mexico
e-mail: hastud2@gmail.com

E. Ruiz-Garcia, MD MSc • A. Meneses-Garcia, MD PhD
Laboratorio de Medicina Traslacional, Instituto Nacional de Cancerología, SS, México DF, Mexico

C. Lopez-Camarillo, PhD
Posgrado en Ciencias Genomicas, Universidad Autonoma de la Ciudad de Mexico, México DF, Mexico

J.G. de la Garza-Salazar, MD
Departamento de Oncología Médica, Instituto Nacional de Cancerología, SS, México DF, Mexico

L. Benitez-Bribiesca, MD
Deparmento of investigation at Instituto Mexicano del Seguro Social (IMSS), Instituto Nacional de Cancerología, Mexico City, Mexico

J.G. de la Garza-Salazar et al. (eds.), *Cervical Cancer*,
DOI 10.1007/978-3-319-45231-9_3

transformation, but future discussion and direction for microbiome in cancer research (oncobioma) and particularly in HPV-associated human cancer could be evaluated as causative causes that modulate initiation, progression, or cancer metastasis.

Keywords HPV • High risk-HPV • Neoplastic transformation • HPV genome integration • C-myc • E6 • pRb • E7 • p53 • Telomerase • Tumor metabolome • Dysbiosis • Oncobioma

3.1 HPV Generalities, Life Cycle and Genome

"To avoid criticism, do nothing, say nothing, be nothing" Elbert Hubbard (writer)

Human papillomaviruses (HPVs) are members of the *papovaviridae* family. The viral structure consists of a 72-capsomere capsid; capsomeres are two structural proteins: 57 kD late protein L1 (80% of the viral particle) and 43–53 kD minor capsid protein L2 [1]. The HPV absence of envelope makes them stable and let them remain infectious for months in hostile environments [2]. The HPVs are present in higher vertebrates, however, they show a species-specificity pattern but the horizontal transmission from non-primates to humans has not been reported. HPV causes a local infection in the stratified epithelia and induces a productive replication with differentiation in a non-acute one, but produces a chronic disease where viral spread and/or viremia do not occur. The life cycle of HPV is associated with the differentiation program of epithelial cells. In normal epithelial cells, the only actively dividing cells are present in the basal layers of the stratified epithelium, which is basically formed by "transit amplifying cells" (TAC) and stem cells. Cells that are proliferating and can terminally differentiate are TAC and cells, which have the potential to proliferate indefinitely, are stem cells, although they divide infrequently in order to replenish the TAC pool [3]. After viral infection, HPVs deposit their double strand DNA genome into nuclei of infected cells and establishes as extra-chromosomal plasmids or episomes [4]. HPV gains entry to cells in the basal layer of the epithelium that becomes exposed through micro-abrasions [4]. The HPV genome has three genomic regions E and L genes, which are numbered according to the size: 4-kb early (E) region that encodes nonstructural proteins, 3-kb late (L) region that encodes two capsid proteins (L1, L2 genes), and 1-kb noncoding long control region (LCR) that regulates viral replication and gene expression (Fig. 3.1). Papillomavirus life cycle is linked to the differentiation program of infected epithelium cells and infects basal epithelial cells in the sole cell layer in the epithelium actively dividing. Although integrin-6 has been related, HPV receptor(s) has not been characterized [5]. Viral HPV-DNA is in the nuclei of infected host cells in a low copy number and lately undergoes differentiation moving toward the epithelium surface. The mechanism changes when the HPV-DNA is present in terminally differentiated cells; the

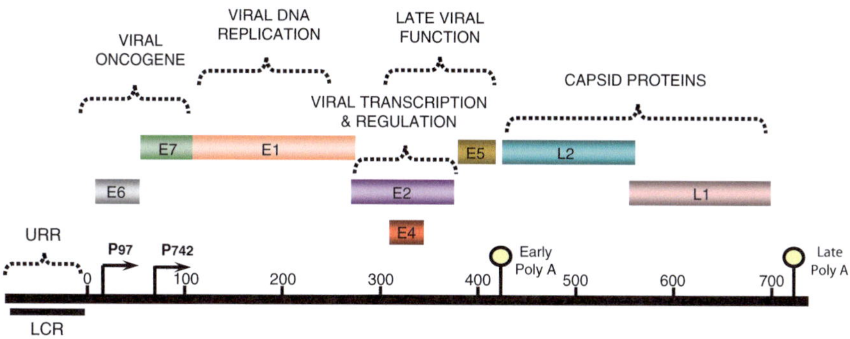

Fig. 3.1 HPV Genome linear arrangement. HPV genome is small (8 kb), circular and with double strand DNA. There are eight open reading frames (ORFs) expressed from a single polycistronic transcript transcribed from a single strand of DNA. The Upstream Regulatory Region (URR) is in the non-coding region and regulates viral transcription and replication. HPV genes are regulated during differentiation by the virus early promoter (P97), the differentiation late-dependent promoter (P742), and tow Polyadenylation signals (PolyA). E6 and E7 are oncogenes responsible of the replication competence. E1 and E2 are genes of viral DNA replication and regulation of viral transcription. E4 and E5 are genes for late viral functions and L1 and L2 are genes for protein capsids

virus replicates in a high number of copies, late genes are expressed, and progeny virus is produced [6]. The HPVs are not lytic viruses and the progeny virus is shed into the environment as a cargo within epithelial squamae. This review discusses the various mechanisms of transformation and the roles HPV plays in cervical carcinogenesis.

3.2 Transforming Mechanisms of HPV Viral Oncoproteins

HPVs potential to promote malignant transformation is the key for the low- and high-risk classification created from observations of HPV types found in cancers as high-risk (HR-HPV) and the ones found in benign lesions as low-risk (LR-HPV), and by experimental evidence that demonstrated their abilities to modify proliferation and genome stability. The general molecular aspects and functions of human papillomavirus proteins are shown in Table 3.1. The most important oncogenic proteins are E6 and E7, because of their immortalizing and transforming high potential, both in animal models and 'in vitro' models. The hallmarks of dysplasia lesions (low and high grade) as precursor of cervical cancer are the expression of HR-HPV E6/E7 genes; the expression of both genes contributes to genomic stability and malignant progression [7]. HPV E6 is a 150-amino acid protein containing two metal binding motifs (PDZ protein-binding motif), which acts as molecular organizing center for cellular signal transduction pathways [8]. There is a cellular defense mechanism that induces synthesis of aberrant and/or viral DNA into differentiated keratinocytes, which eliminates cells by selective and type-specific

Table 3.1 Molecular aspects and transforming functions of human papillomavirus proteins

Viral protein/genomic element	Molecular weight/size	Viral protein function	Host protein interactions
Non-coding elements			
Long Control Region (LCR)	500–1000 bp	Origin of replication and regulation of HPV gene expression	TBX2, TBX3, GATA3, FOXA1, c-Myc
Early proteins			
E1	68–85 kD	Helicase function; essential for viral replication and control of gene transcription	UAF1, USP1, USP12, USP46
E2	48 kD	Viral transcription factor; essential for viral replication and control of gene transcription; genome segregation and encapsidation, apoptosis regulation	Brd4, Nrdp-1, DED-B, CCHCR1
E3	Unknown	Functions not known	None
E1^E4	10–44 kD	Binding to cytoskeletal protein and keratin intermediate filaments	SRPK1, CK-IF
E5	14 kD	Interaction with EGF/PDGF-receptors	Nrdp-1, PDGFR, BAP31
E6	16–18 kD	Integration with several cellular proteins; degradation of p53 and activation of telomerase	Bak, p300/CBP, ADA3, NFX1–91, Paxillin, Gps2, c-Myc, ERC55, IRF-3, Mcm7, p53, XRCC1, β-Catenin, PSD-95, hDlg2, zo-1, SAP97
E7	~10 kD	Integration with several cellular proteins; interaction with pRB and transactivation of E2F-dependent protein	AP1 family, α-glucosidase, Cyclin A, Cyclin E complexes, p300, CBP, Pcaf, IGFBP-3, IRF-1, Mi2β, M2-PK, pRb, pRb-associated pocket proteins, $p21^{CIP-1}$, $p27^{KIP-1}$, TAF110, TATA BOX-bp, HDAC, CK19
E8^-E2C	20 kD	Long-distance transcription and replication repressor protein	NCoR/SMRT complexes, CHD6
Late proteins			
L1	57 kD	Major capsid protein	HSPG, Alpha 6 beta 4 integrin
L2	43–53 kD	Minor capsid protein	SUMO and/or SUMOylated proteins, TRAPPC8, annexin A2, SNX27, TSG101, TBX2, TBX3

processes such as apoptosis, differentiation and senescence; the name of such mechanism is "trophic sentinel response" (TSR) [8]. One of the molecular mechanisms of E6 protein to promote malignancy in epithelial cells is the induction of TP53 ubiquitination and proteasome degradation by retargeting E6-AP [9]. A considerable number of cellular proteins have been reported to associate with E6 (see Table 3.1). HR-HPV E6 proteins eliminate the TSR triggered by E7 expression through inactivation of TP53 [10]. The HPV16 E6/E7 ORF cassette is regulated by the epidermal growth factor (EGF) pathway; there is a natural gradient of EGF and EGFR expression in the stratified epithelium, and it is the reason to assume that EGF modulates E6/E7 splicing during the viral life cycle and transformation [11]. HPV E7 is a low-molecular-weight protein of approximately 100 amino acids without intrinsic enzymatic activities. HPV-16 E7 oncoprotein has an amino-terminal 37-amino-acid residue similar to sequences of CR1 and to CR2 of Adenovirus E1A protein (Ad E1A). CR1 sequences are responsible for the retinoblastoma tumor suppressor protein (pRB) degradation and cellular transformation; CR2 sequences are the pRB-binding site (LXCXE), necessary for cellular transformation. E7 carboxyl terminus contains a metal binding motif for association with host cellular proteins, which include histone-modifying enzymes, in order to contribute toward malignant transformation. Such as AdE1A and SV40 T antigen, the HPV E7 protein interacts with several host cellular proteins (see Table 3.1). The ability of HPV E7, Ad E1A, and SV40 T antigen to associate with pRB is basic for the viral genome replication. HR-HPV-derived E7 proteins interact with pRB more efficiently than the E7 proteins encoded by LR-HPVs [12]. E7-interacting proteins, including transcription factors, cell cycle regulators, and metabolic enzymes, appear to associate with carboxyl-terminal E7 sequences [13]. The HPV E7 amino-terminal pRB binding site protein has been implicated in histone deacetylase binding, a necessary event for the HPV viral life cycle [14]. HPV-16 E6 and E7 oncoproteins over-regulate the TGF-beta1 promoter in cervical tumor cells [15]. The HPV oncoproteins E6 and E7 have been implicated in the regulation of the Wnt/β-catenin pathway [16].

3.3 Genomic Integration of HPV and Host Genomic Instability Induction as Basic Steps toward Malignant Transformation by HPV

Cellular signal transduction pathways are dysfunctional in human solid tumors [17], and it has been proposed the minimally oncogenic steps necessary to generate 'in vitro' transformed human epithelial cells. The expression of simian virus 40 (SV40) large tumor antigen (T), SV40 small tumor antigen (t), inactivates TP53 and pRb tumor suppressors, just like the HPV E6 and E7 oncoproteins work; the catalytic subunit of human telomerase (hTERT) which HPV E6 can activate transcriptionally, and the activated *H-Ras* oncogene are required to transform primary human epithelial cells [18]. Hence, the expression of HR-HPV E6/E7 oncogenes provides the minimal carcinogenic hits for primary human epithelial cells transformation [19].

HPV infects differentiated squamous epithelial cells (growth arrested) incompetent to support genome synthesis, but the HPV genome encodes functions that create and/or maintain a genome replication competence in differentiated keratinocytes. During the HPV life cycle, it is established a mechanism of long-term viral persistence into the squamous epithelia. HR-HPVs have evolved specific molecular mechanisms to maintain the host immune evasion and escape to guaranty viral progeny and not to induce an oncogenic process, which is not the natural function of the HPV infection. One of the events of HPV-induced carcinogenesis is the HPV genome integration into a host chromosome, and it is probably a failed viral mechanism. The HPV genome integration occurs into common fragile sites of the human genome [20], but there are not apparent hot spots for integration and no evidence for insertional mutagenesis [21]. Papillomavirus E1 and E2 proteins play a role in viral replication. The papillomavirus E2 protein works: (i) as a DNA binding transcription factor interacting with specific motifs (ACCN6GGT) in the LCR region [22]; (ii) as a transcriptional activator or transcriptional repressor in keratinocytes [23]; (iii) associated with viral DNA helicase E1 to modulate viral gene expression, in order to increase the recognition of the origin and the viral genome replication [24]; (iv) playing a role in viral genome segregation during cell division by tethering viral genomes to mitotic chromosomes [25]; (v) in association with mitotic chromosomes by interaction with the human bromo-domain protein Brd4 [26]. HPV genome integration to host genome follows a major specific pattern regarding the HPV genome function, and the consequence is the consistently maintained expression of the viral E6 and E7 genes, whereas other DNA viral genome regions (such as E2 region) are deleted and/or their expression is disturbed [27]. The E2 loss expression is significant and results in deregulated E6 and E7 expression; when it happens with HPV-16 an increased E6/E7 expression and stability after genome integration occurs [28], and host cellular specific alterations of gene expression appears [29]. Infected cells with integrated HPV genome that expresses E6/E7 have a selective growth advantage in comparison with infected cells harboring episomal HPV genome. The continued E6/E7 expression in cervical cancer cells is an obligated process for transformed phenotype maintenance [30]. HPV 16 and 18 integrations in high-grade lesions are accompanied by chromosomal abnormalities [31]. HR-HPV genomes are integrated into the host genome in the most invasive cancers, an increased ability of HR-HPV types to integrate into host DNA compared to those with low-risk types [32]. Extra-chromosomal HPV DNA is found in benign and low-grade lesions and HPV integration can be found in premalignant lesions grade 2/3 such as cervical intraepithelial neoplasia (CIN2/3). LR-HPV types are rarely found integrated in tumors, which was demonstrated by the absence of full-length E2 transcripts studies of tissue specimens from patients with a history of benign early-onset recurrent respiratory papillomatosis developing laryngeal cancer [33]. HPV integration disrupts the E2 gene [34], so determination of absent amplification of E2 sequences has been considered a molecular marker of integration or progression in cervical cancer; unfortunately, the results obtained are ambiguous. Detection of early gene transcripts by reverse-transcription PCR is more sensitive in cancers as well as in benign or dysplastic cervical samples, in which the presence of integrated genomes correlates with the severity of the disease, especially for HPV 18 [35]. HPV genomes integration is a failed step that affects both viral and host gene expression. Increased E7 protein synthesis correlate with viral DNA integration where integrated viral DNA confers growth advantages and phenotypic cellular changes with high-grade neoplasia compared to extrachromosomal viral DNA cells. The disruption pattern in the viral genome does not occur in the host genome, in contrast, HPV DNA sequences integration uses preferential sites of human chromosomes and suggests a non-random pattern of integration, for example, in cervical carcinomas it has been observed HPV integration into and around the hTERT gene, which resulted in an increase in hTERT expression [36], or HPV 18 DNA has been found integrated in the proximity of *c-myc* gene in several cervical cancers, but surprisingly not up-regulation of endogenous proto-oncogene expression was observed [37]. HPV 16 and 18 DNA sequences have been found integrated in particular chromosomal loci known as common fragile sites in cervical cancers [37]. An association between the loss of fragile histidine tetrads (FHIT) expression and progression of HPV 16-positive CIN has been demonstrated [38]. Invasive cervical cancers expressing HR-HPV E6 and E7 transcripts contain normal FHIT transcription, while low amount of viral transcripts were detected when FHIT was abnormally expressed, which suggests that E6 and E7 could be repressed in the presence of FHIT aberrations [39]. An intensive review of HPV integration sites in cervical dysplasia and cancer concluded that integration is randomly distributed over the whole host genome with genomic fragile sites predilection [40]. Modification of host cell genes that interfere with the expression or function of viral genes will eventually contribute to immune evasion; the tumor progression and invasion are an important event for malignant cellular transformation [41]. We have to continue looking for the physical and functional relevance of viral and cellular genes in the HPV-mediated transforming mechanisms, since experimental evidence could be an indication that the major function of HPV integration is the conservation and stabilization of HPV gene expression. Human carcinogenesis is considered a genomic instability disease [42]. Human solid tumors display aneuploidy, however; transformed human cells generated 'in vitro' maintain their genome stability [43]. Therefore, genomic instability is not a generic manifestation of oncogenic transformation but represents a tumor cell characteristic to acquire genetic alterations necessary for the survival and clonal expansion within the emergent neoplasia changing microenvironment [44]. Recently, it has been demonstrated that beyond HPV-induced immortalization, the chromosomal aberrations are inversely related to the HPV type immortalization capacity, which means that HR-HPV types with reduced immortalization capacity, needs more genetic host cell aberrations to facilitate immortalization and these could explain the differences in HPV-type prevalence in cervical cancers [45]. The combined expression of HR-HPV E6 and E7 proteins in cervical cancer cells causes inactivation of *p53* and *pRb* tumor suppressor pathways and induces telomerase activation; these signal transduction pathways are disrupted in the majority of human solid tumors and they constitute a minimal subset of oncogenic hits to generate transformed 'in vitro' human cells [17]; complementary oncogenic events as E6/E7 expression are necessary to 'in vivo' and 'in vitro' transformation. Cervical carcinomas show chromosomal abnormalities [41], such as a specific gain at chromosome 3q for transition from HR-HPV-associated severe dysplasia to invasive carcinoma [46]. HPV-16 E7 oncoprotein contributes to genomic instability by the induction of centrosome duplication errors and generation of mitotic defects and aneuploidy in normal human epithelial cells, and also the characteristic multipolar mitoses in cervical lesions [47]. Centrosomic abnormalities emerge as a consequence of cytokinesis and/or cell division defects, thus occurring mostly in cells that have also accumulated nuclear abnormalities [48], also associated mitotic defects are present in cells that express episomal HPV-16 at a low number of copies, similarly to low-grade HPV-associated lesions [49], but the incidence of these alterations increases in cells when HPV genome is integrated to the host genome [50]. HPV E7 expression induces primary centrosome and centriole duplication errors in normal diploid cells but the mechanism remains absent of an explanation [51]. HPV E7 expression has the ability to target pRB family members, and it can explain the reason why the expression of HPV-16 E7 causes an increased incidence of centrosome abnormalities in mouse embryo fibroblasts that lack of pRB, p107, and p130 expression [48]. Centrosome abnormalities have also been detected in cervical lesions [49]. HPV-16 E7 expression works as mitotic mutator due to increased mitotic errors each round of cell division, inducing the genomic plasticity for the acquisition of cellular mutations that contribute to malignant progression [50]. The presence of double-strand DNA breaks in HPV-16 E6/E7- expressing cells is a mechanistic rationalization of what is facilitating HPV genome integration and why it is accompanying malignant progression [52]. However, integration of oncogenic HPV genomes in cervical lesions is a consequence rather than the cause of chromosomal instability induced by deregulated HR-HPV E6-E7 oncogene expression [53], and there is a gain of human telomerase gene TERC as important associated genetic event during the progression of dysplasia to cervical cancer [54].

3.4 Telomerase Activation as Molecular Transformation and Immortalization Mechanisms by HPV

Telomere shortening is a cell-autonomous mechanism that restricts the proliferative capacity of normal somatic cells. The hTERT expression of the catalytic telomerase subunit, in primary human cells, causes life span extension and immortalization. Cell types that must undergo a large number of cell divisions such as stem cells, express telomerase, a ribonucleoprotein that prevents telomere erosion. Many human tumor cells express actively telomerase, suggesting that aberrant telomerase activity is critical for human tumorigenesis. hTERT expression is considered one of the obligatory components for the generation of human tumor-like cells 'in vitro' [55]. HR-HPV E6 proteins and E7 contribute to immortalization of primary human epithelial cells by induction of telomerase activity [56]. HPVs have been shown to integrate in the proximity of *c-myc* gene, which justifies the search for alterations of this proto-oncogene in HPV-associated lesions. Ocadiz et al. [57] described for the first time the amplification of a human oncogene in samples of cervical cancers, such oncogene was *c-myc*. Recently, another group described it but compared it with benign and premalignant cervical lesions [58]. Moreover, a significant association between *c-myc* amplification and HPV 16 infection was observed. Elevated levels of *c-myc* have been found in several HPV-positive cervical carcinoma cell lines [59]. However, the significance of these events in HPV-mediated transformation remains unclear. The involvement of the c-Myc protein in HPV-induced immortalization was recently addressed [60]. HR-HPV E6 was shown to associate with c-Myc complexes (Myc/Max) and activate the hTERT promoter. The specific c-Myc antagonist, Mad, represses E6-transactivation of hTERT. HR-E6 proteins induce hTERT expression at a transcriptional level [61]. The minimal E6 responsive hTERT promoter fragment contains *c-myc* responsive E-boxes that contribute to E6-mediated transcriptional activation, but E6 does not markedly affect *c-myc* expression or the composition of c-Myc transcription factor complexes [62]. In HR-HPV expressing E6, the direct interaction with *c-myc* oncogene form, a c-Myc/E6 complex that activates hTERT expression [63]. An alternative hypothesis that tries to explain forward is that E6 relieves the telomerase promoter repression by inducing NFX1–91 degradation, which is a transcriptional repressor [64]. In E6-positive cells the telomerase activity increases when they become immortalized, although E6 expression levels do not change [65], meaning that other factors are participating in telomerase activation. Other experiments have revealed the E6 immortalization potential in mammary epithelial cells and keratinocytes by inactivation of TP53 [66]. Nowadays there is a scientific evidence that oncogenic types specifically activate the hTERT promoter (a limited set of viruses within the Alphapapillomavirus genus are oncogenic), while non-oncogenic types do not, which that means activation of the hTERT promoter is associated with oncogenic types [67].

3.5 Metabolic Tumor Adaptations as HPV Transforming Mechanisms

Although long-term information is stored almost exclusively in the genome, the proteome is crucial for short-term information storage; and the transcription factor-controlled information retrieval is strongly influenced by the state of the metabolome. The elementary building blocks in the proteome are proteins, but metabolomes are constituted by proteins and metabolites that form different interacting network called metabolic pathways [68, 69]. Nowadays is well knows that tumor cells metabolism (tumor metabolome) is characterized by a high concentration of glycolytic enzymes. About these scope there is an interesting report, where they characterized the metabolism of non-transformed rat kidney cells (NRK cells), showing a high glutaminolytic flux rate and a low (ATP + GTP):(CTP + UTP) ratio, whereas fructose 1,6-biphosphate (FBP) levels and pyruvate kinase isoenzyme type M2 (M2-PK) activity was very low. When a stable oncogenic *ras* and HPV-16 E7 expression were stablish in the NRK cells, an FBP up-regulation and M2-PK activity was detected, these results suggest, that oncogenic *ras* and E7 protein are the perfect conditions to create the ideal tumor metabolome as generally found in tumor cells [70–72]. Folic acid is necessary for the synthesis of *S*-adenosylmethionine, an elementary sustrate in the DNA methylation [73], but low folate levels increase the fragile sites on DNA which also decrease the DNA repair [74] and the DNA methylation process [75, 76], these conditions enhance the risk of DNA attacks by virus and carcinogens [77, 78], which also include HPV [79]. The global DNA methylation increase in the cervical tissue, increase the grade of cervical dysplasia, suggesting that the methylation status is an early event in the cervical transformation mechanisms. About genital HPV types, DNA methylation in the regulatory region, regulate 'in vitro' HR-HPV expression [80, 81]. One of these 'in-vitro' studies demonstrated that methylation of CpG sites in the HPV 18 enhancer region resulted in a down-regulation of transcriptional activity [80]. Other study demonstrates the methylation was found to be more at CpGs within E2 binding sites proximal to the P97 promoter, which means that the E2 binding site methylation in presence of intact E2, cause to loss of E2 repressor activity [82]. The reactive oxygen species (ROS) and their down-regulation by anti-oxidants is the other metabolic point that have relevance during the process of HPV infection. Activation of AP-1 (main transcription factor for the expression of E6 and E7 proteins of HR-HPVs) is down regulated by antioxidants in 'in vitro' models [83–85] and recently by other dietary molecules such as Curcumin (diferuloylmethane), which is an active component of the perennial herb turmeric and a potent anti-oxidant and is well-known for its anti-inflammatory and anti-carcinogenic activity [86]. Experimental evidence demonstrated that pyrrolidine-dithiocarbamate (anti-oxidant) selectively inhibit AP-1-induced by HPV 16 gene expression in immortalized human keratinocytes, suggesting that redox potential manipulation could be a therapeutic approach to interfere with the HR-HPVs transformation mechanisms [87]. Surprisingly, other study demonstrates that using curcumin (diferuloylmethane) in HeLa cells culture it was possible to modulate the transcription of AP-1 and HPV [88, 89]. Retinoic acid indirectly reduces HPV mRNA levels by modification of AP-1 activity [90] and/or transforming growth factor β (TGFβ) expression [91]. The property of cell growth suppression by retinoic acid is lost in the latest stages of HPV 16-induced transformation in cervical tumor cell lines and keratinocytes, the mechanism includes loss of growth inhibition and TGF β sensitivity [92], continued growth stimulation [93, 94] and loss of retinoid receptor expression [95]. In the serum, All Trans Retinoic Acid (ATRA) level highly influences the progression of cervical lesions to invasive cancer [96]. The therapy with retinoic acid does not reduce recurrence rates of advanced cervical cancer [97–99] or the cervical intra-neoplasia grade 3 (CIN3) regression [100], even when is combined with chemotherapy and immunotherapy [101]. All these data suggest that retinoic acid could be effective only in the early stages of cervical dysplasia lesions, modulating the clearance and persistence of HPV. The sequence of events required for the establishment of the tumor metabolome in cervical cancer is presently unknown, but it is clear the participation of specific metabolic pathways, specific modulation of metabolites and the HPV infection event during the malignant transformation mechanisms of the cervical epithelium.

3.6 Cervical Host Infections Patterns (Oncobioma) of Malignant Precursor Lesions and Tumor Microenvironment as Promoters and Enhancers of HPV Transforming Mechanisms

Microbiome research has presented an unprecedented growth over the last decade, due to the great developments in the new DNA sequencing technologies such as Next Generation Sequencing (NGS) [102]. The human microbiome study has been focused on health and disease, the clinical interpretation; however, the ability to understand these studies in the context of disease is less straightforward. Pathological conditions such as cancer have seen an increase in research focused on the microbiome pathogenic role, but the clinical value to interpret and/or use these scientific findings are not still translated. The purpose of this chapter section is to provide an introduction for clinicians to learn about how microbiome research and HPV positive cervical cancer could be associated. Microbiota considers a wide variety of microorganisms (bacteria, viruses, protozoa, fungi, and archaea) and the eclectic ecosystem of every individual, creating a commensal, symbiotic, and pathobiont (microorganisms that normally behave in a symbiotic manner with their host but exhibit pathogenic potential based on changes in their abundance or environmental conditions) relationship that has generated focus on its role in carcinogenesis [103]. The new scientific research focused on the interplay between the human microbiome and cancer development, has been termed the 'oncobiome' (the intricate interplay and study of the human microbiome and its influence on cancer development) [103]. It is clear, that these preliminary studies have demonstrated associative relationships rather than causative ones. But the question of whether this emerging field of research is a 'landscape' without a clear picture yet or it represents a new paradigm for cancer research such as other authors and we refer [104]. We propose the scientific evidence to answer the question and to push the new paradigm forward to bring a new perspective to understand and treat cancer. The mechanisms proposed in which infectious agents are suggested as associated co-factors in HPV malignant transformation is by direct biological interactions, such as modification of HPV replication and transcription, and/or indirect effects, such as inflammation and damage to the epithelial barrier that protects against HPV infection to facilitate the virus access to target epithelial cells. In the 1970's laboratory studies demonstrated the ability of Herpes simplex virus-1 (HSV-1) and Herpes simplex virus-2 (HSV-2) to transform hamster cells [105]. The inconsistent HSV DNA detection in human cervical cancer samples created the 'hit and run' hypotheses, which means that a virus may be involved in the initiation or promotion of malignant transformation, but is not required for the maintenance of the transformed phenotype [106]. HSV-2 is an infectious agent that has been studied as a potential co-factor for cervical cancer. Several studies have demonstrated an interaction between HSV-2 and HPV in 'in vitro' transformation [107]. HSV-2 can suppress HPV gene expression [108]. HSV induce tumorigenic clones in keratinocytes that had been immortalized by HPV [108]. HSV is a co-factor in HPV-associated cervical transforming mechanisms, not an etiological agent. Thus, laboratory data and epidemiological data are not consistent with a possible interaction of HSV-2 in HPV-associated epithelial transformation. A study of 200 human cervical cancer specimens failed to detect HSV-2 sequences using sensitive PCR methods [110]. HSV infection downregulate the secretory leukocyte protease inhibitor (SLPI) levels and may impart a greater susceptibility for HPV16 infection by the annexin A2 heterotetramer cell receptor (A2t), providing a mechanism to explain the etiological link between HSV and HPV-associated cancers [111]. Other herpesviruses are reported to infect the cervix and have been demonstrated to transform epithelial cells in 'in vitro' models, which include cytomegalovirus (CMV) [112], human herpesvirus 6 (HHV-6) [113] and Epstein-Barr virus (EBV) [114], the co-infection with herpesviruses, especially CMV and EBV, may be involved in the integration of the HPV-16 genome and may contribute to the development of cervical cancer [115], but unfortunately there is no strong evidence of the potential role of these viruses in the HPV transforming mechanisms. On the other hand, Adeno-associated virus (AAV) may have a protective effect against HPV-associated transforming mechanisms. AAV is a helper-dependent parvovirus that needs for its replication the co-infection with other DNA viruses, such as adenovirus [116]. In 'in vitro' models, AAV inhibits the transforming effect of HPV and furthermore, HPV can support replication of AAV, a finding that is consistent with possible HPV/AAV co-infection in nature [117]. Scientific reports found that AAV suppressed papillomavirus replication by its protein Rep 78 (an AAV major non-structural regulatory protein), and interferes with transcription factors and HPV promoter activity [118]. Nevertheless, AAV high levels decreased HPV replication, low levels increased it, and certain conditions increase the HPV transforming capacity [117]. By direct interaction between AAV proteins and cellular genes, AAV induces tumor cell differentiation, down-regulates *c-Fos* and *c-Myc* genes, inhibits cell proliferation and reduces carcinogen-induced mutagenicity [119–121]. Finally, extensive experimental and limited epidemiological evidence suggests that adeno-associated viruses (AAV) may have anti-oncogenic activity and has also anti-neoplastic effects that are independent of its proposed biological interaction with HPV [122]. Cervical cancer is increased in women who have human immunodeficiency virus (HIV) [123]; HIV-positive patient biomarkers, such as, HIV RNA level and $CD4^+$ T-cell count, are associated with HPV infection risk and cervical cancer. It has been demonstrated by 'in vitro' models that epithelial cells can be infected by HIV [124, 125], and also have shown that HIV TAT protein can co-activate HPV [126, 127]; but unfortunately, there is not the same correlation when it is used an 'in vivo' infection model system [128–130]. The association between multiple HPV infection, low CD4 count and cytological abnormalities supports the interplay of virological and immunological factors in cervical cancer pathogenesis [131, 132]. HPV infection may predispose to HIV infection and facilitate its progression probably by interaction with HIV proteins enhancing effectiveness of HPV proteins, and perhaps contributing to cell cycle disruption [133]. At this time, it looks improbable that HPV-infected cervical epithelial cells could be co-infected with HIV, which limits the idea that both viruses interact biologically at a molecular level. A microbial agent that has been associated with HPV infected cervical cancer patients by epidemiological studies is *Chlamydia trachomatis* (*C. trachomatis*). Different proposed mechanisms by which *C. trachomatis* increases the risk for cervical cancer have been described such as: (i) an anti-apoptotic effect, since infected cells are resistant to apoptosis by the *C. trachomatis* persistent infection [134, 135]. These anti-apoptotic effects result in an epithelial cells persistence and resistance that HPV co-infection follows the development of chromosomal abnormalities and increase the cervical dysplasia grade [136, 137]; (ii) its infection causes human cervical epithelial cells separate from each other due to the breakdown of the N-cadherin/β-catenin complex junctions in the epithelium and increases the basal cells exposure to HPV [138]; (iii) its infection is associated with squamous metaplasia and hypertrophic ectopy, which is a cervical neoplasia risk factor [139]; (iv) its persistent infection increases the HPV risk infection due to modulate immune factors like the inhibition of interferon (IFN) γ-inducible major histocompatibility complex (MHC) class II, as well as MHC class I expression [140, 141]; (v) by inhibition of NK cell function, decreasing the NK cells lytic capability, reducing TNFα and IFNγ production by NK cells and thereby decreasing antibody-dependent cellular cytotoxicity [142]; (vi) its chronic infection is associated with a predominantly T-helper (Th2) (humoral immune) cytokine pattern, whereas Th1 (cellular immune) cytokines participate in the control of intracellular microbes such as *C. trachomatis* and HPV [143]. A meta-analysis of HPV and *C. thracomatis* co-infection demonstrated that individuals infected with *C. trachomatis* have a higher risk of cervical cancer [144]. Based on this scientific evidence, it could be considered that it occurs an adaptive immune response to facilitate the HPV infection. MHC class I quantitative or qualitative alterations due to the presence of viral antigens can result in stimulation of natural killer (NK) cells that can kill a broad range of intracellular microbial infected cells without prior sensitization. During cervical inflammation, the immune response to microbial infection plays a role in HPV-associated tumorigenesis and explains the associations of precursor lesions and cervical cancer with a wide spectrum of pathogens, which include herpesviruses, *C. trachomatis, Trichomonas vaginalis, Neisseria gonorrhoeae, Candida albicans* and others [145]. The mechanisms by which inflammation might cause an increased risk for cervical cancer have been best described for *C. trachomatis*. Many of the cytokines that are secreted during *C. trachomatis* infection, including TNFα and IFNγ, could cause tissue damage by inducing apoptosis of uninfected cells; infiltrating macrophages releasing reactive oxygen species causes a mayor tissue damage [135, 145]. These effects result in partial disruption of the tissue barrier and exposure of basal cells to HPV infection. Furthermore, the ROS released by infiltrating macrophages could cause host cell DNA damage and increase the risk for malignant precursor lesions and cervical cancer [146, 147], these proposed mechanisms have evolved from the association between inflammatory host responses and oxidative DNA damage [148]. There is no scientific evidence to have a direct effect of *C. trachomatis* on host DNA or on the transcription of HPV genes though. A Korean group recently report that the predominance of *A. vaginae*, *G. vaginalis* and *L. iners* with a concomitant paucity of *L. crispatus* in the cervical microbiota was associated with CIN risk, suggesting that bacterial dysbiosis and its combination with oncogenic HPV may be a risk factor for cervical neoplasia [149]. The following is one of the last observations of the associated mechanisms of HPV multiple infections we want to refer to and what is the potential roles of the microbiome in cervicovaginal diseases. A few years ago, in our institutions we were evaluating an anti-HPV topical drug and using the most advanced methods, we had to detect the HPV pattern infection of these patients; we found a complex association of multiple HR-HPV infections in patients according to the dysplasia grade, which means higher dysplasia grade higher number of HR-HPV types associated with the lesion [150]. We discuss the interpretation of the scientific evidence in a biological and clinical context, for analysis and future discussion and direction for microbiome in cancer research and particularly in human cancer associated to viral pathogens. The genomic medicine for the routine clinical use should be seen as a blueprint for the microbiome or better understood as 'oncobioma'. These scientific evidences suggest that microbial dysbiosis (a biological state whereby host microbial composition is unbalanced toward other micro-organisms compared to 'healthy' host composition) is associated with malignant transformation. Whether these associations are causative and can therefore modulate initiation, progression, or cancer metastasis at this moment remains unclear.

Acknowledgment The contributors of this chapter want to pay homage to Luis Benitez-Bribiesca M.D. who worked in our Institutions as Professor, Mentor, Colleague and Editor for over 40 years. We are extremely grateful to him for all his scientific efforts, teachings, advice and critiques, which were the translational pathway to take our scientific works from basic research to the clinic and patient care, such as he always claimed.

In Memoriam

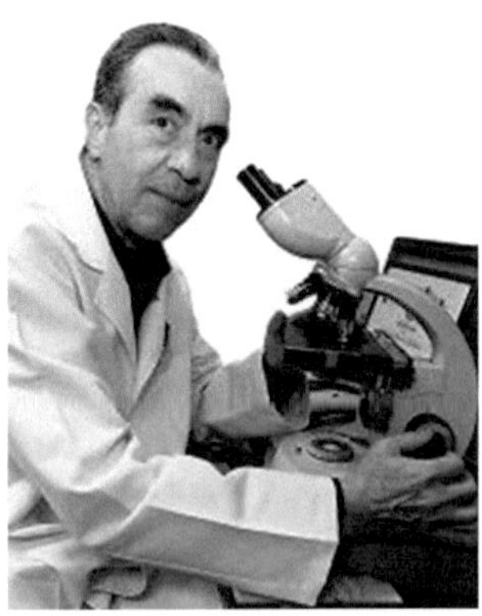

Luis S. Benitez-Bribiesca M.D.
(1934–2015)

References

1. Pfister H, Fuchs PG. Anatomy, taxonomy and evolution of papillomaviruses. Intervirology. 1994;37:143–9.
2. Orth G, Jablonska S, Breitburd F, Favre M, Croissant O. The human papillomaviruses. Bull Cancer. 1978;65:151–64.
3. Bodily J, Laimins LA. Persistence of human papillomavirus infection: keys to malignant progression. Trends Microbiol. 2011;19(1):33–9.
4. Moody CA, Laimins LA. Human Papillomavirus oncoproteins: pathways to transformation. Nat Rev Cancer. 2010;10(8):550–60.
5. Evander M, Frazer IH, Payne E, Qi YM, Hengst K, McMillan NA. Identification of the 6 integrin as a candidate receptor for papillomaviruses. J Virol. 1997;71:2449–56.
6. Stubenrauch F, Laimins LA. Human papillomavirus life cycle: active and latent phases. Semin Cancer Biol. 1999;9:379–86.
7. McCance DJ, Kopan R, Fuchs E, Laimins LA. Human papillomavirus type 16 alters human epithelial cell differentiation in vitro. Proc Natl Acad Sci U S A. 1988;85:7169–73.
8. Evan GI, Vousden KH. Proliferation, cell cycle and apoptosis in cancer. Nature. 2001;411:342–8.
9. Scheffner M, Huibregtse JM, Vierstra RD, Howley PM. The HPV-16 E6 and E6-AP complex functions as a ubiquitin-protein ligase in the ubiquitination of p53. Cell. 1993;75:495–505.
10. Jones DL, Münger K. Analysis of the p53-mediated G1 growth arrest pathway in cells expressing the human papillomavirus type 16 E7 oncoprotein. J Virol. 1997;71:2905–12.
11. Rosenberger S, De-Castro Arce J, Langbein L, Steenbergen RD, Rösl F. Alternative splicing of human papillomavirus type-16 E6/E6* early mRNA is coupled to EGF signaling via Erk1/2 activation. Proc Natl Acad Sci U S A. 2010;107(15):7006–11.
12. Münger K, Phelps WC, Bubb V, Howley PM, Schlegel R. The E6 and E7 genes of the human papillomavirus type 16 together are necessary and sufficient for transformation of primary human keratinocytes. J Virol. 1989;63:4417–21.
13. Münger K, Basile JR, Duensing S, Eichten A, Gonzalez SL, Grace M, Zacny VL. Biological activities and molecular targets of the human papillomavirus E7 oncoprotein. Oncogene. 2001;20:7888–98.
14. Brehm A, Nielsen SJ, Miska EA, McCance DJ, Reid JL, Bannister AJ, Kouzarides T. The E7 oncoprotein associates with Mi2 and histone deacetylase activity to promote cell growth. EMBO J. 1999;18:2449–58.
15. Peralta-Zaragoza O, Bermudez-Morales V, Gutierrez-Xicotencatl L, Alcocer-Gonzalez J, Recillas-Targa F, Madrid-Marina V. E6 and E7 oncoproteins from human papillomavirus type 16 induce activation of human transforming growth factor beta1 promoter throughout Sp1 recognition sequence. Viral Immunol. 2006;19(3):468–80.
16. Bello JO, Nieva LO, Paredes AC, Gonzalez AM, Zavaleta LR, Lizano M. Regulation of the Wnt/β-catenin signaling pathway by human papillomavirus E6 and E7 oncoproteins. Viruses. 2015;7(8):4734–55.
17. Hanahan D, Weinberg RA. The hallmarks of cancer. Cell. 2000;100:57–70.
18. Hahn WC, Weinberg RA. Modelling the molecular circuitry of cancer. Nat Rev Cancer. 2002;2:331–41.
19. Astudillo de la Vega H, Benítez-Bribiesca L. Is it possible to create human malignant cells in the laboratory? Gac Med Mex. 2000;136(2):173–4.
20. Thorland EC, Myers SL, Gostout BS, Smith DI. Common fragile sites are preferential targets for HPV16 integrations in cervical tumors. Oncogene. 2003;22:1225–37.
21. Ziegert C, Wentzensen N, Vinokurova S, Kisseljov F, Einenkel J, Hoeckel M, von Knebel Doeberitz M. A comprehensive analysis of HPV integration loci in anogenital lesions combining transcript and genome-based amplification techniques. Oncogene. 2003;22:3977–84.
22. McBride AA, Romanczuk H, Howley PM. The papillomavirus E2 regulatory proteins. J Biol Chem. 1991;266:18411–4.

23. Demeret C, Desaintes C, Yaniv M, Thierry F. Different mechanisms contribute to the E2-mediated transcriptional repression of human papillomavirus type 18 viral oncogenes. J Virol. 1997;71:9343–9.
24. Chiang CM, Ustav M, Stenlund A, Ho TF, Broker TR, Chow LT. Viral E1 and E2 proteins support replication of homologous and heterologous papillomaviral origins. Proc Natl Acad Sci U S A. 1992;89:5799–803.
25. Skiadopoulos MH, McBride AA. Bovine papillomavirus type 1 genomes and the E2 transactivator protein are closely associated with mitotic chromatin. J Virol. 1998;72:2079–88.
26. You J, Croyle JL, Nishimura A, Ozato K, Howley PM. Interaction of the bovine papillomavirus E2 protein with Brd4 tethers the viral DNA to host mitotic chromosomes. Cell. 2004;117(3):349–60.
27. Baker CC, Phelps WC, Lindgren V, Braun MJ, Gonda MA, Howley PM. Structural and translational analysis of human papillomavirus type 16 sequences in cervical carcinoma cell lines. J Virol. 1987;61:962–71.
28. Jeon S, Lambert PF. Integration of human papillomavirus type 16 DNA into the human genome leads to increased stability of E6 and E7 mRNAs: implications for cervical carcinogenesis. Proc Natl Acad Sci U S A. 1995;92:1654–8.
29. Alazawi W, Pett M, Arch B, Scott L, Freeman T, Stanley MA, Coleman N. Changes in cervical keratinocyte gene expression associated with integration of human papillomavirus 16. Cancer Res. 2002;62:6959–65.
30. Goodwin EC, DiMaio D. Repression of human papillomavirus oncogenes in HeLa cervical carcinoma cells causes the orderly reactivation of dormant tumor suppressor pathways. Proc Natl Acad Sci U S A. 2000;97:12513–8.
31. Hopman AH, Smedts F, Dignef W, Ummelen M, Sonke G, Mravunac M, Vooijs GP, Speel EJ, Ramaekers FC. Transition of high-grade cervical intraepithelial neoplasia to micro-invasive carcinoma is characterized by integration of HPV 16/18 and numerical chromosome abnormalities. J Pathol. 2004;202(1):23–33.
32. Kessis TD, Connolly DC, Hedrick L, Cho KR. Expression of HPV16 E6 or E7 increases integration of foreign DNA. Oncogene. 1996;13:427–31.
33. Reidy PM, Dedo HH, Rabah R, Field JB, Mathog RH, Gregoire L, Lancaster WD. Integration of human papillomavirus type 11 in recurrent respiratory papilloma-associated cancer. Laryngoscope. 2004;114(11):1906–9.
34. Schwarz E, Freese UK, Gissmann L, Mayer W, Roggenbuck B, Stremlau A, zur Hausen H. Structure and transcription of human papillomavirus sequences in cervical carcinoma cells. Nature. 1985;314(6006):111–4.
35. Hudelist G, Manavi M, Pischinger KI, Watkins-Riedel T, Singer CF, Kubista E, Czerwenka KF. Physical state and expression of HPV DNA in benign and dysplastic cervical tissue: different levels of viral integration are correlated with lesion grade. Gynecol Oncol. 2004;92(3):873–80.
36. Ferber MJ, Montoya DP, Yu C, Aderca I, McGee A, Thorland EC, Nagorney DM, Gostout BS, Burgart LJ, Boix L, Bruix J, McMahon BJ, Cheung TH, Chung TK, Wong YF, Smith DI, Roberts LR. Integrations of the hepatitis B virus (HBV) and human papillomavirus (HPV) into the human telomerase reverse transcriptase (hTERT) gene in liver and cervical cancers. Oncogene. 2003;22(24):3813–20.
37. Ferber MJ, Thorland EC, Brink AA, Rapp AK, Phillips LA, McGovern R, Gostout BS, Cheung TH, Chung TK, Fu WY, Smith DI. Preferential integration of human papillomavirus type 18 near the c-myc locus in cervical carcinoma. Oncogene. 2003;22(46):7233–42.
38. Butler D, Collins C, Mabruk M, Leader MB, Kay EW. Loss of Fhit expression as a potential marker of malignant progression in preinvasive squamous cervical cancer. Gynecol Oncol. 2002;86(2):144–9.
39. Segawa T, Sasagawa T, Yamazaki H, Sakaike J, Ishikawa H, Inoue M. Fragile histidine triad transcription abnormalities and human papillomavirus E6-E7 mRNA expression in the development of cervical carcinoma. Cancer. 1999;85(9):2001–10.

40. Wentzensen N, Vinokurova S, von Knebel DM. Systematic review of genomic integration sites of human papillomavirus genomes in epithelial dysplasia and invasive cancer of the female lower genital tract. Cancer Res. 2004;64(11):3878–84.
41. zur Hausen H. Immortalization of human cells and their malignant conversion by high risk human papillomavirus genotypes. Semin Cancer Biol. 1999;9:405–11.
42. Klausner RD. The fabric of cancer cell biology—weaving together the strands. Cancer Cell. 2002;1:3–10.
43. Zimonjic D, Brooks MW, Popescu N, Weinberg RA, Hahn WC. Derivation of human tumor cells in vitro without widespread genomic instability. Cancer Res. 2001;61:8838–44.
44. Cahill DP, Kinzler KW, Vogelstein B, Lengauer C. Genetic instability and Darwinian selection in tumours. Trends Cell Biol. 1999;9:M57–60.
45. Schütze DM, Krijgsman O, Snijders PJ, Ylstra B, Weischenfeldt J, Mardin BR, Stütz AM, Korbel JO, de Winter JP, Meijer CJ, Quint WG, Bosch L, Wilting SM, Steenbergen RD. Immortalization capacity of HPV types is inversely related to chromosomal instability. Oncotarget. 2016;7:37608–21. doi:10.18632/oncotarget.8058.
46. Habermann JK, Hellman K, Freitag S, Heselmeyer-Haddad K, Hellstrom AC, Shah K, Auer G, Ried T. A recurrent gain of chromosome arm 3q in primary squamous carcinoma of the vagina. Cancer Genet Cytogenet. 2004;148:7–13.
47. Storchova Z, Pellman D. From polyploidy to aneuploidy, genome instability and cancer. Nat Rev Mol Cell Biol. 2004;5:45–54.
48. Duensing S, Münger K. Human papillomavirus type 16 E7 oncoprotein can induce abnormal centrosome duplication through a mechanism independent of inactivation of retinoblastoma protein family members. J Virol. 2003;77:12331–5.
49. Riley RR, Duensing S, Brake T, Münger K, Lambert PF, Arbeit JM. Dissection of human papillomavirus E6 and E7 function in transgenic mouse models of cervical carcinogenesis. Cancer Res. 2003;63:4862–71.
50. Duensing S, Münger K. Mechanisms of genomic instability in human cancer: insights from studies with human papillomavirus oncoproteins. Int J Cancer. 2004;109:157–62.
51. Duensing S, Duensing A, Crum CP, Münger K. Human papillomavirus type 16 E7 oncoprotein-induced abnormal centrosome synthesis is an early event in the evolving malignant phenotype. Cancer Res. 2001;61:2356–60.
52. Thomas JT, Laimins LA. Human papillomavirus oncoproteins E6 and E7 independently abrogate the mitotic spindle checkpoint. J Virol. 1998;72:1131–7.
53. Vinokurova S, Wentzensen N, Kraus I, Klaes R, Driesch C, Melsheimer P, Kisseljov F, Dürst M, Schneider A, von Knebel DM. Type-dependent integration frequency of human papillomavirus genomes in cervical lesions. Cancer Res. 2008;68(1):307–13.
54. Hopman AH, Theelen W, Hommelberg PP, Kamps MA, Herrington CS, Morrison LE, Speel EJ, Smedts F, Ramaekers FC. Genomic integration of oncogenic HPV and gain of the human telomerase gene TERC at 3q26 are strongly associated events in the progression of uterine cervical dysplasia to invasive cancer. J Pathol. 2006;210(4):412–9.
55. Blasco MA, Hahn WC. Evolving views of telomerase and cancer. Trends Cell Biol. 2003;13:289–94.
56. Kiyono T, Foster SA, Koop JI, McDougall JK, Galloway DA, Klingelhutz AJ. Both Rb/p16INK4a inactivation and telomerase activity are required to immortalize human epithelial cells. Nature. 1998;396:84–8.
57. Ocadiz R, Sauceda R, Cruz M, Graef AM, Gariglio P. High correlation between molecular alterations of the c-myc oncogene and carcinoma of the uterine cervix. Cancer Res. 1987;47(15):4173–7.
58. Abba MC, Laguens RM, Dulout FN, Golijow CD. The c-myc activation in cervical carcinomas and HPV 16 infections. Mutat Res. 2004;557(2):151–8.
59. Dürst M, Croce CM, Gissmann L, Schwarz E, Huebner K. Papillomavirus sequences integrate near cellular oncogenes in some cervical carcinomas. Proc Natl Acad Sci U S A. 1987;84(4):1070–4.

60. Veldman T, Liu X, Yuan H, Schlegel R. Human papillomavirus E6 and Myc proteins associate in vivo and bind to and cooperatively activate the telomerase reverse transcriptase promoter. Proc Natl Acad Sci U S A. 2003;100(14):8211–6.
61. McMurray HR, McCance DJ. Human papillomavirus type 16 E6 activates TERT gene transcription through induction of c-Myc and release of USF-mediated repression. J Virol. 2003;77(18):9852–61.
62. Gewin L, Galloway DA. E box-dependent activation of telomerase by human papillomavirus type 16 E6 does not require induction of c-myc. J Virol. 2001;75(15):7198–201.
63. Liu X, Dakic A, Zhang Y, Dai Y, Chen R, Schlegel R. HPV E6 protein interacts physically and functionally with the cellular telomerase complex. Proc Natl Acad Sci U S A. 2009;106(44):18780–5.
64. Gewin L, Myers H, Kiyono T, Galloway DA. Identification of a novel telomerase repressor that interacts with the human papillomavirus type-16 E6/E6-AP complex. Genes Dev. 2004;18(18):2269–82.
65. Fu B, Quintero J, Baker CC. Keratinocyte growth conditions modulate telomerase expression, senescence, and immortalization by human papillomavirus type 16 E6 and E7 oncogenes. Cancer Res. 2003;63(22):7815–24.
66. McMurray HR, McCance DJ. Degradation of p53, not telomerase activation, by E6 is required for bypass of crisis and immortalization by human papillomavirus type 16 E6/E7. J Virol. 2004;78(11):5698–706.
67. Van Doorslaer K, Burk RD. Association between hTERT activation by HPV E6 proteins and oncogenic risk. Virology. 2012;433(1):216–9.
68. Oltvai ZN, Barabási AL. Systems biology. Life's complexity pyramid. Science. 2002;298(5594):763–4.
69. Hughes TR, Robinson MD, Mitsakakis N, Johnston M. The promise of functional genomics: completing the encyclopedia of a cell. Curr Opin Microbiol. 2004;7(5):546–54.
70. Mazurek S, Zwerschke W, Jansen-Dürr P, Eigenbrodt E. Metabolic cooperation between different oncogenes during cell transformation: interaction between activated ras and HPV-16 E7. Oncogene. 2001;20(47):6891–8.
71. Mazurek S, Eigenbrodt E. The tumor metabolome. Anticancer Res. 2003;23(2A):1149–54.
72. Mazurek S. Pyruvate kinase type M2: a key regulator of the metabolic budget system in tumor cells. Int J Biochem Cell Biol. 2011;43(7):969–80.
73. Poirier LA. The effects of diet, genetics and chemicals on toxicity and aberrant DNA methylation: an introduction. J Nutr. 2002;132(8 Suppl):2336S–9S.
74. Ames BN, Wakimoto P. Are vitamin and mineral deficiencies a major cancer risk? Nat Rev Cancer. 2002;2(9):694–704.
75. Wainfan E, Kilkenny M, Dizik M. Comparison of methyltransferase activities of pair-fed rats given adequate or methyl-deficient diets. Carcinogenesis. 1988;9(5):861–3.
76. Kim YI, Giuliano A, Hatch KD, Schneider A, Nour MA, Dallal GE, Selhub J, Mason JB. Global DNA hypomethylation increases progressively in cervical dysplasia and carcinoma. Cancer. 1994;74(3):893–9.
77. Hsieh LL, Wainfan E, Hoshina S, Dizik M, Weinstein IB. Altered expression of retrovirus-like sequences and cellular oncogenes in mice fed methyl-deficient diets. Cancer Res. 1989;49(14):3795–9.
78. Davis CD, Uthus EO. DNA methylation, cancer susceptibility, and nutrient interactions. Exp Biol Med (Maywood). 2004;229(10):988–95.
79. Flatley JE, Sargent A, Kitchener HC, Russell JM, Powers HJ. Tumour suppressor gene methylation and cervical cell folate concentration are determinants of high-risk human papillomavirus persistence: a nested case control study. BMC Cancer. 2014;14:803. doi:10.1186/1471-2407-14-803.
80. Rösl F, Arab A, Klevenz B, zur Hausen H. The effect of DNA methylation on gene regulation of human papillomaviruses. J Gen Virol. 1993;74(Pt 5):791–801.
81. Thain A, Jenkins O, Clarke AR, Gaston K. CpG methylation directly inhibits binding of the human papillomavirus type 16 E2 protein to specific DNA sequences. J Virol. 1996;70(10):7233–5.

82. Bhattacharjee B, Sengupta S. CpG methylation of HPV 16 LCR at E2 binding site proximal to P97 is associated with cervical cancer in presence of intact E2. Virology. 2006;354(2):280–5.
83. Cripe TP, Alderborn A, Anderson RD, Parkkinen S, Bergman P, Haugen TH, Pettersson U, Turek LP. Transcriptional activation of the human papillomavirus-16 P97 promoter by an 88-nucleotide enhancer containing distinct cell-dependent and AP-1-responsive modules. New Biol. 1990;2(5):450–63.
84. Offord EA, Beard P. A member of the activator protein 1 family found in keratinocytes but not in fibroblasts required for transcription from a human papillomavirus type 18 promoter. J Virol. 1990;64(10):4792–8.
85. Velazquez Torres A, Gariglio Vidal P. Possible role of transcription factor AP1 in the tissue-specific regulation of human papillomavirus. Rev Invest Clin. 2002;54(3):231–42.
86. Mishra A, Kumar R, Tyagi A, Kohaar I, Hedau S, Bharti AC, Sarker S, Dey D, Saluja D, Das B. Curcumin modulates cellular AP-1, NF-kB, and HPV16 E6 proteins in oral cancer. Ecancermedicalscience. 2011;9:525.
87. Rösl F, Das BC, Lengert M, Geletneky K, zur Hausen H. Antioxidant-induced changes of the AP-1 transcription complex are paralleled by a selective suppression of human papillomavirus transcription. J Virol. 1997;71(1):362–70.
88. Prusty BK, Das BC. Constitutive activation of transcription factor AP-1 in cervical cancer and suppression of human papillomavirus (HPV) transcription and AP-1 activity in HeLa cells by curcumin. Int J Cancer. 2005;113(6):951–60.
89. Date AA, Destache CJ. Natural polyphenols: potential in the prevention of sexually transmitted viral infections. Drug Discov Today. 2016;21(2):333–41.
90. Schüle R, Rangarajan P, Yang N, Kliewer S, Ransone LJ, Bolado J, Verma IM, Evans RM. Retinoic acid is a negative regulator of AP-1-responsive genes. Proc Natl Acad Sci U S A. 1991;88(14):6092–6.
91. Batova A, Danielpour D, Pirisi L, Creek KE. Retinoic acid induces secretion of latent transforming growth factor beta 1 and beta 2 in normal and human papillomavirus type 16-immortalized human keratinocytes. Cell Growth Differ. 1992;3(11):763–72.
92. Borger DR, Mi Y, Geslani G, Zyzak LL, Batova A, Engin TS, Pirisi L, Creek KE. Retinoic acid resistance at late stages of human papillomavirus type 16-mediated transformation of human keratinocytes arises despite intact retinoid signaling and is due to a loss of sensitivity to transforming growth factor-beta. Virology. 2000;270(2):397–407.
93. Sizemore N, Choo CK, Eckert RL, Rorke EA. Transcriptional regulation of the EGF receptor promoter by HPV16 and retinoic acid in human ectocervical epithelial cells. Exp Cell Res. 1998;244(1):349–56.
94. Rorke EA, Zhang D, Choo CK, Eckert RL, Jacobberger JW. TGF-beta-mediated cell cycle arrest of HPV16-immortalized human ectocervical cells correlates with decreased E6/E7 mRNA and increased p53 and p21(WAF-1) expression. Exp Cell Res. 2000;259(1):149–57.
95. Bartsch D, Boye B, Baust C, zur Hausen H, Schwarz E. Retinoic acid-mediated repression of human papillomavirus 18 transcription and different ligand regulation of the retinoic acid receptor beta gene in non-tumorigenic and tumorigenic HeLa hybrid cells. EMBO J. 1992;11(6):2283–91.
96. Berlin Grace VM, Niranjali Devaraj S, Radhakrishnan Pillai M, Devaraj H. HPV-induced carcinogenesis of the uterine cervix is associated with reduced serum ATRA level. Gynecol Oncol. 2006;103(1):113–9.
97. Wadler S, Schwartz EL, Haynes H, Rameau R, Quish A, Mandeli J, Gallagher R, Hallam S, Fields A, Goldberg G, McGill F, Jennings S, Wallach RC, Runowicz CD. All-trans retinoic acid and interferon-alpha-2a in patients with metastatic or recurrent carcinoma of the uterine cervix: clinical and pharmacokinetic studies. New York Gynecologic Oncology Group. Cancer. 1997;79(8):1574–80.
98. Weiss GR, Liu PY, Alberts DS, Peng YM, Fisher E, Xu MJ, Scudder SA, Baker Jr LH, Moore DF, Lippman SM. 13-cis-retinoic acid or all-trans-retinoic acid plus interferon-alpha in recurrent cervical cancer: a Southwest Oncology Group phase II randomized trial. Gynecol Oncol. 1998;71(3):386–90.

99. Keefe KA, Schell MJ, Brewer C, McHale M, Brewster W, Chapman JA, Rose GS, McMeeken DS, Lagerberg W, Peng YM, Wilczynski SP, Anton-Culver H, Meyskens FL, Berman ML. A randomized, double blind, Phase III trial using oral beta-carotene supplementation for women with high-grade cervical intraepithelial neoplasia. Cancer Epidemiol Biomarkers Prev. 2001;10(10):1029–35.
100. Meyskens Jr FL, Surwit E, Moon TE, Childers JM, Davis JR, Dorr RT, Johnson CS, Alberts DS. Enhancement of regression of cervical intraepithelial neoplasia II (moderate dysplasia) with topically applied all-trans-retinoic acid: a randomized trial. J Natl Cancer Inst. 1994;86(7):539–43.
101. Braud AC, Gonzague L, Bertucci F, Genre D, Camerlo J, Gravis G, Goncalves A, Moutardier V, Viret F, Maraninchi D, Viens P. Retinoids, cisplatin and interferon-alpha in recurrent or metastatic cervical squamous cell carcinoma: clinical results of 2 phase II trials. Eur Cytokine Netw. 2002;13(1):115–20.
102. Ash C, Mueller K. Manipulating the Microbiota. Science. 2016;352(6285):530–1.
103. Thomas RM, Jobin C. The microbiome and cancer: is the 'Oncobiome' mirage real? Trends Cancer. 2015;1(1):24–35.
104. de Martel C, Ferlay J, Franceschi S, Vignat J, Bray F, Forman D, Plummer M. Global burden of cancers attributable to infections in 2008: a review and synthetic analysis. Lancet Oncol. 2012;13:607–15.
105. Duff R, Rapp F. Properties of hamster embryo fibroblasts transformed in vitro after exposure to ultraviolet-irradiated herpes simplex virus type 2. J Virol. 1971;8(4):469–77.
106. Galloway DA, McDougall JK. The oncogenic potential of herpes simplex viruses: evidence for a 'hit-and-run' mechanism. Nature. 1983;302(5903):21–4.
107. Dhanwada KR, Garrett L, Smith P, Thompson KD, Doster A, Jones C. Characterization of human keratinocytes transformed by high risk human papillomavirus types 16 or 18 and herpes simplex virus type 2. J Gen Virol. 1993;74(Pt 6):955–63.
108. Fang L, Ward MG, Welsh PA, Budgeon LR, Neely EB, Howett MK. Suppression of human papillomavirus gene expression in vitro and in vivo by herpes simplex virus type 2 infection. Virology. 2003;314(1):147–60.
109. DiPaolo JA, Woodworth CD, Popescu NC, Koval DL, Lopez JV, Doniger J. HSV-2-induced tumorigenicity in HPV16-immortalized human genital keratinocytes. Virology. 1990;177(2):777–9.
110. Tran-Thanh D, Provencher D, Koushik A, Duarte-Franco E, Kessous A, Drouin P, Wheeler CM, Dubuc-Lissoir J, Gauthier P, Allaire G, Vauclair R, Dipaolo JA, Gravitt P, Franco E, Coutlée F. Herpes simplex virus type II is not a cofactor to human papillomavirus in cancer of the uterine cervix. Am J Obstet Gynecol. 2003;188(1):129–34.
111. Skeate JG, Porras TB, Woodham AW, Jang JK, Taylor JR, Brand HE, Kelly TJ, Jung JU, Da Silva DM, Yuan W, Kast WM. Herpes simplex virus downregulation of secretory leukocyte protease inhibitor enhances human papillomavirus type 16 infection. J Gen Virol. 2016;97(2):422–34.
112. Doniger J, Muralidhar S, Rosenthal LJ. Human cytomegalovirus and human herpesvirus 6 genes that transform and transactivate. Clin Microbiol Rev. 1999;12:367–82.
113. Kashanchi F, Araujo J, Doniger J, Muralidhar S, Hoch R, Khleif S, Mendelson E, Thompson J, Azumi N, Brady JN, Luppi M, Torelli G, Rosenthal LJ. Human herpesvirus 6 (HHV-6) ORF-1 transactivating gene exhibits malignant transforming activity and its protein binds to p53. Oncogene. 1997;14:359–67.
114. Thompson MP, Kurzrock R. Epstein-Barr virus and cancer. Clin Cancer Res. 2004;10:803–21.
115. Szostek S, Zawilinska B, Kopec J, Kosz-Vnenchak M. Herpesviruses as possible cofactors in HPV-16-related oncogenesis. Acta Biochim Pol. 2009;56(2):337–42.
116. Leonard CJ, Berns KI. Adeno-associated virus type 2: a latent life cycle. Prog Nucleic Acid Res mol Biol. 1994;48:29–52.
117. Meyers C, Alam S, Mane M, Hermonat PL. Altered biology of adeno-associated virus type 2 and human papillomavirus during dual infection of natural host tissue. Virology. 2001;287:30–9.

118. Prasad CK, Meyers C, Zhan DJ, You H, Chiriva-Internati M, Mehta JL, Liu Y, Hermonat PL. The adeno-associated virus major regulatory protein Rep78-c-Jun-DNA motif complex modulates AP-1 activity. Virology. 2003;314:423–31.
119. Bantel-Schaal U. Growth properties of a human melanoma cell line are altered by adenoassociated parvovirus type 2. Int J Cancer. 1995;60:269–74.
120. Walz C, Schlehofer JR. Modification of some biological properties of HeLa cells containing adeno-associated virus DNA integrated into chromosome 17. J Virol. 1992;66:2990–3002.
121. Schlehofer JR, Heilbronn R. Infection with adeno-associated virus type 5 inhibits mutagenicity of herpes simplex virus type 1 or 4-nitroquinoline-1-oxide. Mutat Res. 1990;244:317–20.
122. Al-Daraji WI, Smith JH. Infection and cervical neoplasia: facts and fiction. Int J Clin Exp Pathol. 2009;2(1):48–64.
123. Mbulaiteye SM, Biggar RJ, Goedert JJ, Engels EA. Immune deficiency and risk for malignancy among persons with AIDS. J Acquir Immune Defic Syndr. 2003;32:527–33.
124. Moore JS, Rahemtulla F, Kent LW, Hall SD, Ikizler MR, Wright PF, Nguyen HH, Jackson S. Oral epithelial cells are susceptible to cell-free and cell-associated HIV-1 infection in vitro. Virology. 2003;313:343–53.
125. Yeaman GR, Howell AL, Weldon S, Demian DJ, Collins JE, O'Connell DM, Asin SN, Wira CR, Fanger MW. Human immunodeficiency virus receptor and coreceptor expression on human uterine epithelial cells: Regulation of expression during the menstrual cycle and implications for human immunodeficiency virus infection. Immunology. 2003;109:137–46.
126. Vernon SD, Hart CE, Reeves WC, Icenogle JP. The HIV-1 *tat* protein enhances E2dependent human papillomavirus 16 transcription. Virus Res. 1993;27:133–45.
127. Buonaguro FM, Tornesello ML, Buonaguro L, Del Gaudio E, Beth-Giraldo E, Giraldo G. Role of HIV as cofactor in HPV oncogenesis: in vitro evidences of virus interactions. Antibiot Chemother. 1994;46:102–9.
128. Greenhead P, Hayes P, Watts PS, Laing KG, Griffin GE, Shattock RJ. Parameters of human immunodeficiency virus infection of human cervical tissue and inhibition by vaginal virucides. J Virol. 2000;74:5577–86.
129. Miller CJ, Shattock RJ. Target cells in vaginal HIV transmission. Microbes Infect. 2003;5:59–67.
130. Wu Z, Chen Z, Phillips DM. Human genital epithelial cells capture cell-free human immunodeficiency virus type 1 and transmit the virus to CD4+ cells: Implications for mechanisms of sexual transmission. J Infect Dis. 2003;188:1473–82.
131. Garbuglia AR, Piselli P, Lapa D, Sias C, Del Nonno F, Baiocchini A, Cimaglia C, Agresta A, Capobianchi MR. Frequency and multiplicity of human papillomavirus infection in HIV-1 positive women in Italy. J Clin Virol. 2012;54(2):141–6.
132. Strickler HD, Burk RD, Fazzari M, Anastos K, Minkoff H, Massad LS, Hall C, Bacon M, Levine AM, Watts DH, Silverberg MJ, Xue X, Schlecht NF, Melnick S, Palefsky JM. Natural history and possible reactivation of human papillomavirus in human immunodeficiency virus-positive women. J Natl Cancer Inst. 2005;97(8):577–86.
133. Clarke B, Chetty R. Postmodern cancer: the role of human immunodeficiency virus in uterine cervical cancer. Mol Pathol. 2002;55(1):19–24.
134. Fan T, Lu H, Hu H, Shi L, McClarty GA, Nance DM, Greenberg AH, Zhong G. Inhibition of apoptosis in chlamydia-infected cells: Blockade of mitochondrial cytochrome c release and caspase activation. J Exp Med. 1998;187:487–96.
135. Perfettini JL, Hospital V, Stahl L, Jungas T, Verbeke P, Ojcius DM. Cell death and inflammation during infection with the obligate intracellular pathogen, *Chlamydia*. Biochimie. 2003;85:763–9.
136. Lorenzato M, Clavel C, Masure M, Nou JM, Bouttens D, Evrard G, Bory JP, Maugard B, Quereux C, Birembaut P. DNA image cytometry and human papillomavirus (HPV) detection help to select smears at high risk of high-grade cervical lesions. J Pathol. 2001;194:171–6.
137. Melsheimer P, Klaes R, von Knebel-Doeberitz M, Bastert G. Prospective clinical study comparing DNA flow cytometry and HPV typing as predictive tests for persistence and progression of CIN I/II. Cytometry. 2001;46:166–71.

138. Prozialeck WC, Fay MJ, Lamar PC, Pearson CA, Sigar I, Ramsey KH. *Chlamydia trachomatis* disrupts N-cadherin-dependent cell–cell junctions and sequesters β-catenin in human cervical epithelial cells. Infect Immun. 2002;70:2605–13.
139. Moscicki AB, Burt VG, Kanowitz S, Darragh T, Shiboski S. The significance of squamous metaplasia in the development of low grade squamous intraepithelial lesions in young women. Cancer. 1999;85:1139–44.
140. Zhong G, Liu L, Fan T, Fan P, Ji H. Degradation of transcription factor RFX5 during the inhibition of both constitutive and interferon γ-inducible major histocompatibility complex class I expression in chlamydia-infected cells. J Exp Med. 2000;191:1525–34.
141. Hook CE, Telyatnikova N, Goodall JC, Braud VM, Carmichael AJ, Wills MR, Gaston JSH. Effects of *Chlamydia trachomatis* infection on the expression of natural killer (NK) cell ligands and susceptibility to NK cell lysis. Clin Exp Immunol. 2004;138:54–60.
142. Mavoungou E, Poaty-Mavoungou V, Touré FS, Sall A, Delicat A, Yaba P, Mandeme Y, Nabias R, Lansoud-Soukate J. Impairment of natural killer cell activity in *Chlamydia trachomatis* infected individuals. Trop Med Int Health. 1999;4:719–27.
143. Stephens RS. The cellular paradigm of chlamydial pathogenesis. Trends Microbiol. 2003;11:44–51.
144. Zhu H, Shen Z, Luo H, Zhang W, Zhu X. Chlamydia Trachomatis Infection-Associated Risk of Cervical Cancer: A Meta-Analysis. Medicine (Baltimore). 2016;95(13):e3077.
145. Castle PE, Giuliano AR. Genital tract infections, cervical inflammation, and antioxidant nutrients — Assessing their roles as human papillomavirus cofactors. J Natl Cancer Inst Monogr. 2003;31:29–34.
146. Gravitt PE, Castle PE. *Chlamydia trachomatis* and cervical squamous cell carcinoma (Letter to the Editor). JAMA. 2001;285:1703–4.
147. Smith JS, Bosetti C, Muñoz N, Herrero R, Bosch FX, Eluf-Neto J, Meijer CJLM, van den Brule AJC, Franceschi S, Peeling RW. *Chlamydia trachomatis* and invasive cervical cancer: a pooled analysis of the IARC multicentric case–control study. Int J Cancer. 2004;111:431–9.
148. Touati E, Michel V, Thiberge JM, Wuscher N, Huerre M, Labigne A. Chronic Helicobacter pylori infections induce gastric mutations in mice. Gastroenterology. 2003;124(5):1408–19.
149. Oh HY, Kim BS, Seo SS, Kong JS, Lee JK, Park SY, Hong KM, Kim HK, Kim MK. The association of uterine cervical microbiota with an increased risk for cervicalintraepithelial neoplasia in Korea. Clin Microbiol Infect. 2016;21(7):674.e1–9.
150. Munoz D, Cantu D, Gonzalez A, Meneses A, Mohar A, Astudillo-de la Vega H, Nguyen B. A phase II trial of the use of 4, 4'-dihydroxybenzophenone-2, 4-dinitrophenyl-hydrazone (A-007) topical gel in the treatment of high-grade squamous intraepithelial lesions (HSIL) of the cervix. ASCO Annual Meeting Proceedings. *J Clin Oncol*. 2006;25(18_suppl):5593.

Chapter 4
Transcriptome Studies Reveal Altered Signaling Pathways in Cervical Cancer

Carlos Pérez-Plasencia, Jorge Fernández-Retana, and Jaime G. de la Garza-Salazar

Abstract Transcriptome analysis provides a global idea of the molecular mechanisms affected in different pathologies. Characterization of over- or under-expressed genes constitutes an initial step in this type of analysis. The integration of the information acquired by these global expression profiles regarding signaling pathways or organized modules that work according to specific cellular responses has made it possible for us to understand the development and progression of almost every type of neoplasia. In the case of cervical cancer, transcriptome studies have allowed us to comprehend the viral-mediated carcinogenic process, i.e., human papillomavirus (HPV). In spite of the great progress that has been accomplished regarding radiotherapy and chemotherapy, its impact in cervical cancer in limited; approximately 40% of the patients develop resistance to the conventional treatment schemes, and the disease will eventually recur, leading to the patient's death. For this reason, knowing which signaling pathways present altered expression in this neoplasia opens a window of opportunity for those patients whose tumors display certain resistance to conventional treatment, further progression or even recurrence. In this chapter, we will summarize the main signaling pathways that are found to be altered in this neoplasia, pathways that have been described in various works in which the cervical cancer transcriptome was analyzed.

C. Pérez-Plasencia, PhD (✉)
Genomics Laboratory, Department of Investigation, Instituto Nacional de Cancerología-México, Av. San Fernando No 22, Col. Sección XVI, Mexico City 14080, Mexico

Laboratory of Funtional Genomics, Unidad de Biomedicina, FES-IZTACALA, UNAM, Tlalnepantla, Mexico
e-mail: carlos.pplas@gmail.com

J. Fernández-Retana, PhD
Laboratory of Funtional Genomics, Unidad de Biomedicina, FES-IZTACALA, UNAM, Tlalnepantla, Mexico

Posgrado en Ciencias Biológicas, Facultad de estudios superiores Iztacala, Universidad Nacional Autónoma de México, México, Mexico

J.G. de la Garza-Salazar, MD
Department of Clinical Investigation, Instituto Nacional de Cancerología-México, Mexico City, Mexico

J.G. de la Garza-Salazar et al. (eds.), *Cervical Cancer*,
DOI 10.1007/978-3-319-45231-9_4

Keywords Human Papilloma Virus • Cervical Carcinoma • Molecular Pathogenesis • Transcriptional Profile

4.1 Introduction

Carcinogenesis is a complicated process that involves progressive and accumulative genomic alterations that include mutations (deletions, insertions, duplications, and others) and complex genomic re-arrangements caused by chromosome instability, an intrinsic characteristic of cancer. These changes at the genomic level can affect the expression profile of certain genes, which enables the deregulation of the cell mechanisms responsible for cell cycle control, apoptosis, extracellular matrix degradation, invasion, angiogenesis, and other processes [1, 2]. Different molecular mechanisms involved in the initiation, progression and maintenance of the tumoral phenotype have been described in cervical cancer (CC). Some of the latter have been identified and characterized using genomic analysis resources, primarily expression microarrays [3]. The use of genomics-derived resources, especially microarrays, has enabled not only the characterization and description of different neoplasias but also the discovery of new diagnosis, prognosis and clinical follow-up markers. In breast cancer, microarrays have made possible the clinical classification of histopathologically similar tumors based on molecular criteria [4, 5]. Expression microarrays have been successfully employed in the prediction of progressive breast [6, 7], prostate [8], colon and rectum [9] and head and neck cancers [10], among other neoplasias, thus demonstrating the potential of microarrays as clinical oncological resources.

In CC, different studies have focused mainly on the analysis of the expression profiles induced upon infection with HPV [11–14]; nonetheless, there are few studies in which the analysis of the different expression profiles of the tumors is associated with the patient's clinical history or clinical outcome [15–17]. In this chapter, we will review the molecular pathways involved in the pathogenesis of CC that have been analyzed by means of global expression experiments, focusing on the analysis of molecular mechanisms associated with the development and progression of CC. These mechanisms include the NF-κB, TGF-β/Smads, WNT/β-catenin and MAP kinases (MAPK) pathways, which are involved in different stages of the carcinogenesis process.

4.2 Nuclear Factor Kappa B (NF-κB) Pathway

The NF-κB pathway is ubiquitous in different cell types. Under normal conditions, this pathway plays an important role in immune response regulation. NF-κB transcription factor activation controls the activation of genes involved in development, cell differentiation, cytoskeleton reorganization, cell adhesion, cell survival and apoptosis evasion. This pathway also activates the immune response and the chronic inflammation necessary to sustain several chronic diseases, including cancer [18].

Signals leading to NF-κB activation have been associated with the promotion and progression of cancer development. Furthermore, NF-κB has also been associated with chemotherapy and radiotherapy resistance; thus, it has been proposed as a potential therapeutic target. NF-κB activation is a clear example of a tumorigenic mechanism of cervical carcinogenesis that can be activated by HPV infection.

NF-κB activation occurs through two main mechanisms, which are referred to as the canonical and the non-canonical pathways. The former is activated by several factors, including tumor necrosis factor receptors (TNFRs), Toll-like receptors and the interleukin ß receptor (IL-ßR), all three of which are involved in the promotion of inflammation. The non-canonical pathway is activated by a sub-family of the TNF receptors, such as CD40, Lymphotoxin-b (LTBR) and B cell activating factor (BAFF), all of which are associated with the NF-κB innate immune response and inflammation [18].

4.2.1 HPV Infection Induces NF-κB Activation

Different global expression experiments have shown that HPV infection in cell lines induces the aberrant activation of several up-stream proteins of the TNFRL/NF-κB signaling pathway, which is associated with the apoptosis evasion process. These molecules are TRAIL and its ligand, CD27 (CD27L). It has been suggested that CD27 initiates NF-κB activating signals by means of its specific association with TRAF-2, which promotes the proliferation of cells and increases the expression of genes involved in apoptosis inhibition, such as cIAP-1 and cIAP-2. These proteins promote NF-κB activation in response to TNF-α, inhibiting apoptosis and allowing cell cycle progression. NF-κB activation is an apoptosis resistance mechanism that is also induced by other viruses, such as Epstein-Barr, Hepatitis B and SV40 [19, 20].

In cervical cancer biopsies, it has been demonstrated that serum amyloid A1 (SAA1) can activate the NF-κB pathway [21]. SAA1 is a protein that increases in expression by hundreds of times upon inflammatory stimulus, suppressing apoptosis [22]. In contrast, SAA regulates metastasis and invasion by increasing the production of TNF-α and the activity of extracellular matrix-degrading enzymes [23].

In short, the induction of gene expression mediated by HPV infection uses the same mechanisms that NF-κB signaling activates in order to evade the immune response and to control the cell cycle of the infected epithelial tissues.

4.3 Regulation of Tumor Growth Factor ß (TGF-ß)

TGF-ß belongs to a multifunctional super-family of highly conserved cytokines that can be involved in activities such as cell proliferation, differentiation, morphogenesis, tissue homeostasis and regeneration. Extracellular ligands of the TGF-ß family

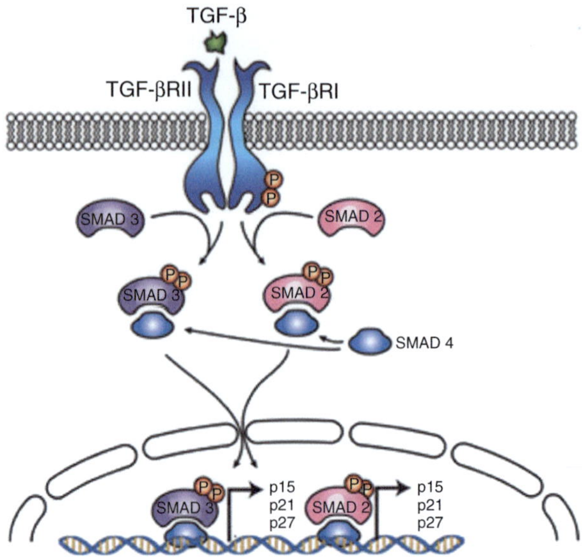

Fig. 4.1 TGF-ß/SMAD signaling cascade. The association of TGF-ß with its membrane receptors TGF-ßRI and II induces kinase domain activation, allowing heterodimeric complex formation with Smad2 or Smad3 with Smad4, which subsequently activates target genes

relay their signal by associating with type I receptors (TGF-ßRI), which form heterodimers with type II receptors (TGF-ßRII), and inducing the phosphorylation of serine/threonine residues. Finally, SMAD-like transcription factors translocate to the nucleus for the transcription of target genes (Fig. 4.1) [24].

SMAD factors activate transcription programs that vary according to cell type and context; therefore, they integrate and relay signals from different ligands of the TGF-ß superfamily. In cancer, TGF-ß/SMAD signaling has a dual role. In early stages of the oncogenic process, this signaling can inhibit the growth of epithelial cells and induce apoptosis, functioning as a tumor suppressor pathway. It is common for human tumors to escape this TGF-ß/SMAD-induced proliferation inhibition and apoptosis by means of mutations or deletions in the key components of this pathway, such as specific receptors (TGFBRI and TGFBRII) [25]. In advanced stages of the oncogenic process, however, TGF-ß/SMAD signaling promotes tumor progression by stimulating the reverse differentiation of epithelial cells into invasion-capable, metastatic cells [26].

4.3.1 Differential Expression Profiles in the TGF-β Pathway

In cervical carcinogenesis, the changes induced by HPV infection can elicit different molecular mechanisms depending on the type of virus infecting the epithelial cells of the cervix. It has been shown that cultured human keratinocytes infected

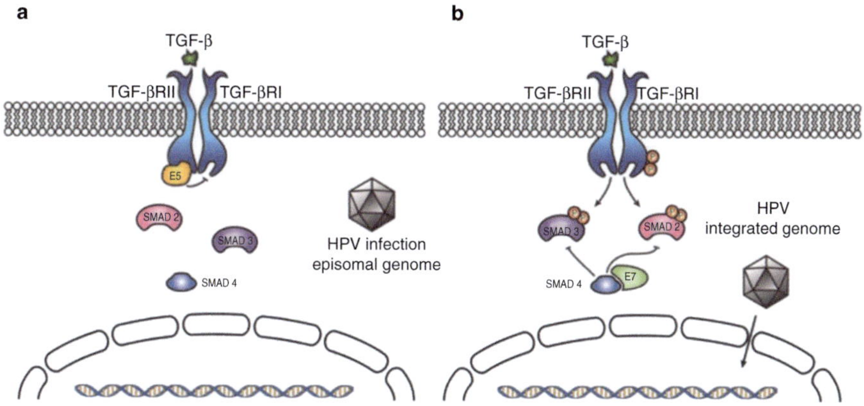

Fig. 4.2 TGF-ß inactivation by HPV oncoproteins. (**a**) After infection, viral DNA is found in its episomal state, so E5 expression blocks the kinase domains of dimerized TGF-ßRI and TGF-ßRII receptors. This blockade impedes the TGF-ß/Smad signaling cascade. (**b**) Viral genome integration disrupts the open reading frame of the E5 gene; E7 expression is increased, and E7 associates with Smad4, recruiting and inhibiting the function of the Smad2/3 and Smad4 complexes, respectively. This mechanism enables the cell to progress along the cell cycle and evade the immune response

with low-risk HPV (types 6 and 11) display different expression profiles than those infected with high-risk HPV (types 16 and 18). Low-risk HPV types induced the over-expression of the TGF-ß superfamily genes but did not suppress the expression of interferon-inducible genes [27]. In contrast, high-risk HPVs reduced the expression of TGF-ß response genes [28, 29]. These findings suggest that the TGF-ß signaling pathway acts in order to suppress tumor formation, while the interferon response helps to counteract infection by viruses of low carcinogenic potential.

The dual role of TGF-ß as a tumor suppressor and promoter of tumor progression is well documented in the work of several groups investigating cervical cancer. At the beginning of tumor progression, TGF-ß loses its tumor suppressor activity, apparently when the viral genome is still episomal; the HPV protein E5 reduced the activity of the TGF-ßRII receptor [30], thus preventing the signal generated by the ligand TGF-ß I from inducing the dimerization of the Smad3/4 complex (Fig. 4.2a). In advanced stages, the integration of the viral genome into that of the cell enables the over-expression of the oncogenic proteins E6 and E7 [31]. It has been shown that E7 blocks TGF-ß signaling by associating with Smad2, Smad3 and Smad4, which subsequently affects their roles as negative regulators of the cell cycle (Fig. 4.2b). Some expression studies performed with microarrays have demonstrated the low expression of Smad2, Smad3 and Smad4 in tumoral tissues, which leads to cell immortalization and unregulated proliferation [13, 32]. When different expression profiles induced by TGF-ßI in cervical cancer cell lines that display a different sensitivity to these ligands are compared, it has been shown that the cell lines least sensitive to this ligand over-express genes involved in different signaling pathways that favor tumorigenesis (i.e., both TNFα and MAPK pathways and, interestingly, genes that participate in the Wnt/ß-catenin pathway [33]). These results show the importance of TGF-ß as an oncogenic suppressor/activator and its capacity to interact with other signaling pathways that promote the tumoral phenotype. TGF-ß is a crucial mechanism against viral infections, which is why this pathway is either a direct or an indirect target of several proteins encoded by oncogenic viruses, such as E7. TGF-ß inactivation in the early stages of the viral infection favors the establishment of the tumoral phenotype, and eventually, its re-activation induces angiogenesis and metastasis, both of which are regulated by angiogenic proteins such as VEGF and IL-8 [34].

Global expression profile analysis of cells and tissues in different stages of the carcinogenic process makes it possible for us to comprehend the functional role of different signaling pathways and the interactions they establish in complex signaling networks. It has been reported that TGF-ß regulation also has an effect on other pathways, such as Wnt, whose aberrant activation in cancer contributes to epithelial-mesenchymal transition (EMT), which is fundamental for the TGF-ß-regulated processes of migration and metastasis [35].

4.4 Wnt/ß-Catenin Pathway Activation in CxCa

Wnt/ß-catenin has an important role in cell cycle control, differentiation, embryogenesis, stem phenotype maintenance, cell migration, and other processes. This pathway plays a fundamental role in cancer because practically every tumor analyzed displays alterations in this signaling pathway [36]. In 1982, the fundamental work of Nusse and Varmus established the relation between Wnt and carcinogenesis by identifying IntI (WntIa) as a virus-related locus that induces breast cancer in mice (murine mammary tumor virus, MMTV) [37]. Subsequent studies showed that the genes activated by the Wnt signaling cascade participate in cell cycle progression. Cyclin D is activated by this cascade; the Cyclin D protein regulates the serine/threonine kinase activity of Cdk4 and Cdk6 and regulates the cell cycle by inducing its progression into G1 phase, favoring the replication of malignant cells [38]. Although Cyclin D is a key protein for the progression of the cell cycle, it is not the only protein induced by the Wnt signaling cascade. Several agonists and antagonists participate in modulating this signaling pathway and its effect on the cell cycle (Fig. 4.3). Other studies have demonstrated that the antagonists of this pathway are either suppressed by hyper-methylation of their promoter regions or mutated in different tumor types [39]. The effects elicited by Wnt ligands are relayed by three well-studied signaling pathways. First, activation of the Wnt/ß-catenin pathway, also known as the canonical pathway, leads to stabilization of ß-catenin in the cytoplasm and its subsequent delocalization into the nucleous, where it functions as a transcriptional co-factor, activating cell proliferation-associated genes. The Wnt/ß--catenin pathway is activated in practically every type of cancer. The second pathway is known as the planar cell polarity pathway (Wnt/PCP). This pathway is involved in the differentiation processes of the epithelial planes and cytoskeletal re-organization. Finally, the third pathway is the calcium-dependent pathway, which is

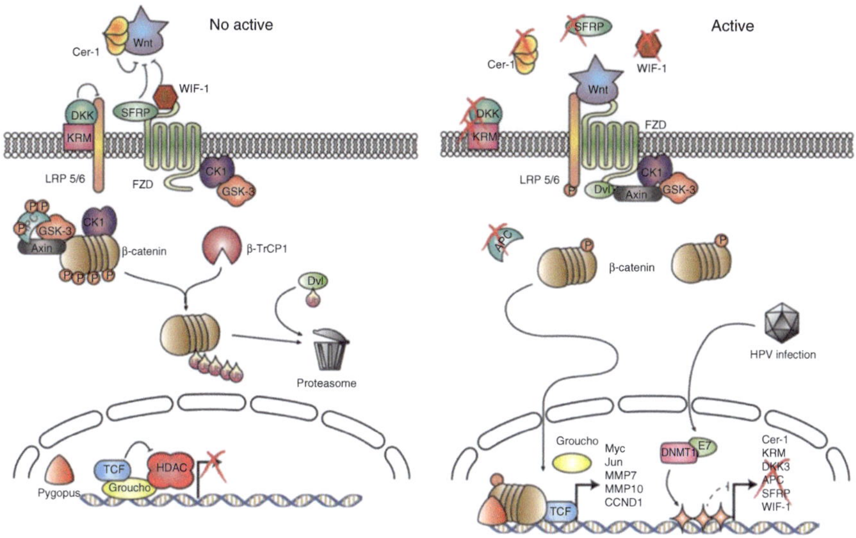

Fig. 4.3 Wnt/ß-catenin-regulated signaling cascade. (**a**) Inactive form. When the signaling cascade is off because of the absence of ligands or because of the over-expression of extracellular (CER1, WIF1 and SFRP) or membrane-bound negative regulators (DKK and KRM), ß-catenin associates with the degradation complex formed by APC, Axin, CK1γ and GSK3. This protein is then marked by the ubiquitin-ligase ß-TRPC1 and degraded by the proteasome. (**b**) Active form. Upon associating with its FZD receptors, Wnt induces the uncoupling of the degradation complex, allowing ß-catenin to accumulate in the cytoplasm and translocate to the nucleus, where it transactivates genes involved in proliferation, extracellular matrix degradation, invasion and metastasis. In contrast, the viral oncoprotein E7 can bind DNA methyltransferase 1 (DNMT1) and induce the methylation of the negative regulators of this signaling cascade

not very well understood, and it is not yet clear whether this pathway is involved in the tumorigenic process (Fig. 4.4) [40].

In cervical carcinogenesis, aberrant activation of the Wnt pathway is a phenomenon that has been observed since the first stages of neoplastic development. Over-expression of the frizzled receptors has been shown (FZD2 and FZD4), as has the inhibition of negative regulators such as SFRP4 and DKK133. Furthermore, it is now possible to analyze the methylation state in the promoters of different Wnt negative regulators, such as sFRPs, Axin, Dickkopf, Klotho and APC, which are found to be hyper-methylated during the malignant progression of CC, which would account for their low expression levels [33, 41]. Coordinated inactivation of both negative regulators permits the Wnt/ß-catenin pathway to keep the cell replication and transformation signals activated, thus promoting the tumoral phenotype.

Cytoskeletal reorganization is an important process for cell motility, invasion and metastasis. p120 is a member of a family of proteins that have an armadillo repeat domain, which regulates the activity of small GTPases, in particular, the Rho, Rac and Cdc42 families that participate in the Wnt/PCP pathway (Fig. 4.4a). In a previous study, p120 was found to be over-expressed in early stages in patients with

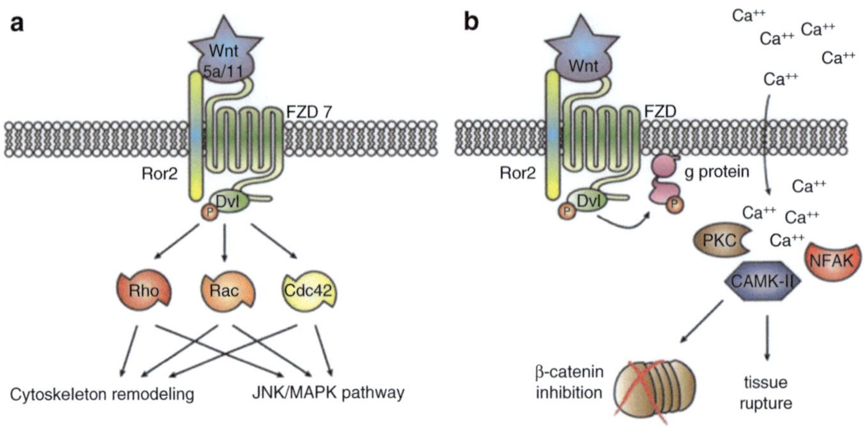

Fig. 4.4 Non-canonical Wnt signaling pathways. (**a**) Wnt/PCP pathway. Its activation depends on the interaction of the ligand Wnt5a with the receptor FZD7 and the co-receptor ROR2, which transduces the signal to the Dvl protein, which inactivates GTPases of the Rho family, such as EhoA, Rac1 and Cdc42. This mechanism induces cytoskeletal rearrangements, producing changes in cell polarity and stimulating the epithelium-mesenchymal transition (EMT), which results in the activation of invasion and metastasis. (**b**) Wnt/Ca^{2+} pathway. The activation of the pathway is regulated by G proteins that are activated by the Wnt/Fzd/Dvl complex. G proteins increase the intracellular levels of Ca^{2+}, which in turn activate the calcium-dependent kinase (CAMKII), protein kinase C (PKC) and the NFAK transcription factor

lymph node metastasis [35]. This evidence suggests that the Wnt/PCP pathway promotes cell migration by means of Rho family small GTPase activation.

Because of the notorious importance of the Wnt pathway in the development and its promotion of the tumoral phenotype of cervical cancer, it has been proposed that after HPV infection, the activation of this pathway becomes the second hit toward carcinogenesis (according to the classical hypothesis of Alfred Knudson) [41, 42].

TGF-ß inhibition and the high-risk HPV-induced coordinated activation of different genes that promote the Wnt/ß-catenin pathway favor constant proliferation and chromosomic instability, both of which are necessary characteristics to induce carcinogenesis [43]. In short, it is evident that the activation of the canonical pathway is necessary to establish the tumoral phenotype and that activation of the non-canonical Wnt/PCP pathway is associated with acquisition of the invasive and metastatic phenotypes.

4.5 Role of the Mitogen-Activated Protein Kinase (MAPK) Pathway

Oncogenic virus infection is associated with alterations in different signaling pathways, and MAPK, one of the classical pathways in cell homeostasis, is one of them. The MAPK pathway regulates the communication between extracellular signals and the cell machinery that controls functional processes such as cell growth, proliferation, apoptosis, differentiation, migration and invasion [44]. This pathway is

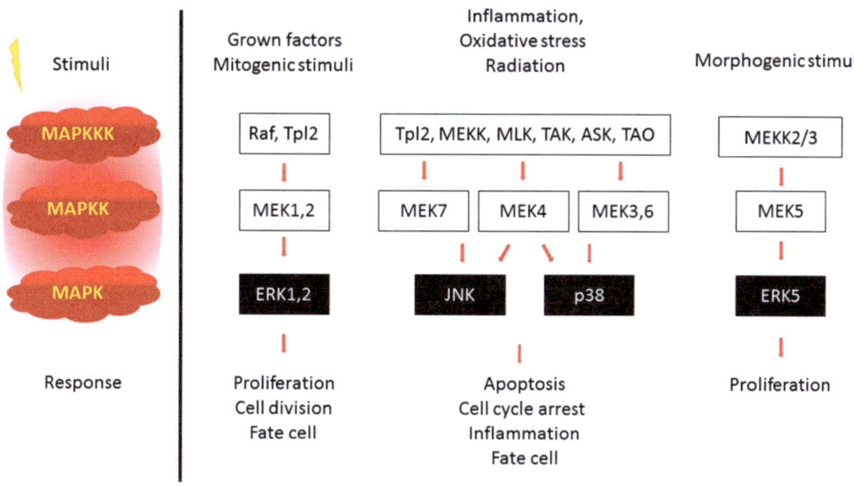

Fig. 4.5 Schematic summary of the main elements involved in the MAPK signaling pathway. For a more detailed explanation, please refer to the text

regulated in three levels of phosphorylation cascades (Fig. 4.5), in which one MAPK is activated upon phosphorylation by another MAPK of the same family (MAPKK), which in turn will be activated by another such kinase (MAPKKK). In this manner, six different types of MAPKs have been described, which are the extracellular regulation kinases (ERK1/2, ERK3/4, ERK5, ERK7/8), the amino-terminal kinase of JUN 1/2/3 (JNK) and the p38 isoform ERK6 [45, 46]. The differential activation of the MAPK pathways grants different properties to the cells in the malignant transformation process. For example, the activation of the Ras/ERK pathway, which is responsible for the control of cell survival, differentiation, proliferation, metabolism and motility in response to extracellular signals, is known to confer proliferative capacity, whereas the JNK and p38 pathways, which are involved in the cellular stress response, confer protection against neoplastic pharmaceuticals [47]. Therefore, some researchers have suggested drug resistance and senescence evasion as intrinsic characteristics or hallmarks of cancer [48].

In the context of drug resistance and senescence evasion, the interaction between the TGF-ß and MAPK pathways is the key. In cell lines derived from cervical tumors resistant to proliferation inhibition and TGF-ß1 ligand-induced apoptosis, several genes were found to be over-expressed, such as MEF2C (a target gene pf p38), MEK6 (which regulates p38 upstream in the pathway), and ATF4 (a transcription factor involved in the MAPK signaling pathway), in addition to other target genes of Smads/MAPK, such as AFT3, CDKN1A and GADD45B [33, 46]. These results show that cells answer coordinately to induced stress by over-expressing genes in the TGF-ß and MAPK pathways. These results will help to explain the mechanisms of evasion of conventional therapy in locally advanced and advanced cases in which radiotherapy and cisplatin-based conventional treatment induce cellular stress by generating reactive oxygen species and DNA damage.

4.5.1 MAPK Signaling Pathway Component Expression in Cervical Cancer

Expression profile comparison between cisplatin-resistant and cisplatin-sensitive tumors did not show differences in the expression levels of MAPK components [49]. MAP3K2 over-expression has only been observed in radio-sensitive tumors [50]. This kinase is involved in activation of the transcription factor NF-κB. These results suggest that MAPKs are generally activated in cervical cancer, which explains why the comparison of the expression profiles of chemo- and radiosensitive tumors with resistant tumors did not reveal any difference in the expression levels of these genes.

4.6 Conclusions

During cervical carcinogenesis, the changes in the global expression profiles are induced early by HPV infection of epithelial cells. These changes occur in a gradual fashion and involve different signaling pathways, which enable the transition of pre-malignant lesions to the establishment of the tumoral phenotype. Transcriptome characterization, mainly by expression microarray analysis, has demonstrated the role of particular genes that participate in specific signaling pathways. In several reports, the association between carcinogenic progression and signaling pathways, such as TGF-ß, WNT (canonical and the non-canonical), and MAPKs, among others, has been quite evident. These findings allow us to suggest a space-time model that represents key events during cervical carcinogenesis (Fig. 4.6). In this model, the role of the viral protein E5 has a higher relevance than has been previously acknowledged mainly because of activation of the TGF-ß/Smad pathway. The interaction between high-risk HPV E5 and the TGF-ßRII receptor prevents the onset of signaling; hence, the infected cells are not eliminated via apoptosis. The pathological effect of E5 is lost afterward, when the viral genome integrates into that of the cell in later stages of the carcinogenic process, because the open reading frame of E5 becomes discontinuous once the viral genome has been linearized.

During the progression of cervical lesions to in situ carcinoma, some components of the Wnt and MAPK pathways modify their expression levels. In the case of Wnt, there is negative regulation of various suppressors of the same pathway mainly through epigenetic regulation. This negative regulation is how Cerverus, Kremen, Dkk3 and APC reduce their expression levels, allowing activation of the canonical Wnt/ß-catenin pathway.

In spite of the evidence that the viral oncoproteins E6 and E7 activate a signaling cascade that leads to the activation of MAPKs, it seems that this activation is TGF-ß-dependent and that its main targets are the JNK and p38 pathways, which are activated upon cell stress. The activation of these pathways is important because it provides a cyto-protective tumor environment, granting the tumor cells resistance to conventional therapy.

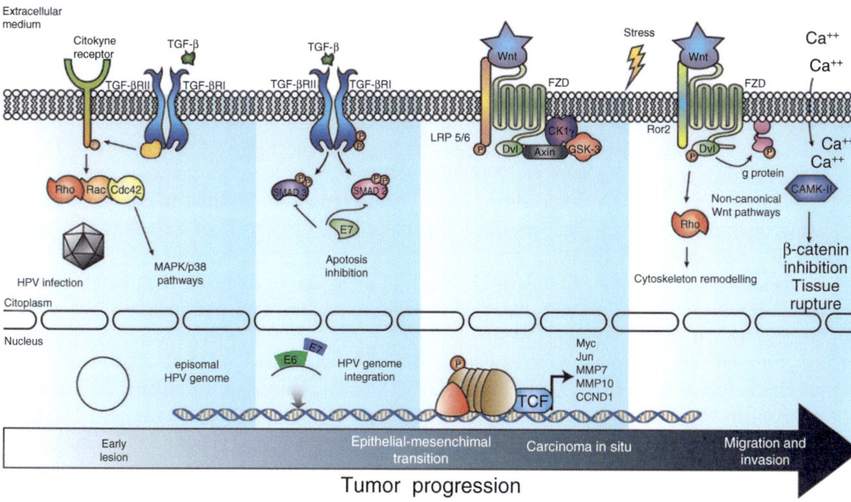

Fig. 4.6 Integral model of the TGF-ß, Wnt and MAPK pathways. At the beginning of high-risk HPV infection, the genes of the TGF-ß and MAPK/p38 pathways are over-expressed to activate defense mechanisms against the viral infection. However, the viral protein E5 blocks the signal transduction of TGF-ß, resulting in the aberrant activation of cellular stress components by means of p38. In this way, ATM/ATR-mediated DNA recombination mechanisms become activated. After viral integration, the canonical Wnt/ß-catenin pathway becomes activated in response to the inhibition of the negative regulators of this pathway, favoring the nuclear translocation of ß-catenin and inducing the expression of genes involved in the progression of the cell cycle, such as c-Jun, CCND1 and Myc

A method for evaluating the complexity of the changes presented during a tumorigenic process is the use of genome analysis resources. The description and integration of molecular processes are more complex than they appear; however, these approximations make it possible for us to comprehend at a holistic level the changes that occur during cervical carcinogenesis.

References

1. Fearon ER, Vogelstein B. A genetic model for colorectal tumorigenesis. Cell. 1990;61:759–67.
2. Sherr CJ. Cancer cell cycles. Science. 1996;274:1672–7.
3. Clarke PA, te Poele R, Wooster R, Workman P. Gene expression microarray analysis in cancer biology, pharmacology, and drug development: progress and potential. Biochem Pharmacol. 2001;62:1311–36.
4. Yeoh E-J, Ross ME, Shurtleff SA, et al. Classification, subtype discovery, and prediction of outcome in pediatric acute lymphoblastic leukemia by gene expression profiling. Cancer Cell. 2002;1:133–43.
5. Perou CM, Sørlie T, Eisen MB, et al. Molecular portraits of human breast tumours. Nature. 2000;406:747–52. doi:10.1038/35021093.

6. van t Veer LJ, Dai H, van de Vijver MJ, et al. Gene expression profiling predicts clinical outcome of breast cancer. Nature. 2002;415:530–6. doi:10.1038/415530a.
7. van de Vijver MJ, He YD, van't Veer LJ, et al. A gene-expression signature as a predictor of survival in breast cancer. N Engl J Med. 2002;347:1999–2009. doi:10.1056/NEJMoa021967.
8. Augustin H, Hammerer PG, Graefen M, et al. Characterisation of biomolecular profiles in primary high-grade prostate cancer treated by radical prostatectomy. J Cancer Res Clin Oncol. 2003;129:662–8. doi:10.1007/s00432-003-0496-9.
9. Nannini M, Pantaleo MA, Maleddu A, et al. Gene expression profiling in colorectal cancer using microarray technologies: results and perspectives. Cancer Treat Rev. 2009;35:201–9. doi:10.1016/j.ctrv.2008.10.006.
10. Roepman P, Wessels LFA, Kettelarij N, et al. An expression profile for diagnosis of lymph node metastases from primary head and neck squamous cell carcinomas. Nat Genet. 2005;37:182–6. doi:10.1038/ng1502.
11. Fragoso-Ontiveros V, Maria Alvarez-Garcia R, Contreras-Paredes A, et al.. Gene expression profiles induced by E6 from non-European HPV18 variants reveals a differential activation on cellular processes driving to carcinogenesis. Virology. 2012. doi:10.1016/j.virol.2012.05.029.
12. Backsch C, Rudolph B, Steinbach D, et al. An integrative functional genomic and gene expression approach revealed SORBS2 as a putative tumour suppressor gene involved in cervical carcinogenesis. Carcinogenesis. 2011;32:1100–6. doi:10.1093/carcin/bgr093.
13. Pérez-Plasencia C, Vázquez-Ortiz G, López-Romero R, et al. Genome wide expression analysis in HPV16 cervical cancer: identification of altered metabolic pathways. Infect Agent Cancer. 2007;2:16. doi:10.1186/1750-9378-2-16.
14. López J, Poitevin A, Mendoza-Martínez V, et al. Cancer-initiating cells derived from established cervical cell lines exhibit stem-cell markers and increased radioresistance. BMC Cancer. 2012;12:48. doi:10.1186/1471-2407-12-48.
15. Wong YF, Selvanayagam ZE, Wei N, et al. Expression genomics of cervical cancer: molecular classification and prediction of radiotherapy response by DNA microarray. Clin Cancer Res Off J Am Assoc Cancer Res. 2003;9:5486–92.
16. Zempolich K, Fuhrman C, Milash B, et al. Changes in gene expression induced by chemoradiation in advanced cervical carcinoma: a microarray study of RTOG C-0128. Gynecol Oncol. 2008;109:275–9. doi:10.1016/j.ygyno.2008.01.027.
17. Borkamo ED, Schem B-C, Fluge O, et al. cDNA microarray analysis of serially sampled cervical cancer specimens from patients treated with thermochemoradiotherapy. Int J Radiat Oncol Biol Phys. 2009;75:1562–9. doi:10.1016/j.ijrobp.2009.08.007.
18. Karin M, Greten FR. NF-kappaB: linking inflammation and immunity to cancer development and progression. Nat Rev Immunol. 2005;5:749–59. doi:10.1038/nri1703.
19. Ruutu M, Peitsaro P, Johansson B, Syrjänen S. Transcriptional profiling of a human papillomavirus 33-positive squamous epithelial cell line which acquired a selective growth advantage after viral integration. Int J Cancer J Int Cancer. 2002;100:318–26. doi:10.1002/ijc.10455.
20. Mahoney DJ, Cheung HH, Mrad RL, et al. Both cIAP1 and cIAP2 regulate TNFalpha-mediated NF-kappaB activation. Proc Natl Acad Sci U S A. 2008;105:11778–83. doi:10.1073/pnas.0711122105.
21. Peng G, Dan W, Jun W, et al. Transcriptome profiling of the cancer and adjacent nontumor tissues from cervical squamous cell carcinoma patients by RNA sequencing. Tumour Biol J Int Soc Oncodevelopmental Biol Med. 2015; doi:10.1007/s13277-014-2963-0.
22. Uhlar CM, Whitehead AS. The kinetics and magnitude of the synergistic activation of the serum amyloid A promoter by IL-1 beta and IL-6 is determined by the order of cytokine addition. Scand J Immunol. 1999;49:399–404.
23. Lee HY, Kim M-K, Park KS, et al. Serum amyloid a stimulates matrix-metalloproteinase-9 upregulation via formyl peptide receptor like-1-mediated signaling in human monocytic cells. Biochem Biophys Res Commun. 2005;330:989–98. doi:10.1016/j.bbrc.2005.03.069.
24. Massagué J. TGFβ signalling in context. Nat Rev Mol Cell Biol. 2012;13:616–30. doi:10.1038/nrm3434.

25. Massagué J. TGFβ in cancer. Cell. 2008;134:215–30. doi:10.1016/j.cell.2008.07.001.
26. Ikushima H, Miyazono K. TGF-β signal transduction spreading to a wider field: a broad variety of mechanisms for context-dependent effects of TGF-β. Cell Tissue Res. 2012;347:37–49. doi:10.1007/s00441-011-1179-5.
27. Thomas JT, Oh ST, Terhune SS, Laimins LA. Cellular changes induced by low-risk human papillomavirus type 11 in keratinocytes that stably maintain viral episomes. J Virol. 2001;75:7564–71. doi:10.1128/JVI.75.16.7564-7571.2001.
28. Nees M, Geoghegan JM, Munson P, et al. Human papillomavirus type 16 E6 and E7 proteins inhibit differentiation-dependent expression of transforming growth factor-beta2 in cervical keratinocytes. Cancer Res. 2000;60:4289–98.
29. Duffy CL, Phillips SL, Klingelhutz AJ. Microarray analysis identifies differentiation-associated genes regulated by human papillomavirus type 16 E6. Virology. 2003;314:196–205.
30. French D, Belleudi F, Mauro MV, et al. Expression of HPV16 E5 down-modulates the TGFbeta signaling pathway. Mol Cancer. 2013;12:38. doi:10.1186/1476-4598-12-38.
31. Wan F, Miao X, Quraishi I, et al. Gene expression changes during HPV-mediated carcinogenesis: a comparison between an in vitro cell model and cervical cancer. Int J Cancer J Int Cancer. 2008;123:32–40. doi:10.1002/ijc.
32. Jakowlew SB. Transforming growth factor-beta in cancer and metastasis. Cancer Metastasis Rev. 2006;25:435–57. doi:10.1007/s10555-006-9006-2.
33. Kloth JN, Fleuren GJ, Oosting J, et al. Substantial changes in gene expression of Wnt, MAPK and TNFalpha pathways induced by TGF-beta1 in cervical cancer cell lines. Carcinogenesis. 2005;26:1493–502. doi:10.1093/carcin/bgi110.
34. Toussaint-Smith E, Donner DB, Roman A. Expression of human papillomavirus type 16 E6 and E7 oncoproteins in primary foreskin keratinocytes is sufficient to alter the expression of angiogenic factors. Oncogene. 2004;23:2988–95. doi:10.1038/sj.onc.1207442.
35. Noordhuis MG, Fehrmann RSN, Wisman GBA, et al. Involvement of the TGF-beta and beta-catenin pathways in pelvic lymph node metastasis in early-stage cervical cancer. Clin Cancer Res Off J Am Assoc Cancer Res. 2011;17:1317–30. doi:10.1158/1078-0432.CCR-10-2320.
36. Clevers H. Wnt/beta-catenin signaling in development and disease. Cell. 2006;127:469–80. doi:10.1016/j.cell.2006.10.018.
37. Nusse R, Varmus HE. Many tumors induced by the mouse mammary tumor virus contain a provirus integrated in the same region of the host genome. Cell. 1982;31:99–109.
38. Shtutman M, Zhurinsky J, Simcha I, et al. The cyclin D1 gene is a target of the beta-catenin/LEF-1 pathway. Proc Natl Acad Sci U S A. 1999;96:5522–7.
39. Katoh M. WNT/PCP signaling pathway and human cancer (review). Oncol Rep. 2005;14:1583–8.
40. Janssens N, Janicot M, Perera T. The Wnt-dependent signaling pathways as target in oncology drug discovery. Investig New Drugs. 2006;24:263–80. doi:10.1007/s10637-005-5199-4.
41. Perez-Plasencia C, Duenas-Gonzalez A, Alatorre-Tavera B. Second hit in cervical carcinogenesis process: involvement of wnt/beta catenin pathway. Int Arch Med. 2008;1:10. doi:10.1186/1755-7682-1-10.
42. Uren A, Fallen S, Yuan H, et al. Activation of the canonical Wnt pathway during genital keratinocyte transformation: a model for cervical cancer progression. Cancer Res. 2005;65:6199–206. doi:10.1158/0008-5472.CAN-05-0455.
43. Niehrs C, Acebron SP. Mitotic and mitogenic Wnt signalling. EMBO J. 2012;31:2705–13. doi:10.1038/emboj.2012.124.
44. Dhillon AS, Hagan S, Rath O, Kolch W. MAP kinase signalling pathways in cancer. Oncogene. 2007;26:3279–90. doi:10.1038/sj.onc.1210421.
45. Kyriakis JM, Avruch J. Mammalian mitogen-activated protein kinase signal transduction pathways activated by stress and inflammation. Physiol Rev. 2001;81:807–69.
46. Krens SFG, Spaink HP, Snaar-Jagalska BE. Functions of the MAPK family in vertebrate-development. FEBS Lett. 2006;580:4984–90. doi:10.1016/j.febslet.2006.08.025.

47. Mendoza MC, Er EE, Blenis J. The Ras-ERK and PI3K-mTOR pathways: cross-talk and compensation. Trends Biochem Sci. 2011;36:320–8. doi:10.1016/j.tibs.2011.03.006.
48. Hanahan D, Weinberg RA. Hallmarks of cancer: the next generation. Cell. 2011;144:646–74. doi:10.1016/j.cell.2011.02.013.
49. Iwakawa M, Ohno T, Imadome K, et al. The radiation-induced cell-death signaling pathway is activated by concurrent use of cisplatin in sequential biopsy specimens from patients with cervical cancer. Cancer Biol Ther. 2007;6:905–11.
50. Kitahara O, Katagiri T, Tsunoda T, et al. Classification of sensitivity or resistance of cervical cancers to ionizing radiation according to expression profiles of 62 genes selected by cDNA microarray analysis. Neoplasia N Y N. 2002;4:295–303. doi:10.1038/sj.neo.7900251.

Chapter 5
Pre-invasive Lesions of the Cervix

Aarón González-Enciso, Salim Abraham Barquet-Muñoz, David Francisco Cantú-de-León, and Cristian Yaoska Corea-Urbina

Abstract Invasive Cervical carcinoma o Cervical Cancer (CCa) is the fourth leading cause of death among women. CCa is preceded by dysplastic alterations in the epithelial cells of the cervix that do not compromise the stroma. The most significant risk factor is one that is also required for the development of pre-invasive cervical lesions: persistent infection with a strain of human papilloma virus (HPV) that has a viral genotype. Timely detection programs consist of methods aimed at identifying women with asymptomatic pre-malignant lesions that can be healed with treatment. Current screening tests to detect CCa include cervical cytology, either conventional or liquid-based, and assays to detect high and low risk viruses or specific serotypes. Furthermore, because HPV is an etiological factor and because we know that primary prevention of HPV is a health-promoting strategy, prophylactic vaccines have been developed for this virus. Treatments for pre-malignant lesions depend on the degree of the lesion, the availability of medical resources, the experience of the surgeons in performing specific procedures and patient choice.

Keywords Human papilloma virus • Intra-epithelial lesion • Low-grade • High-grade

A. González-Enciso, MD (✉) • S.A. Barquet-Muñoz, MD • C.Y. Corea-Urbina, MD
Gynecologic Tumors Department, Instituto Nacional de Cancerología-México,
Av. San Fernando No 22, Col. Sección XVI México, D.F, Mexico City 14080, Mexico
e-mail: agencisonco@hotmail.com

D.F. Cantú-de-León, PhD
Gynecologic Tumors Department, Instituto Nacional de Cancerología-México,
Av. San Fernando No 22, Col. Sección XVI México, D.F, Mexico City 14080, Mexico

Clinical Research Department, Instituto Nacional de Cancerología-México,
Mexico City, Mexico

J.G. de la Garza-Salazar et al. (eds.), *Cervical Cancer*,
DOI 10.1007/978-3-319-45231-9_5

5.1 Introduction

CCa is the fourth leading cause of death in women. A total of 528,000 new cases were reported on 2012, resulting in an estimated mortality of 266,000. This represents 7.5% of all cancer deaths in women around the world [1]. CCa is known to be preceded by dysplastic alterations in the cells of the cervical epithelium that do not compromise the stroma. The most important risk factors for CCa are linked to sexual behavior, and of these, HPV infection is fundamental to the development of these lesions. In recent decades, our understanding of the biology of HPV and its epidemiology has increased exponentially, leading to the creation of new screening methods and recommendations in addition to vaccines against HPV that serve to prevent CCa. Being aware of the natural history of these lesions provides us with a wide window of time in which to detect this condition early and to therefore treat affected patients in a timely and efficient manner.

5.2 Epidemiology

VPH infection is relatively common and it is thought that the risk of infection during a person's life is approximately 75%. The population under 30 years old has an HPV prevalence of roughly 58.9%. It is estimated that approximately 291 million women around the world have had contact with the virus at least once in their life, corresponding to a prevalence of 10.4%. In Latin America there is a second peak in prevalence at approximately 55 years of age, when the incidence is 52.8% for HPV 16 and 9.4% for HPV 18 [2].

5.3 Risk Factors for the Development of Pre-invasive Lesions

The most important and fundamental risk factors for the development of pre-invasive cervical lesions are persistent infection with HPV and its viral genotype. However, other co-factors have also been shown to increase the risk of infection and the risk of progression to malignant transformation.

The best known factors are an early onset of sexual activity, multiparity, potentially infective sexual partners, multiple sexual partners, and immunodeficiency [2]. These co-factors increase the risk of progressing to a high-grade intraepithelial lesion. Out of all of the previously mentioned co-factors, the most important factor is immunodeficiency. This is especially true in HIV-infected women because infection increases the risk of persistent infection with HPV at all ages [3]. Similarly, smoking and the prolonged use of oral contraceptives promote the development of squamous metaplasia by promoting persistent HPV infection [2].

Table 5.1 HPV classification

Low-risk: 6, 11, 40, 42, 54, 57
High-grade: 16, 18, 26, 31, 33, 35, 39, 45, 51, 52, 53, 56, 58, 59, 66, 68

5.4 Human Papilloma Virus

The causal link between HPV and the development of cervical cancer was first identified in 1970, when Dr. Harald zur Hausen suggested that the viral particles that were observed in genital warts were also responsible for malignant neoplasia of the cervix [4]. HPV 16 and 18 were later identified as being responsible for 70% of all CCa cases.

HPV belongs to the Papillomaviridae family, the members of which have a high affinity for mucous tissues and epithelia and are capable of inducing strong epithelial proliferation at the site of infection. There are at least 120 different HPV serotypes, and of these, at least 40 infect the genitals [5]. The latter group is classified as either low or high risk according to their contribution to the development of malignant neoplasia (Table 5.1). Low-risk HPV viruses are associated with genital warts, whereas high-risk HPV viruses are associated with intraepithelial high-grade lesions and CCa.

The HPV viral genome is DNA-based, consisting of a circular double-helix. It is divided into a series of early open reading frames (ORFs) (E1–E7) and late ORFs (L1–L2) that are encoded in approximately 8000 bp. VPH has a protein capsule that is formed by 72 capsomeres that are made of the proteins encoded in the L1 and L2 ORFs. These capsomeres serve as protection and a means of interaction with the proteins in the host cell. Early ORFs encode replication, regulation and cell proliferation proteins [6]. The precise functions of E6 and E7 are worth mentioning. Over-expressing the E6 ORF promotes the ubiquitination and subsequent degradation of the regulator protein p53, which results in the progression of the cell cycle and avoidance of apoptosis, which allows the transformed cells to replicate. Similarly, the oncoprotein E7 promotes the degradation of the Rb gene, which results in the disruption of the cell cycle [2]. Both of these events inhibit apoptosis, resulting in the promotion of carcinogenesis.

5.5 Vaccines

Because HPV as an etiological factor and it is known that preventing the spread of HPV is a significant health strategy, prophylactic vaccines have been developed. In 2006, the United States Food and Drug Administration (FDA) approved the first vaccine against HPV. Gardasil® is a quadrivalent vaccine that was developed by Merck laboratories to protect individuals against HPV serotypes 6, 11, 16 and 18. In 2009, the FDA approved a second bivalent vaccine (Cervarix® by GlaxoSmithKline) that was specific to HPV serotypes 16 and 18 [7]. Both vaccines were developed using the recombinant expression of proteins obtained from the viral capsid (L1), which self-assembles upon expression to form structures called virus-like particles

(VLPs) that are similar to those found in complete virions. These VLPs induce a substantial antigenic effect without also inducing infection, and they attain antibody levels 100-fold higher than those observed in natural infections [16]. Table 5.2 lists the most important characteristics of these two vaccines.

Routine administration has been recommended for both vaccines in girls and boys between 11 and 12 years old; however, administration can begin in children as young as 9 years old. The administration of these vaccines is also recommended in women between 13 and 26 years old who have not been previously vaccinated or who have not completed the three recommended doses. If a woman turns 26 years old before completing the three doses, the pending doses can be administered after she turns 26 years old. Ideally, the vaccine should be administered before the onset of sexual activity [10].

Several randomized studies have demonstrated the efficacy of HPV vaccinations. The efficacy of the quadrivalent vaccine was established in the FUTURE I and FUTURE II studies. In both of these studies, an efficacy of 100% was obtained for the prevention of HPV lesions 6/11/16/18. The vaccine also showed an efficacy of 75% for preventing intraepithelial vaginal neoplasias. A similarly high efficacy was found for its ability to prevent benign lesions of the vulva and the vagina that can be caused by HPV types not related to the vaccine [11].

The efficacy of the bivalent vaccine was evaluated in the randomized, double-blinded PATRICIA study. In the PATRICIA study, vaccinated patients showed a 100% efficacy for preventing lesions caused by HPV 16 and 18. Additionally, it demonstrated 100% efficacy in preventing in situ adenocarcinomas and reduced the risk of high-grade intra-epithelial lesions caused by HPV types that are not related to the vaccine [12].

The fact that a woman receives the full vaccination scheme does not exempt her from regular cytological analyses of the cervix and the vaginal, which favor the early detection of lesions of any kind [13].

Table 5.2 Characteristics of vaccines against human papilloma virus (HPV)

	Gardasil®	Cervarix®
Name	Quadrivalent vaccine against HPV	Bivalent vaccine against HPV
Pharmaceutical company	Merck & Co	GlaxoSmithKline Biologicals
HPV serotypes	6, 11, 16 and 18	16 and 18
Adjuvant	225 μmg Phosphate Hydroxysulphate amorphous of aluminum	500 μmg aluminum hydroxide,50 μmg de 3-O- deacetylated -4 –Lipid A mono-phosphorylated
Virus-like particles (VLPs)	20/40/40/20 μmg	20/20 μmg
Production	Leaven (saccharomyces cerevisiae)	Insect cells (SF9)/baculovirus
Doses and schemes	0, 2, 5 months; 0.5 mL; Intramuscular	0,1, 6 months; 0.5 mL; Intramuscular
Antibodies quantitation	1–19 times more than the natural infection	14–17 times more than the natural infection

5.6 Natural History of HPV Infection

In most infected women, the infection is asymptomatic, and immune responses result in the spontaneous disappearance of the infection after 12–18 months in 80% of cases. A strong relationship exists between persistent HPV infections and squamous intraepithelial lesions (SIL) incidence, particularly for HPV types 16 and 18, the risk of developing a neoplastic lesion is higher. In the beginning of this disease, the cells exhibit only signs of the viral infection, but they then turn into cervical intra-epithelial neoplasias (CINs) and ultimately progress to invasive cancer [14].

Most CINs develop in the transformation zone of the cervix, which is located in the squamous-columnar junction between the columnar epithelium of the endocervix and the squamous epithelium of the ectocervix. CINs make up a continuous spectrum of neoplastic cells that display changes in their cytoplasm and the loss of nuclear polarization, pleomorphism and mitotic index. They are divided into three types: CIN I, or mild dysplasia (Fig. 5.1), in which only one-third of the lower epithelium is affected; CIN II, or moderate dysplasia (Fig. 5.2), in which the lesion extends up to the middle third of the epithelium; and CIN III, or severe dysplasia, which is in situ carcinoma (Fig. 5.3), in which the lesion extends through the full thickness of the epithelium [15]. CIN I represents a transitory manifestation of a viral infection, during which the infected epithelium differs from a normal epithelium only in some slight cellular alterations. In CINs II and III, HPV prevents the maturation and differentiation of the infected basal cells, resulting in the generation of one or several clones of neoplastic cells. It is currently thought that CIN I is the only benign HPV infection-related process, and these cases are therefore called

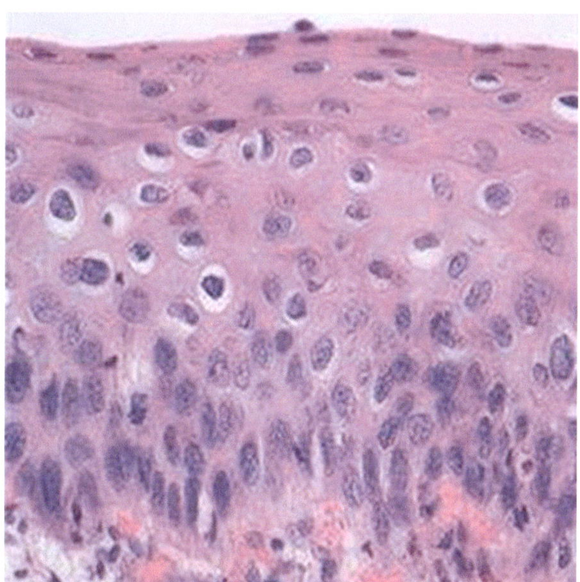

Fig. 5.1 Intra-epithelial cervical neoplasia (CIN) I. Immature epithelial cells are found only in the lower one-third of the epithelium

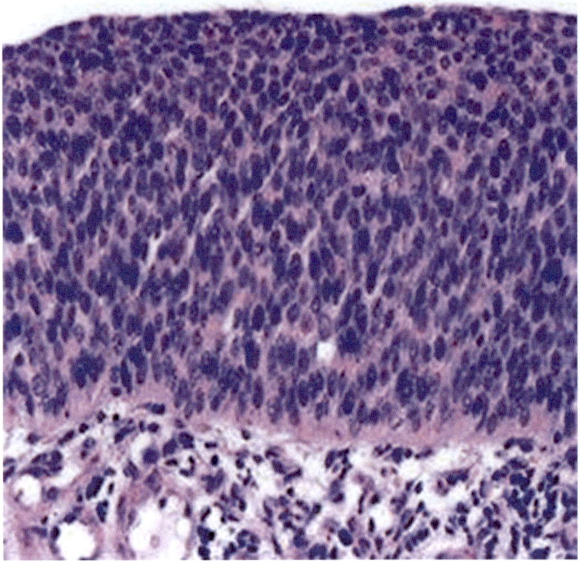

Fig. 5.2 Intra-epithelial cervical neoplasia (CIN) II. Immature epithelial cells are found in the two lower two-thirds of the epithelium

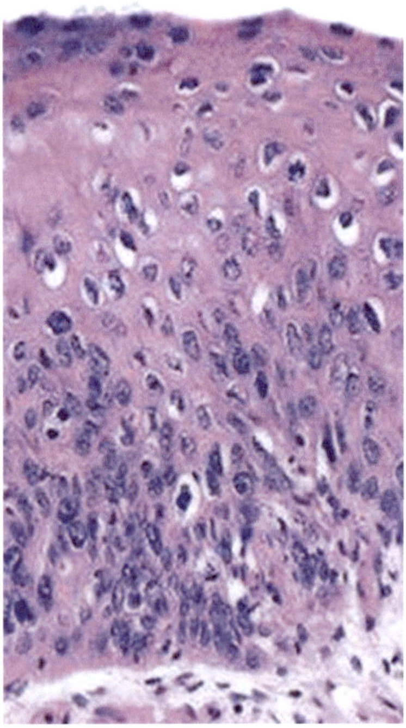

Fig. 5.3 Intra-epithelial cervical neoplasia (CIN) III. Immature epithelial cells are observed through the full thickness of the epithelium but do not extend beyond the basal lamina. This category includes cases of in situ carcinoma

low-grade intra-epithelial lesions. CINs II and III comprise the premalignant lesions, and they are referred to as high-grade intra-epithelial lesions. CIN I can be produced by both low-risk and high-risk viral serotypes, whereas CINs II and III are produced only by serotypes with high oncological risk.

Most low-grade intra-epithelial lesions disappear spontaneously after a period of 2 years, especially in patients found to be positive for low-risk HPVs. Only a small percentage (15%) of cases progress to high-grade intra-epithelial lesions over a 24 month period, and this is especially likely if the patient is positive for a high-risk HPV (17.3%) [16].

5.7 Screening

Timely detection programs consist of identifying asymptomatic women with pre-malignant lesions in whom treatment can lead to healing. When screening studies are routinely performed, there is an up to two to tenfold lower risk of developing invasive CCa than in patients who never submit themselves to this type of evaluation [16]. Current screening tests to detect CCa include cervical cytology, either conventional or liquid-based, and assays to detect high- versus low-risk viruses or specific serotypes.

In March 2012, the American Cancer Society (ACS), the American Society for Colposcopy and Cervical Pathology (ASCCP) and the American Society for Clinical Pathology (ASCP) reviewed their recommendations for Cervical Cancer screening. Simultaneously, the US Preventive Services Task Force (USPSTF) and the American Congress of Obstetricians and Gynecologists also reviewed their clinical practices [17].

The screening recommendations they proposed are summarized as follows:

- Screening must not be performed in patients younger than 21 years old.
- Cytological screening must be performed every 3 years in patients between 21 and 29 years old. The use of HPV-detecting tests is not advised for this group of young women.
- HPV-detecting tests and cytology must be performed every 5 years on patients between 30 and 65 years old. It is acceptable to perform the cytological screening only every 3 years.
- Screening can be suspended in patients who are older than 65 years old provided they have previously undergone appropriate and negative screenings. If they were previously diagnosed with CIN II, the screening must continue for at least 20 years because there was a diagnosis of a pre-invasive lesion.
- After a hysterectomy, patients must not be screened if the cervix was removed and there is no clinical history of CIN II or III.
- Women who were previously immunized with a bivalent or quadrivalent vaccine must follow the same recommendations as those made for non-immunized women [17].

5.8 Nomenclature

Cytology reports were first introduced in 1998 and subsequently revised in 2001 in the city of Bethesda, at which time both the terminology and the diagnosis reporting protocols were standardized. The Bethesda system was developed via a process that involved a literature revising omit, expert opinions and a discussion of the proposed changes [18]. Some of the terms that were revised in 2001 according to the Bethesda system are included in Table 5.3.

The classification of cervical epithelial alterations according to their histological characteristics differentiates groups of women based on the state of cellular maturation and the thickness of the affected area in the squamous epithelium, as has already been described in this chapter.

Table 5.3 Summary of the Bethesda system 2001 terminology [18]

Interpretation/Result
Negative for intraepithelial lesion or malignancy
Organisms: trichomonas vaginalis, fungal organisms, etc
Cellular changes:
consistent with herpes simplex virus other non-neoplastic findings (Optional to report; list not comprehensive)
Reactive cellular changes:
Inflammation (includes typical repair)
Radiation
Intrauterine contraceptive device
Glandular cells
Status posthysterectomy
Atrophy
Epithelial cell abnormalities:
Squamous cell atypical squamous cells (ASC)
ASC of undetermined significance (ASC-US)
ASC cannot exclude HSIL (ASC-H)
Low-grade squamous intraepithelial lesion (LSIL) encompassing: human papillomavirus/mild dysplasia/cervical intraepithelial neoplasia (CIN) 1
High-grade squamous intraepithelial lesion (HSIL) encompassing: moderate (CIN 2) and severe dysplasia (CIN 3) and carcinoma in situ
Glandular cell
Atypical glandular cell (AGC) (specify endocervical, endometrial, or not otherwise specified)
Atypical glandular cells, favor neoplastic (specify endocervical or not otherwise specified)
Endocervical adenocarcinoma in situ (AIS)
Adenocarcinoma
Endometrial cells in a woman with 40 years of age automated review and ancillary testing (Include as appropriate)

5.9 Approach and Treatment of Pre-invasive Lesions

5.9.1 Colposcopic Evaluation

Colposcopy is not a screening method because performing it adequately requires a large amount of resources and preparation. However, every cytological anomaly is considered an indication that prompts an Colposcopy. The objective is to reveal any anomalies that may direct the biopsy sampling to dismiss invasive cancer. Colposcopic evaluations are advised in patients with a macroscopically normal cervix but in whom abnormal cytology has been observed. Colposcopic characteristics are classified according to appearance and increase in value of a potentially subjacent malignity post-application of acetic acid, which is used to dissolve the cervical mucous and reveal the lesioned tissue, which is whiter than the surrounding epithelium. The more anomalies that are observed, the higher the possibility of a high-grade lesion or an invasive cancer. Using this method, a well-defined acetic-white lesion that does not display point markings, is not mosaic and has a normal vascular pattern is most likely to indicate a secondary lesion of HPV or a low-grade intra-epithelial lesion (Fig. 5.1). An anomaly that reveals itself as a thick acetic-white epithelium, a thick mosaic and an increased vascular pattern may correspond to a high-grade intra-epithelial lesion (Fig. 5.2) or an invasive carcinoma (Figs. 5.3, 5.4, 5.5 and 5.6) [19].

5.9.2 Treatment Generalities

The applied procedures depend mainly on the histological diagnosis. Nevertheless, this choice is influenced by the cytological diagnosis, the age and future fertility plans of the patient, and the presence of colposcopic findings or evidence of

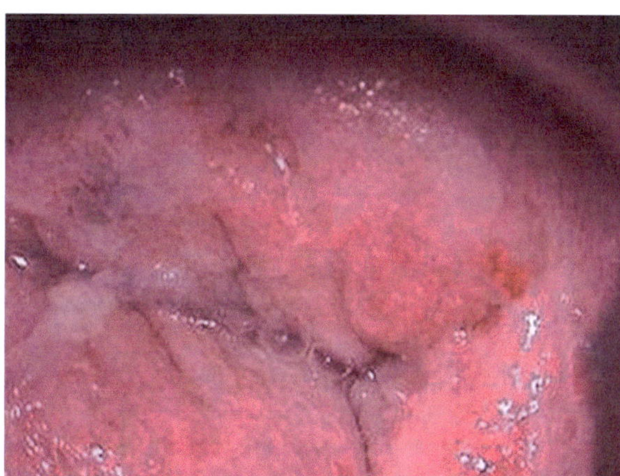

Fig. 5.4. Low-grade intra-epithelial lesion. Fine point markings can be seen that have poorly defined borders and a mild acetic-white epithelium

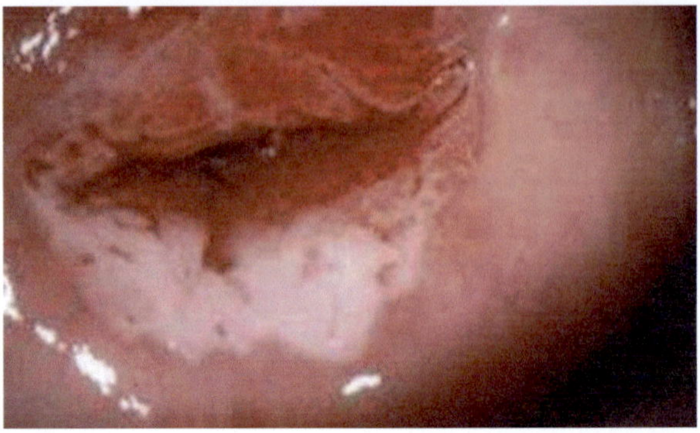

Fig. 5.5. High-grade intra-epithelial lesion. A thick acetic-white epithelium with regular and well-defined borders and a thick mosaic is shown

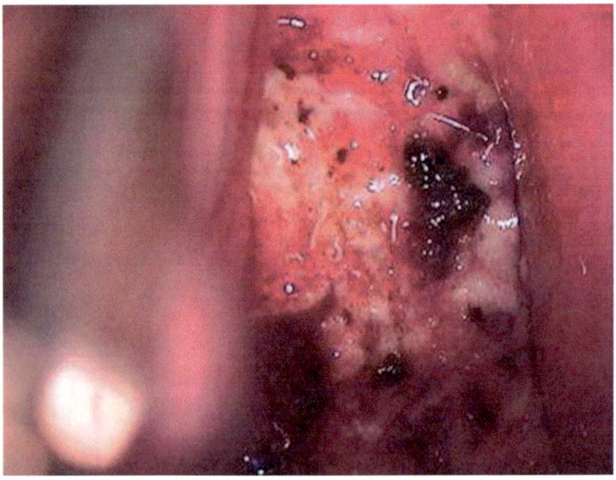

Fig. 5.6 Invasive Cervical carcinoma o Cervical Cancer (CCa)

endocervical dysplasia. The treatment also depends on the degree of the lesion, the availability of medical resources, the experience of the surgeons in performing specific procedures and the patient's choice.

5.9.3 Atypical Squamous Cells of Uncertain Significance (ASC-US) and Low-Grade Intra-epithelial Lesions

Most lesions undergo spontaneous resolution within a period no longer than 24 months. This is why surveillance is necessary as long as the results of colposcopy are satisfactory. In general terms, surveillance includes observing the patient for cervicovaginal cytologies every 6 months [16]. Hysterectomy is not a valid treatment option [16, 20]. Current recommendations for low-grade intra-epithelial lesions that are diagnosed by cytology are based on the results of a co-test. Low-grade intra-epithelial lesion diagnoses are indirect indicators of HPV seropositivity because approximately 80% of such cases will have a positive HPV test. Still, there are women who have a negative HPV test with positive cytology for a low-grade intra-epithelial lesion. In these cases, it is advised that the practitioner perform a co-test after 1 year. If both tests are negative, then the co-test must be performed in 3 years. In women between 21 and 24 years old who have positive cytology for a low-grade intra-epithelial lesion, the tests must be performed annually for 2 years. The risk of cervical cancer in women younger than 25 years old is very low (1.4 in every 100 thousand women per year), and they frequently have a positive HPV test, even though their HPV-related lesions tend to be in regression [21]. If, upon repeating this tests on a patient, an ASC-H or high-grade intra-epithelial lesion is found, colposcopy is advised. If the patient has ASC-US or high-grade intra-epithelial lesions that become higher after two cytological assays, colposcopy is advised. In post-menopausal patients, low-grade intra-epithelial lesions can be monitored every 6 months using co-trials or by performing colposcopy. If an HPV test is negative or no dysplasia is identified in the colposcopy, the co-test can be performed after 1 year. If the result is ASC-US or a high-grade intra-epithelial lesion, a colposcopy must be performed [22].

In patients in whom a CIN I biopsy was detected that was preceded by a low-grade intra-epithelial lesion or ASC-US, a co-test must be performed after 1 year; if both are negative, the patient must return to a normal screening schedule. If a diagnosis of CIN I persists for 2 years, it is acceptable to continue with the follow-up or to treat the lesion as if it had a higher grade. In cases where the result of the second revision is CIN II or worse, the lesion must be treated. In patients in whom a diagnosis of CIN I is preceded by ASC-H or a high-grade intra-epithelial lesion, the follow-up must be more thorough, including an excisional biopsy, a follow-up and a review of the findings.

In patients between 21 and 24 years old, it is advised that the case is handled using a conservative approach. If such a biopsy is preceded by a high-grade intra-epithelial lesion or ASC-H, a cytological assay must be performed every 6 months, and colposcopies should be performed every two. If CIN II or worse is suspected, then a biopsy must be taken. If, after 2 years, the cytology-detected high-grade lesion persists without evidence of the same in the biopsy, then an excision process is advised. CIN I patients between 21 and 24 years old must never be treated [22].

5.9.4 *High-Grade Intra-epithelial Lesion*

High-grade intra-epithelial lesion are relatively rare, representing only 0.6% of such specimens [23]. However, if a high-grade intra-epithelial lesion is detected by cytology, there is a probability of approximately 70–75% that a CIN II or III will be found in a colposcopy, biopsy or excision [24]. Given the elevated rate of persistence and progression of these conditions, surveillance is mandatory, independent of the age of the patient or her menopause stage. In patients with a CIN II or III diagnosis that has been confirmed by biopsy with discarded invasion and a satisfactory colposcopy, ablative methods (e.g., cryotherapy, electro-coagulation, or laser vaporization) and excision methods (e.g., loop diathermy, laser or cold knife cone biopsy, or total hysterectomy) are the approved therapies [16].

The present recommendations suggest that colposcopy must be performed whenever there is a cytological diagnosis of ASC-US with a positive HPV test, a high-grade intra-epithelial lesion, ASC-H or AGC [22]. After performing a cytological assay to detect high-grade intra-epithelial lesions with an inadequate colposcopy or a positive endocervical curettage, it is recommended that the practitioner perform an excision procedure both to obtain a sample for a more precise diagnosis and to treat the patient. Any histological CIN II or III diagnosis in the cervical biopsy must be directed to excision or the ablation of the transformation zone unless the patient is pregnant. The "see-and-treat" option is recommended in geographical zones with difficult access or very low economical resources or when a poor follow-up scheme is conducted in patients with a high-grade intra-epithelial lesion cytology in whom a biopsy was not performed. In patients between 21 and 25 years old with CIN II, the regression rate is high, i.e. 28% in 1 year, 63% in 2 years and 68% in 3 years [21]. If a CIN II is detected in a young women and was preceded by ASC-H or a high-grade intra-epithelial lesion, either an ablative or excision procedure could be considered to remove the transformation zone, or simply colposcopic observation every 6 months, especially in CIN II cases. If it persist after 2 years, excision is advised.

In patients with satisfied parity, if the excision reveals positive borders, a definitive surgical procedure is necessary (extrafascial hysterectomy) because the most important marker for recurrence/persistence is the state of the cervical cone margins 16. The incidence/recurrence rates in these cases can reach 16% in cases with positive margins, while a negative margin is associated with a risk of only 4% [16].

5.9.5 *Glandular Lesions*

For any kind of glandular lesion, the recommendation is to perform a colposcopy and endocervical curettage independent of the HPV test result. Moreover, endometrial curettage is recommended in women older than 35 years old with atypical glandular cell cytology (AGC) and adenocarcinoma in situ (AIS). In cases of AGC in which a CIN II or more is cytologically discarded, the patient can remain under surveillance every 12–24 months. If both results are negative, surveillance must continue for 3 years. In cases of AGC with CIN II or high-grade intra-epithelial lesions but without glandular neoplasia, if the AGC occurs with neoplastic risk or AIS in patients with satisfied parity and a histological diagnosis, a hysterectomy can be performed. Conservative treatments are performed in patients that are considering a future maternity, and an excision procedure is performed if the endocervical cancer sample has CIN or AIS. An incision is then performed and re-evaluated in 6 months using the co-test and colposcopy plus endocervical sampling [22].

5.10 Treatment Options

Treatment options consist of two types: excision (e.g., loop diathermy, laser or cold knife cone biopsy) and ablative (e.g., cryotherapy and laser). In a review, Cochrane 2010, analyzed 29 randomized, controlled studies that included 5441 women with CIN and found no evidence showing that any one procedure was better that any other [25]. In particular, the treatment must be selected in accordance with factors that benefit the patient, her diagnosis and the gynecologist's training. For ablative treatments, it must be certain that there was a satisfying colposcopy with a benign result from an endocervical curettage, the absence of invasion and a fully visible lesion. Some of the advantages of this procedure are its reduced cost and the fact that it does not increase the risk of pre-term delivery. However, it should be considered that there will be no sample available for histologic review. Regarding laser ablation, its requisites are similar to those for cryotherapy, and it is especially recommended for high-grade intra-epithelial lesions. Its main disadvantage is its elevated cost.

Excision procedures, or cone biopsies, are generally performed for diagnosis and therapeutic purposes and consist of removing a large cone-like portion of the cervix that includes the exocervical opening and various portions of the endocervical canal. It is important to mention that the surgeon's experience is fundamental to achieving the success of the procedure and a low rate of complications. This represents, in general, the second diagnosis option, right after colposcopy and biopsy.

Cold knife cone biopsies require local-regional or even general anesthesia and hospitalization, is associated with more complications and produces a more evident anatomic distortion. For these reasons, it is performed with much lower frequency. In contrast, CO^2 -laser cone biopsy can be performed in an ambulatory fashion. It usually preserves the reproductive integrity of the patient, is associated with minimum complications and an excellent healing rate, and facilitates follow-up. Its disadvantages are the fact that it involves thermal damage, the cost of the equipment is high, it requires extensive training, and the time of surgery is long. The loop diathermy cone biopsy (Fig. 5.7) method is based on the principle of monopolar procedures. Its

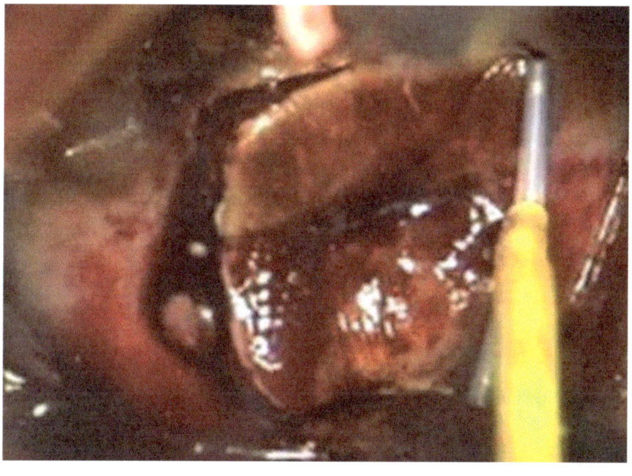

Fig. 5.7 Performance of a loop diathermy cone biopsy

advantages include the fact that it allows a sample to be obtained for histopathological analysis; it is an ambulatory, quick and economic procedure; it is relatively easy to learn; and it is associated with a high healing rate. Nonetheless, inadequate training and the apparent simplicity of the procedure can lead to incomplete excisions, which occurs 44% of the time. Another disadvantage is the high percentage of negative cones (ranging between 14 and 30%), which means that the surgery involves a high number of unnecessary treatment 16 however, there is a risk of removing too much cervical tissue, which would compromise the fertility of the patient.

5.11 Conclusion

Improving the diagnosis and treatment of cervical cancer is a priority for health systems, especially in developing countries. Both the etiology and the natural history of this neoplasia are known. The role of timely detection to identify premalignant lesions with healing potential, which facilitates efficacious and practical procedures, has also been extensively supported. The options for achieving the timely detection of these conditions are various and are focused on cytological analyses and the detection of HPV using molecular assays. Implementing measures that increase the rate of timely detection has lowered both the incidence and the mortality of cervical cancer.

References

1. Ferlay J, Soerjomataram I, Ervik M, Dikshit R, Eser S, Mathers C, Rebelo M, Parkin DM, Forman D, Bray F. GLOBOCAN 2012 v1.0, Cancer Incidence and Mortality Worldwide: IARC CancerBase No. 11 [Internet]. Lyon, Fr Int Agency Res Cancer. 2013. http://globocan.iarc.fr. Accessed on day/month/yea.
2. Crosbie EJ, Einstein MH, Franceschi S, Kitchener HC. Human papillomavirus and cervical cancer. Lancet. 2013;382:889–99. doi:10.1016/S0140-6736(13)60022-7.
3. Moscicki AB, Schiffman M, Burchell A, et al. Updating the natural history of human papillomavirus and anogenital cancers. Vaccine. 2012;30. doi:10.1016/j.vaccine.2012.05.089.
4. Zur Hausen H. Papillomaviruses in anogenital cancer as a model to understand the role of viruses in human cancers. Cancer Res. 1989;49:4677–81.
5. Bernard HU, Burk RD, Chen Z, van Doorslaer K, zur Hausen H, de Villiers EM. Classification of papillomaviruses (PVs) based on 189 PV types and proposal of taxonomic amendments. Virology. 2010;401:70–9. doi:10.1016/j.virol.2010.02.002.
6. Tornesello ML, Buonaguro L, Giorgi-Rossi P, Buonaguro FM. Viral and cellular biomarkers in the diagnosis of cervical intraepithelial neoplasia and cancer. Biomed Res Int. 2013;2013:519619. doi:10.1155/2013/519619.
7. Szarewski A. Prophylactic HPV vaccines. Eur J Gynaecol Oncol. 2007;28:165–9. doi:10.2298/AOO0904068M.
8. Harper DM, Franco EL, Wheeler C, et al. Efficacy of a bivalent L1 virus-like particle vaccine in prevention of infection with human papillomavirus types 16 and 18 in young women: a randomised controlled trial. Lancet. 2004;364:1757–65. doi:10.1016/S0140-6736(04)17398-4.

9. Villa LL, Costa RLR, Petta CA, et al. High sustained efficacy of a prophylactic quadrivalent human papillomavirus types 6/11/16/18 L1 virus-like particle vaccine through 5 years of follow-up. Br J Cancer. 2006;95(11):1459–66.
10. CDC. Recommendations on the use of quadrivalent human papillomavirus vaccine in males--Advisory Committee on Immunization Practices (ACIP). 2011. Available at: http://www.ncbi.nlm.nih.gov/pubmed/22189893.
11. Garland SM, Hernandez-Avila M, Wheeler CM, et al. Quadrivalent vaccine against human papillomavirus to prevent anogenital diseases. N Engl J Med. 2007;356(19):1928–43.
12. Lehtinen M, Paavonen J, Wheeler CM, et al. Overall efficacy of HPV-16/18 AS04-adjuvanted vaccine against grade 3 or greater cervical intraepithelial neoplasia: 4-year end-of-study analysis of the randomised, double-blind PATRICIA trial. Lancet Oncol. 2012;13:89–99. doi:10.1016/S1470-2045(11)70286-8.
13. Workowski KA, Berman S. Sexually transmitted diseases treatment guidelines, 2010. MMWR Recomm Rep. 2010;59:1–110.
14. Schlecht NF, Kulaga S, Robitaille J, et al. Persistent human papillomavirus infection as a predictor of cervical intraepithelial neoplasia. JAMA. 2001;286:3106–14. doi:10.1001/jama.286.24.3106.
15. Galgano MT, Castle PE, Atkins KA, Brix WK, Nassau SR, Stoler MH. Using biomarkers as objective standards in the diagnosis of cervical biopsies. Am J Surg Pathol. 2010;34:1077–87. doi:10.1097/PAS.0b013e3181e8b2c4.
16. Duarte-Franco E, Franco EL. Cancer of the Uterine Cervix. BMC Womens Health. 2004;4:S13. doi:10.1186/1472-6874-4-S1-S13.
17. Karjane N, Chelmow D. New cervical cancer screening guidelines, again. Obstet Gynecol Clin N Am. 2013;40:211–23. doi:10.1016/j.ogc.2013.03.001.
18. Solomon D, Davey D, Kurman R, et al. The 2001 Bethesda System: terminology for reporting results of cervical cytology. JAMA J Am Med Assoc. 2002;287:2114–9. doi:10.1097/00006254-200208000-00015.
19. Tatti S, Bornstein J, Prendiville W. Colposcopy: a global perspective. introduction of the new IFCPC colposcopy terminology. Obstet Gynecol Clin N Am. 2013;40:235–50. doi:10.1016/j.ogc.2013.02.002.
20. Wright TC, Massad LS, Dunton CJ, Spitzer M, Wilkinson EJ, Solomon D. 2006 consensus guidelines for the management of women with cervical intraepithelial neoplasia or adenocarcinoma in situ. Am J Obstet Gynecol. 2007;197:340–5. doi:10.1016/j.ajog.2007.07.050.
21. Moscicki AB, Hills N, Shiboski S, et al. Risks for incident human papillomavirus infection and low-grade squamous intraepithelial lesion development in young females. JAMA. 2001;285:2995–3002. doi:10.1001/jama.285.23.2995.
22. Massad LS, Einstein MH, Huh WK, et al. 2012 updated consensus guidelines for the management of abnormal cervical cancer screening tests and cancer precursors. J Low Genit Tract Dis. 2013;17:S1–S27. doi:10.1097/LGT.0b013e318287d329.
23. Castle PE, Glass AG, Rush BB, et al. Clinical human papillomavirus detection forecasts cervical cancer risk in women over 18 years of follow-up. J Clin Oncol. 2012;30:3044–50. doi:10.1200/JCO.2011.38.8389.
24. Padilla-Paz LA, Carlson J, Twiggs LB, et al. Evidence supporting the current management guidelines for high-grade squamous intraepithelial lesion cytology. J Low Genit Tract Dis. 2004;8:139–46. doi:10.1097/00128360-200404000-00010.
25. Martin-Hirsch PP, Keep SL, Bryant A. Interventions for preventing blood loss during the treatment of cervical intraepithelial neoplasia. Cochrane Database Syst Rev. 2010:CD001421. doi:10.1002/14651858.CD001421.pub2.

Chapter 6
Control and Prevention in Cervical Cancer

Eduardo Lazcano-Ponce, Leith León-Maldonado, Betania Allen-Leigh, Jorge Salmerón, and Mauricio Hernández-Ávila

Abstract Cervical cancer (CC) remains one of the most frequent types of neoplasia and in developing countries is the second most common cause of reported cases, after breast cancer. In Mexico, improvements have been made in defining and perfecting public policies related to this disease and, more importantly, innovative strategies aimed at increasing primary and secondary prevention have been implemented. Beginning in 1974, annual cervical cytology with referral to colposcopy was used for diagnosis and control of CC. In 1994 a histopathological registry was created, in 1996 a cancer information system set up and in 1998 the program transitioned to triennial cytology testing in women with two previous consecutive negative results. In 2007 HPV vaccination began for girls 9–12 years, and the high-risk HPV test (hrHPV) was incorporated as the primary screening test for women 35–64 years. Since 2008, regional molecular biology laboratories for hrHPV test analysis were set up, and 23 out of the 32 states currently have such a laboratory. Extending vaccination programs to include women up to 30 years old (and in some cases up to 45–50 years old) and performing at least one hrHPV test on women ≥30 years old has been proposed. Introduction of an alternative 2-dose HPV vaccination scheme with a periodicity of 6–12 months between doses is recommended for women younger than 15 years old. To improve the results of CC detection programs, it is necessary to: employ appropriate and timely triage alternatives for hrHPV-positive patients, professionalize healthcare personnel and guarantee the quality of program processes, increase screening coverage of the hrHPV test, improve information systems and use a combination of vaccination and screening to accelerate the reduction in the burden of disease associated with CC.

E. Lazcano-Ponce, MD, DrSc (✉) • B. Allen-Leigh, PhD
Centro de Investigación en Salud Poblacional, Instituto Nacional de Salud Pública, Cuernavaca, Morelos, Mexico

L. León-Maldonado, DrPH
CONACYT-Instituto Nacional de Salud Pública, Cuernavaca, and Mexico City, Mexico

J. Salmerón, MD, DrSc
Unidad de Investigación Epidemiológica y en Servicios de Salud, Instituto Mexicano del Seguro Social, Cuernavaca, Morelos, Mexico

M. Hernández Ávila, MD, DrSc
Instituto Nacional de Salud Pública, Cuernavaca, Morelos, and Mexico City, Mexico

J.G. de la Garza-Salazar et al. (eds.), *Cervical Cancer*,
DOI 10.1007/978-3-319-45231-9_6

Keywords cervical cancer • healthcare policy • HPV test • primary screening • HPV vaccination policy • Mexico • middle-income countries

6.1 Introduction

Cervical cancer (CC) is a part of the care plan for addressing central health problems around the world, especially in the least-developed countries. CC remains one of the most frequent neoplasias [1], with half a million new cases diagnosed around the world every year [2]. While in more developed regions, cases of CC may be overshadowed by cases of breast, colorectal, lung, uterine and thyroid cancer, in developing countries, CC remains the second most common cause of reported cases, right after breast cancer. By the year 2012, an adjusted rate of 15.7 cases per 100,000 was estimated for less developed countries, whereas there were 9.9 cases for every 100,000 in developed regions [2].

In all, 16% of cancer cases are attributed to an infectious agent, with a greater proportion of cancer cases attributable to infections occurring in less developed countries (22.9%). The attributable percentage varies according to the region, from 3.3% in Australia to 32.7% in Sub-Saharan Africa. It is worth mentioning that infection with *Helicobacter pylori*, Hepatitis B and C or Human Papilloma Virus (HPV) is responsible for 1.9 million cases of gastric, liver and cervical cancer around the world [3].

CC mortality is a problem that is directly related to poverty and marginalization and that affects the most vulnerable women, who live with greater disadvantages. In Mexico, the highest frequency and mortality rates are found in the southern states (Chiapas, Guerrero and Oaxaca) which present higher levels of poverty and marginalization [4]. The risk of death by CC is three-fold higher in the countryside than in urbanized areas [5].

There is currently an approximately 5% annual reduction in CC mortality rates [6]. Regarding this matter it must be mentioned that in 2006, CC stopped being the leading cause of death as a result of malignant tumors in women. It was displaced at that time by breast cancer [7]. This change can be attributed to a reduction in the birth rate and an increase in the availability of cervical cytological studies [8].

The consolidation of internationally influential research groups in addition to their work and the improvements derived from it have made it possible to offer an organized and integral social response to this problem. Because it involves fields of science and of specialized legislation, the battle against this disease is won through successive approaches that translate into, first, improvements in both diagnosis and treatment, and second, the issuing of laws and standards that contribute to better controlling the problem in terms of regulation.

For those who have closely followed the steps taken by the Mexican government regarding public health, especially over the last four decades, it is evident that although the problem may be far from solved, improvements have been made in defining and perfecting public policies related to this disease and, more importantly, innovative strategies aimed at increasing primary and secondary prevention have been implemented among the population. These will doubtlessly yield a reduction in the number of CC cases in the near future.

A large amount of effort has been made to reduce the disparities that exist within the country and the fact that this disease severely affects more vulnerable populations. Important achievements have been made in broadening coverage and improving the quality of services available to detect and treat CC. However, it is imperative to acknowledge that there remains a need to intensify and complement the actions that have already been taken to control its spread because the persistence of this disease has serious implications for public health. Controlling CC remains an important topic on the public political agenda.

6.2 Review of the Governmental Response in Recent Years

The first steps to promote the early detection of CC were taken at the General Hospital of Mexico by the Health Secretariat (SS) in 1974. Twenty years later, the Official Mexican Normative NOM-014-SSA2–1994 was established [9], in which it was agreed that cervical cytology would be the base diagnostic test for the creation of a CC prevention and control program within the National Health System.

According to this Normative, cytology would be performed on an annual basis, and the women that were diagnosed with an HPV infection would be referred to a colposcopy service. However, it was not yet known at that time that there was no treatment for cases of HPV that did not present lesions and that referring a woman with a morphological image suggesting an HPV infection to a colposcopy clinic would unnecessarily increase expenses, leading to over-diagnoses and a negative psychological impact on the patients.

In 1994, the histopathological register of malignant neoplasms was created by pathologists, hematologists, dermatologists and epidemiologists (this register would later become the cancer histopathological register). In 1996, a system was created to keep records regarding the results of cervical cytology screening activities that comprised the CC prevention and control program, which is now called the Women's cancer information system (SICAM).

Because the evidence indicates that performing a single cytology test every 3 years offers the same benefit as performing an annual test, it was decided in 1998 that triennial tests would be performed on women with two consecutive negative results for dysplasia or cancer. However, patients who tested positive for dysplasia would be subjected to a follow-up in a dysplasia clinic. After being discharged from the clinic, they would resume the triennial schedule of detection tests. At that time, the population selected for screening was women between 25 and 64 years old [10].

In 2007, the Official Mexican Normative NOM-014-SSA2–1994 was modified to improve the prevention, detection, diagnosis, treatment, control and epidemiological surveillance of CC [11]. In this norm, it was explicitly established that there was a need to privilege the detection of this disease in indigenous women and those who reside in rural areas and marginalized urban areas. Similarly, primary and secondary prevention strategies were defined, and both the concept and the practice of counseling were introduced to the healthcare program.

The Weekly Notification System for New Cases is currently part of the System for Research and Epidemiological Surveillance. In this system, the indicators that identify cervical cancer, breast, lung and stomach cancer have been recorded by institutions in the health sector. However, the National System for Health Information gathers the data related to hospital discharges and detection activities, and consultations are granted and tests are performed using this data. Meanwhile the Epidemiological and Statistical Death Record System keeps a record of all deaths that occur in the country and the reason for death. Cancer is naturally among these causes, and also registered are the sex, age group and place of residence of each individual.

6.3 Incorporation of hrHPV as a Primary Test and Its Role as a Milestone in the Fight Against CC

It is worth mentioning that the fight against CC has increased in intensity over the last 10 years. During this same time, a new governmental initiative was issued in support of the 125 municipalities with the lowest human development index. The initiative seeks to eliminate the inequalities that prevent women from attaining access to integral health facilities and proposes the broadening of coverage and improvements in health service conditions as a way to achieve it [12]. The next year, the Health Secretariat, via the National Center for Gender Equality and Reproductive Health, undertook an integral strategy aimed at preventing CC that was called "All women, for each a prevention alternative" [13]. Within the framework of this policy, which was oriented towards improving the quality of life of women living in marginal municipalities, HPV vaccination was recommended for girls between 12 and 16 years of age, and the High-risk HPV test (hrHPV, VPHar is the abbreviation in Spanish) was recommended for women between 35 and 64 years of age. As a result, a total of 82 thousand individuals were vaccinated, and 105 thousand hrHPV tests were performed.

The use of the hrHPV test has been widely recommended as a primary screening method given that its high sensitivity makes it possible for it to identify more cases of grade II or higher intra-epithelial neoplasia (NIC 2+) than a cytological test. It was foreseen that this would result in a reduction in the number of visits to health institutions, which would, in turn, result in an increase in coverage and reliability [14–16].

Several studies have compared the sensitivity and specificity of hrHPV tests to those of cervical cytology [17–20]. The results showed that when detecting NIC 2+ cases, the hrHPV test had higher sensitivity than conventional cytology (96.1% vs. 53.0%). However, the former was also less specific (90.7% vs. 96.3%) [19]. In

Mexico, the sensitivity of the cytological test for detecting histologically confirmed NIC2/3 cases was 40.0%, while that of the hrHPV test was 93.3%. However, the specificity of the cytology assay was 97%, while that of the hrHPV test was 89.2%[20]. These results support the use of the hrHPV test as a primary screening test. This strategy can be used to improve CC prevention programs in places where cervical cytology is inadequate for detecting cancer precursor lesions.

Another advantage of the hrHPV test is that it allows the patient to collect the sample to be analyzed on her own. This is, however, recommended only when there is no qualified technician to take the cervical sample and when there are no risks related to the patient performing the sampling [21]. It is worth noting that the first studies evaluated the acceptability of vaginal self-sampling, the advantages of using this option to eventually overcome the obstacles that complicate the screening process and the suitability of using this alternative for diagnosing women with higher risk [22–24]. These studies found that its greatest advantage is that it offers the possibility of screening women who live in areas with difficult access, marginal regions, or those with other barriers against cervical screening.

Although the hrHPV test may show a clear advantage as a primary test, it is important to keep in mind that a large number of women will have a positive test because HPV infection is relatively common. This is why it is of utmost importance to have alternatives that can be used to identify the women that will require further diagnosis and confirmation, because it will reduce patient anxiety [25] and avoid both unnecessary treatments and expenses for the women with a low risk of progressing to cancer. The use of triage tests, such as the hrHPV genotyping (16/18/45), the use of the E6 protein as a marker of neoplastic progression, the use of cytology to detect morphological changes and the use of immunocytochemistry to detect markers of neoplastic progression, such as p16INK4a/Ki67, could reduce the number of required visits to health institutions, patient expenses and the anxiety that is derived from a positive detection result [26].

This is why it has been recommended that practitioners resort to triage alternatives for women with a positive hrHPV test, including the systematic collection of at least four cervical biopsies and a diagnosis by a group of pathologists. This proposition would not only reduce the number of visits to the physician but would also make the process more efficient and bring down the costs of the program. Furthermore, delaying the initial screening age by 10 years (from 25 to 35 years old) will help to reduce the incidence of this disease in young women [26].

The resources available in the fight against CC increase with time and now include the HPV vaccines, which offer protection against the HPV16 and HPV18 serotypes. Similarly, people who have become infected with these specific serotypes can be protected by these vaccines against other types of HPV and reinfection by the same serotype.

In relation to the recommendations suggesting the formulation of a vaccination policy in Mexico [27], this strategy is part of the primary prevention scheme that has been implemented since 2007 and is aimed at girls between 9 and 12 years of age. Additionally, it includes innovative proposals that could benefit older women.

Bear in mind that using vaccines for primary prevention of CC does not replace screening. On the contrary, the combination of both resources is currently one of the most promising innovations. Additionally, it has been proposed that we extend the vaccination programs to include women up to 30 years old (and in some cases up to 45–50 years old) and that we perform at least one hrHPV test on individuals who are ≥30 years old. This promising proposal, which includes a combination of resources, will extend the use of HPV vaccines and widen the use of the hrHPV test in detection programs and could thereby accelerate the reduction of CC incidence [28].

Because encouraging results have been found for combinations including both vaccination and detection methods, it is widely recommended that we broaden the screening intervals in favor of programs with a more effective cost-benefit ratio, to offer a better quality of life to women, and to reduce the burden of this disease on society as a whole. Within the framework of the recommended strategy for countries where there is a high incidence of CC, our country is currently undertaking efforts to evaluate the benefits of using a combined strategy including both vaccination and screening in women between 25 and 45 years old [29]. This has already set in motion detection programs that use the hrHPV test.

Regarding the availability of resources, a related point to consider is that since 2008, regional molecular biology laboratories have been opened in several states, and those in Puebla, Veracruz, Campeche, Guerrero and Michoacan were the first that had the means to perform the hrHPV tests. According to the most recent reports of the Health Secretary, 23 out of the 32 Mexican federal states already have a molecular biology laboratory, and there is also a reference center at the National Institute of Public Health.

6.4 Incorporation of the Vaccine Against HPV

An HPV vaccine was approved for commercial use in Mexico for the first time in 2006. Currently, 80 countries have integrated these vaccines into their national vaccination programs, and 37 more have evaluation and/or regional programs to facilitate its introduction [30].

There are three HPV vaccines today. One of them is bivalent, and this vaccine offers protection against the HPV16 and 18 serotypes. It has an AS04 adjuvant system that consists of 0.5 mg $Al3+$ hydrated aluminum hydroxide and 50 μg of 3-O-deacyl-4′-monophosphoryl lipid A (MPL) and is approved for use in women from 9 and older. In addition, a tetravalent vaccine also exists, with markers for HPV L1 virus-like particle (VLP) protection for types 6, 11, 16 and 18. This contains an adjuvant that contains 225 μg of amorphous aluminum hydroxyphosphate sulfate and has been approved for women from 9 to 45 years old. The use of this vaccine has also been approved in men from 9 to 26 years old [31].

The reported efficiency of this vaccine against the HPV6, 11, 16 and 18 serotypes in cases with a grade 2 or higher cervical intraepithelial neoplasia (NIC2+) is estimated to be 100% according to the FUTURE 1 and 2 studies, which were performed on women and men between 16 and 26 years of age (95%CI 94–100) [32]. Additionally, in the sentinel cohort of Nordic countries, no NIC2+ cases have been associated with the previously mentioned serotypes [33, 34].

From a population-based point of view, the experience of Australia in 2007 with the introduction of the tetravalent vaccine, which has a coverage of about 70% in women younger than 26 years old, is a good example of the impact of this type of intervention. The sentinel event used to evaluate the effect of the vaccine was the prevalence of genital warts in a Center for Sexual Transmitted Diseases in Sydney and Melbourne. The effect of the vaccine against HPV was observed in both vaccinated women and in unvaccinated heterosexual men in the same age group. These results indicate that there is a "herd effect" in heterosexual men between 21 and 32 years of age that was not observed in homosexual men [35]. Regarding the bivalent vaccine, high efficiency was also reported for its ability to prevent HPV16 and 18 NIC2+ in women between 15 and 25 years old [36].

Additionally, women older than 25 years old are vulnerable to a new HPV infection and could therefore be vaccinated. Today, novel proposals are being considered to expand the HPV vaccination age range. It has been proposed that we vaccinate women between 25 and 45 years of age, which would provide protection to women who are not infected and protect already infected women from future reinfections [29].

Population-wide HPV vaccination programs have been recently modified at an international level. The main change consists of the introduction of an alternative 2-dose vaccination scheme with a periodicity of 6 months between doses in women younger than 15 years old. The available evidence suggests that the effect of two doses on girls between 9 and 14 years old is not less in terms of immunogenicity than the effect achieved with three doses at approximately 18–24 years of age [37]. These immunogenicity studies have also established that the size of the immune response is inversely proportional to the age at which the vaccine was first given, that giving two doses is recommended only in groups between 9 and 14 years of age and that the shortest interval between two doses should be 6 months, whereas the longest should be 12 months. This modification of the HPV vaccination scheme provides advantages, from a public health perspective. In particular, it reduces costs, provides operational benefits when there is a flexible interval between the doses (from 6 to 12 months) and allows for an increase in vaccination coverage in people older than 15 years old.

Concerning the initial schemes used with the first generation of vaccines against HPV, the Advisory Committee on Immunization Practices (ACIP) of the United States recommended using a nonavalent vaccine to continue with or complete any schemes that were initiated using any other HPV vaccine. However, it does not recommend the application of additional vaccines to already completed schemes [38]. In terms of safety, the percentage is very similar to that reported previously for the first HPV vaccines [38].

As a side note, there is a new recommendation in the 2016 ACIP (Advisory Committee on Immunization Practices) guidelines, which advises vaccinating boys and girls approximately 9 years of age when there is a history of sexual abuse because it has been shown that there is a higher risk of HPV infection in these individuals [39]. Similarly, the Centers for Disease Control and Prevention (CDC) of the United States recommends HPV vaccination in immunosuppressed and HIV-infected women in addition to homosexual men [40].

6.5 Final Considerations

To improve the results of CC detection programs, it is necessary to identify and orchestrate triage alternatives that can improve the optimal handling of hrHPV-positive patients, professionalize the personnel who work in the screening programs, guarantee the quality of all steps that are involved and above all, establish mechanisms that make it possible to maintain follow-up of patients to guarantee their correct diagnosis.

According to the national health surveys, the preventive program coverage, which is evaluated in relation to a patient's cytological history over the previous 12 months, increased from 27.4% to 36.1% between the years 2000 and 2005 and from 36.1% to 42.8% between 2006 and 2012, when the survey was performed [41, 42].

Increasing the coverage of the hrHPV test will be an important challenge for the program in the coming years because it represents an opportunity for early detection, which translates into saved lives, the better use of resources and the availability of infrastructure to perform these tests across the country.

Information systems are fundamental to following up on the results of changes in public policies related to health. These instruments are currently facing basic problems: a lack of articulation at all levels of care can result in the numbers not matching or make it impossible to cross-reference information to increase our understanding of the problem, and a lack of access to all of the data that is collected in private medical institutions. As a consequence, we can achieve only a partial view of the problem, to the detriment of the program and the assignment of resources to attend to them.

After 10 years of intensifying the fight against CC, the greatest challenge has been recognition of this issue as a universal problem in which we consider new triage alternatives that will permit the identification of patients that require the confirmation of a positive diagnosis and timely handling of these tests. It is also recommended that the health system assume the challenge of broadening the coverage of preventive measures to facilitate the control of CC. These should use a combination of vaccination and screening to accelerate the reduction in this disease's burden.

These data indicate that it is critical that we consider governmental investment to address CC and that we prioritize related campaigns and preventive activities, such as vaccination and timely detection. This is because in the absence of the former, it is necessary to care for patients with CC when they reach advanced stages, which are associated with a much higher social cost.

References

1. World Health Organization. Media centre [on line]: Cancer Fact sheet N°297: 2015 (consulted march 17th 2016) http://www.who.int/mediacentre/factsheets/fs297/en/.
2. International Agency for Research on Cancer. World Health Organization. Cancer. GLOBOCAN 2012: Estimated cancer incidence, mortality and prevalence worldwide in 2012 (consulted march 17th 2016) http://globocan.iarc.fr/Pages/fact_sheets_population.aspx.
3. de Martel C, Ferlay J, Franceschi S, Vignat J, Bray F, Forman D, Plummer M. Global burden of cancers attributable to infections in 2008: a review and synthetic analysis. Lancet Oncol. 2012;13(6):607–15.
4. Secretaría de Salud. Dirección General de Información en Salud. Bases de datos estándar. Defunciones Generales 2014 [on line]: Sistema Nacional de Información en Salud (SINAIS). México: SSA (consulted january 22th 2016) http://www.dgis.salud.gob.mx/contenidos/basesdedatos/std_defunciones.html
5. Palacio-Mejía LS, Rangel-Gómez G, Hernández-Avila M, Lazcano-Ponce E. Cervical cancer, a disease of poverty: mortality differences between urban and rural areas in Mexico. Salud Pública Méx. 2003;45(Suppl 3):S315–25.
6. Torres-Sánchez LE, Rojas-Martínez R, Escamilla-Núñez C, de la Vara-Salazar E, Lazcano-Ponce E. Cancer mortality trends in Mexico, 1980-2011. Salud Pública Méx. 2014;56(5):473–91.
7. Palacio-Mejía LS, Lazcano-Ponce E, Allen-Leigh B, Hernández-Ávila M. Regional differences in breast and cervical cancer mortality in Mexico between 1979-2006. Salud Púb Méx. 2009;5(Suppl 2):s208–19.
8. Lazcano-Ponce E, Palacio-Mejía LS, Allen-Leigh B, Yunes-Diaz E, Alonso P, Schiavon R, Hernández-Avila M. Decreasing cervical cancer mortality in México: effect of Papanicolaou coverage, birthrate, and the importance of diagnostic validity of cytology. Cancer Epidemiol Biomark Prev. 2008;17(10):2808–17.
9. Norma Oficial Mexicana NOM-014-SSA2–1994, para la Prevención, Tratamiento y Control de Cáncer del Cuello del Útero y de la Mama en la Atención Primaria. (publicada originalmente en el Diario Oficial de la Federación el 26 de abril de 1994). Disponible en: http://www.salud.gob.mx/unidades/cdi/nom/014ssa24.html.
10. Secretaría de Salud. Modificación a la Norma Oficial Mexicana NOM-014-SSA2–1994, para la Prevención, Detección, Diagnóstico, Tratamiento, Control y Vigilancia Epidemiológica del Cáncer Cérvico Uterino. (1998). http://www.salud.gob.mx/unidades/cdi/nom/m014ssa24.html.
11. Secretaría de Salud. Modificación a la Norma Oficial Mexicana NOM-014-SSA2–1994, para la Prevención, Detección, Diagnóstico, Tratamiento, Control y Vigilancia Epidemiológica del Cáncer Cérvico Uterino. (2007). Disponible en: http://www.salud.gob.mx/unidades/cdi/nom/m014ssa294.pdf.
12. Instituto Nacional de las Mujeres. Respuestas al Cuestionario enviado a los gobiernos por la División para el Adelanto de la Mujer de las Naciones Unidas sobre la aplicación de la Plataforma de Acción de Beijing (1995) y los resultados del vigésimo tercer periodo extraordinario de sesiones de la Asamblea General (2000). México: INMUJERES, abril 2009. p. 9.
13. Informe de México sobre el cumplimiento del consenso de Quito. Comisión Económica para América Latina y El Caribe (CEPAL). XI Conferencia Regional sobre la Mujer de América Latina y el Caribe, Brasilia, Brasil, 13 a 16 de julio de 2010.
14. Flores Y, Bishai D, Lazcano E, Shah K, Lörincz A, Hernández M, Salmerón J. Improving cervical cancer screening in Mexico: results from the Morelos HPV Study. Salud Pública Méx. 2003;45(Suppl 3):S388–98.
15. Flores YN, Bishai DM, Lorincz A, Shah KV, Lazcano-Ponce E, Hernández M, Granados-García V, Pérez R, Salmerón J. HPV testing for cervical cancer screening appears more cost-effective than Papanicolaou cytology in Mexico. Cancer Causes Control. 2011;22(2):261–72.

16. Beal CM, Salmerón J, Flores YN, Torres L, Granados-García V, Dugan E, Lazcano-Ponce E. Cost analysis of different cervical cancer screening strategies in Mexico. Salud Pública Méx. 2014;56(5):429–501.
17. Franco EL. Chapter 13: primary screening of cervical cancer with human papillomavirus tests. J Natl Cancer Inst Monogr. 2003;31:89–96.
18. Lörincz AT. Screening for cervical cancer: new alternatives and research. Salud Pública Méx. 2003;45(Suppl 3):S376–87.
19. Cuzick J, Clavel C, Petry KU, Meijer CJ, Hoyer H, Ratnam S, Szarewski A, Birembaut P, Kulasingam S, Sasieni P, Iftner T. Overview of the European and North American studies on HPV testing in primary cervical cancer screening. Int J Cancer. 2006;119(5):1095–101.
20. Lazcano-Ponce E, Lörincz AT, Salmerón J, Fernández I, Cruz A, Hernández P, Mejia I, Hernández-Avila M. A pilot study of HPV DNA and cytology testing in 50,159 women in the routine Mexican Social Security Program. Cancer Causes Control. 2010;21(10):1693–700.
21. Salmerón J, Lazcano-Ponce E, Lörincz A, Hernández M, Hernández P, Leyva A, Uribe M, Manzanares H, Antunez A, Carmona E, Ronnett BM, Sherman ME, Bishai D, Ferris D, Flores Y, Yunes E, Shah KV. Comparison of HPV-based assays with Papanicolaou smears for cervical cancer screening in Morelos State. Mexico Cancer Causes Control. 2003;14(6):505–12.
22. Dzuba IG, Díaz EY, Allen B, Leonard YF, Lazcano Ponce EC, Shah KV, Bishai D, Lorincz A, Ferris D, Turnbull B, Hernández Avila M, Salmerón J. The acceptability of self-collected samples for HPV testing vs. the pap test as alternatives in cervical cancer screening. J Women's Health Gend Based Med. 2002;11(3):265–75.
23. Gravitt PE, Belinson JL, Salmerón J, Shah KV. Looking ahead: a case for human papillomavirus testing of self-sampled vaginal specimens as a cervical cancer screening strategy. Int J Cancer. 2011;129(3):517–27.
24. Lazcano-Ponce E, Lörincz AT, Torres L, Salmerón J, Cruz A, Rojas R, Hernández P, Hernández M. Specimen self-collection and HPV DNA screening in a pilot study of 100,242 women. Int J Cancer. 2014;135(1):109–16.
25. León-Maldonado L, Allen-Leigh B, Lazcano-Ponce E. Counseling for HPV detection when used to screen for cervical cancer: a qualitative study on the needs of women from Michoacán, México. Salud Pública Méx. 2014;56(5):519–27.
26. Torres-Ibarra L, Lazcano-Ponce E, Franco EL, Cuzick J, Hernández M, Lorincz A, Rivera B, Ramírez P, Mendiola-Pastrana I, Rudolph SE, León-Maldonado L, Hernández R, Barrios E, Gravitt P, Moscicki AB, Schmeler KM, Flores YN, Méndez-Hernández P, Salmerón J, FRIDA Study Group. Triage strategies in cervical cancer detection in Mexico: methods of the FRIDA Study. Salud Pública Méx. 2016;58:197–210.
27. Lazcano-Ponce E, Salmerón-Castro J, García-Carrancá A, Aranda-Flores C, Madrid-Marina V, Gómez-Altamirano CM, Martínez-Montañez OG. Recommendations for the definition of a policy on vaccination against papillomavirus in Mexico. Strategic Advisory Group of Experts of the World Health Organization. Salud Pública Méx. 2009;51(4):336–41.
28. Bosch FX, Robles C, Díaz M, Arbyn M, Baussano I, Clavel C, Ronco G, Dillner J, Lehtinen M, Petry KU, Poljak M, Kjaer SK, Meijer CJ, Garland SM, Salmerón J, Castellsagué X, Bruni L, de Sanjosé S, Cuzick J. HPV-FASTER: broadening the scope for prevention of HPV-related cancer. Nat Rev Clin Oncol. 2016;13(2):119–32.
29. Salmerón J, Torres-Ibarra L, Bosch FX, Cuzick J, Lörincz A, Wheeler CM, Castle PE, Robles C, Lazcano-Ponce E. HPV vaccination impact on a cervical cancer screening program: methods of the FASTER-Tlalpan Study in Mexico. Salud Pública Méx. 2016;58:211–9.
30. Cervical Cancer Action. A global coalition to STOP carvical cancer [on line]: cervical cancer action (consulted on march 17th 2016) http://www.cervicalcanceraction.org/.
31. Joura EA, Giuliano AR, Iversen OE, Bouchard C, Mao C, Mehlsen J, Moreira Jr ED, Ngan Y, Petersen LK, Lazcano-Ponce E, Pitisuttithum P, Restrepo JA, Stuart G, Woelber L, Yang YC, Cuzick J, Garland SM, Huh W, Kjaer SK, Bautista OM, Chan IS, Chen J, Gesser R, Moeller E, Ritter M, Vuocolo S, Luxembourg A, Broad Spectrum HPV Vaccine Study. A 9-valent HPV vaccine against infection and intraepithelial neoplasia in women. N Engl J Med. 2015;372(8):711–23.

32. Kjaer SK, Sigurdsson K, Iversen OE, Hernandez-Avila M, Wheeler CM, Perez G, Brown DR, Koutsky LA, Tay EH, García P, Ault KA, Garland SM, Leodolter S, Olsson SE, Tang GW, Ferris DG, Paavonen J, Lehtinen M, Steben M, Bosch FX, Dillner J, Joura EA, Majewski S, Muñoz N, Myers ER, Villa LL, Taddeo FJ, Roberts C, Tadesse A, Bryan J, Maansson R, Lu S, Vuocolo S, Hesley TM, Saah A, Barr E, Haupt RM. A pooled analysis of continued prophylactic efficacy of quadrivalent human papillomavirus (Types 6/11/16/18) vaccine against high-grade cervical and external genital lesions. Cancer Prev Res (Phila). 2009;2(10):868–78.
33. Nygård M, Saah A, Munk C, Tryggvadottir L, Enerly E, Hortlund M, Sigurdardottir LG, Vuocolo S, Kjaer SK, Dillner J. Evaluation of the long-term anti-human papillomavirus 6 (HPV6), 11, 16, and 18 immune responses generated by the quadrivalent HPV vaccine. Clin Vaccine Immunol. 2015;22(8):943–8.
34. FUTURE II Study Group. Quadrivalent vaccine against human papillomavirus to prevent high-grade cervical lesions. N Engl J Med. 2007;356(19):1915–1927.
35. Chow EP, Read TR, Wigan R, Donovan B, Chen MY, Bradshaw CS, Fairley CK. Ongoing decline in genital warts among young heterosexuals 7 years after the Australian human papillomavirus (HPV) vaccination programme. Sex Transm Infect. 2015;91(3):214–9.
36. Skinner SR, Apter D, De Carvalho N, Harper DM, Konno R, Paavonen J, Romanowski B, Roteli-Martins C, Burlet N, Mihalyi A, Struyf F. Human papillomavirus (HPV)-16/18 AS04-adjuvanted vaccine for the prevention of cervical cancer and HPV-related diseases. Expert Rev Vaccines. 2016;15(3):367–87.
37. Lazcano-Ponce E, Stanley M, Muñoz N, Torres L, Cruz-Valdez A, Salmerón J, Rojas R, Herrero R, Hernández-Ávila M. Overcoming barriers to HPV vaccination: non-inferiority of antibody response to human papillomavirus 16/18 vaccine in adolescents vaccinated with a two-dose vs. a three-dose schedule at 21 months. Vaccine. 2014;32(6):725–32.
38. Supplemental information and guidance for vaccination providers regarding use of 9-valent HPV vaccine. Advisory Committee on Immunization Practices Recommended Immunization Schedules. Centers for Disease Control and Prevention. July, 2015. http://www.cdc.gov/hpv/downloads/9vhpv-guidance.pdf.
39. Advisory Committee on Immunization Practices Recommended Immunization Schedules for Persons Aged 0 Through 18 Years — United States, 2016. Centers for Disease Control and Prevention. MMWR, Early Release/Vol.65. February 2, 2016. http://www.cdc.gov/mmwr/volumes/65/wr/pdfs/mm6504a4er.pdf.
40. Centers for Disease Control and Prevention (CDC). Content source: National Center for Immunization and Respiratory Diseases [en línea]: vaccines that might be indicated for adults aged 19 years or older based on medical and other indications (consulted on march 17th 2016) http://www.cdc.gov/vaccines/schedules/hcp/imz/adult-conditions-shell.html.
41. Encuesta Nacional de Salud y Nutrición 2006. Resultados Nacionales. Segunda Edición, 2006. Instituto Nacional de Salud Pública.
42. Encuesta Nacional de Salud y Nutrición 2012. Resultados Nacionales. Segunda Edición, 2013e. Instituto Nacional de Salud Pública.

Chapter 7
Cervical Cancer Cytology and Pathology

José G. Chanona Vilchis, Mónica Lizzette Serrano Arévalo, Lidia Faridi Villegas González, and Ana María Cano Valdez

Abstract In the first part of the present chapter, we will review each one of the sections that constitute the Bethesda system for the interpretation of cervical/vaginal cytology, including recommendations for a proper cytologic report. Furthermore, the main cytologic criteria used in the diagnosis of squamous and glandular invasive cervical neoplasia precursor lesions are included. In the final part of the cytology section, some advantages and drawbacks of liquid-based cytology are discussed. In the second part of the chapter, the main histopathological aspects of the squamous and glandular cervical neoplasias are discussed. We begin with in situ epidermoid carcinoma, followed by microinvasive epidermoid carcinoma, and then present various histologic subtypes of epidermoid invasive carcinoma. Among glandular neoplasias, in situ adenocarcinoma, early adenocarcinoma, and some subtypes of invasive adenocarcinoma will be reviewed. Adenosquamous carcinoma and neuroendocrine cervix neoplasias are also included in the present chapter.

Keywords Bethesda System • Squamous lesion • Low-grade squamous intraepithelial lesion (LSIL) • High-grade squamous intraepithelial lesion (HSIL) • Cervical intraepithelial neoplasia (CIN) • Epidermoid carcinoma • Endocervical adenocarcinoma • Neuroendocrine carcinoma

J.G. Chanona Vilchis (✉) • A.M. Cano Valdez
Department of Pathology, Instituto Nacional de Cancerología-México, Av. San Fernando No 22, Col. Sección XVI, Tlalpan, Mexico City, Mexico, 14080
e-mail: chabapat@gmail.com

M.L. Serrano Arévalo • L.F. Villegas González
Department of Cytopathology, Instituto Nacional de Cancerología-México, Mexico City, Mexico

J.G. de la Garza-Salazar et al. (eds.), *Cervical Cancer*,
DOI 10.1007/978-3-319-45231-9_7

7.1 Cytology and Cervical Cancer

Cervico-vaginal cytology is an accessible, simple, sensitive, and specific test. In Mexico, the cervical cancer detection program was implemented in 1974, with the aim of detecting precursor lesions, as well as decreasing the number of invasive carcinomas [1].

The sensitivity of this test is very high (90–95%), although its specificity is low (50–75%) given the great percentage of false-negative results. Such results are caused by inadequate sampling, processing and interpretation. Poor-quality sample acquisition is due to the lack of sample transformation area, poor extension technique, and improper sample fixation or processing. Errors in interpretation are due to deficient tracking and a lack of personnel training. Quality sampling is crucial to eliminate false-negative and false-positive diagnoses and is therefore the most important factor in improving the sensitivity of cytologic testing [2].

Cervical cytology sampling must be performed when active sexual life starts and then every 2 years; as long as the results are negative, testing should then be performed every 3 years until the patient turns 65 years old.

7.1.1 Cytology Report and the Bethesda System

Since it began in the 1940s, the cervical cytology report has been evolving, from the Papanicolaou classification up to the current day Bethesda system in 1988, when a group of professionals gathered for the first time with the goal of developing a system to report Papanicolaou results, which would report the cytologic interpretation to the gynecologist in a clear, relevant mode.

The Bethesda system has two main objectives: to specify the sample quality and build a unified system to inform or interpret cytologic data in the context of clinical findings and to provide an efficient and clear communication to the physician [3].

The system has three sections: the first is the **sample quality** (satisfactory or unsatisfactory for evaluation); the second is the **general classification**, where the existence of anomalies in epithelial (squamous or glandular) cells is reported; and the third corresponds to the **results** or **interpretation** section, which specifies whether there is a diagnosis of an intraepithelial lesion or malignancy, be it squamous or glandular (in this section, we can include the presence of microorganisms or other non-neoplastic findings), as well as other neoplasias, such as metastasis or lymphomas [3].

(a) **Sample quality.** This depends on various factors, such as adequate cellularity; for conventional cytology, a minimum of 8000–12,000 cells from the squamous epithelium are required; for liquid-based cytology, the minimum is 5000 cells. Another important factor is the presence of cells from the transformation zone; these are the endocervical and metaplasia cells, and a minimum of 10 properly conserved cells is acceptable, isolated or in groups. Two situations that impair proper sample evaluation are when more than 75% of the squamous cells are not clearly visible (thick smear) or when the smear has more than 75% hemorrhage, inflammation or necrosis, which impairs squamous cell evaluation.

(b) **General classification.** When there are no signs of neoplasia, the term "**negative for intraepithelial lesion or malignancy**" is used; this classification includes observations concerning microorganisms, radiotherapy-induced changes, atrophy, DIU (Dispositive intra-uterine)-induced changes, and unspecific inflammation; when a lesion or atypia is observed in the squamous epithelium, either associated with atypia of undetermined significance or even to epidermoid carcinoma, the term "**squamous cell abnormalities**" is used; when there is a lesion or atypia in the glandular epithelium, the term "**glandular cells anomalies**" is used; this includes glandular cell atypia (endocervical, endometrial, or unspecific) up to adenocarcinoma.

(c) **Results or interpretation.** In this section, we briefly describe intraepithelial lesions and malignancy diagnosis, as well as their clinical significance and recommended management according to the last review of the Bethesda system and the last consensus of the American Society of Colposcopy and Cervical Pathology (ASCCP) [3].

7.1.2 Squamous Epithelial Lesions

Atypical Squamous Cells of Undetermined Significance (ASC-US) This represents cytological changes suggestive of an intraepithelial lesion that are qualitatively and quantitatively insufficient to diagnose a low-grade squamous intraepithelial lesion. The 5-year risk of developing a high-grade squamous intraepithelial lesion and cancer with an ASC-US in addition to a positive molecular HPV test is 1.1%; for ASC-US with a positive HPV study, it increases to 18%. The suggested initial management consists of performing a molecular HPV test; if the results are negative, it is recommended to repeat the test and make a co-test (HPV test and cytology); if the test yields positive HPV results, it is recommended to perform a colposcopy [3, 4].

Atypical squamous cells, for which it is not possible to rule out a high-grade intraepithelial lesion (ASC-H) A lesion is observed in immature squamous cells: the cells are usually scarce, and they can show various patterns, including cells with atypical metaplasia, 3D cell clumps, marked atypical repair, severe atrophy, and post-radiotherapy changes suggestive of recurrence. The 5-year risk of a high-grade intraepithelial lesion and cancer, with an ASC-H diagnosis and a negative HPV test, is 12%; for an ASC-H with a positive HPV test, the risk increases to 45%. The suggested management for women with an ASC-H diagnosis is colposcopy regardless of the HPV test results. It is not recommended to perform a molecular HPV test once the ASC-H cytologic diagnosis is performed. There are guides specific for special populations established in the last consensus of the ASCCP [3, 4].

Low-grade squamous intraepithelial lesion (LSIL) This represents changes in mature squamous cells (superficial or intermediate) associated with HPV, and the morphological changes are equivalent to mild dysplasia or low-grade intraepithelial lesion (NIC1) (Fig. 7.1). The 5-year risk of a high-grade intraepithelial lesion or cancer is 18%, similar to ASC-US with positive HPV results. The suggested management is as follows: women without an HPV study must have cytology testing within 12 months; for women with a positive HPV test, colposcopy is recommended; women older than 25 years must be followed-up with cytology testing within 12 months [3, 5].

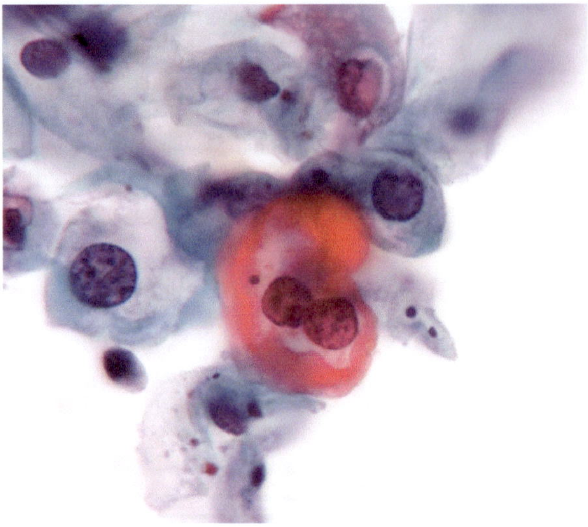

Fig. 7.1 Low-grade intraepithelial lesion (NIC1)

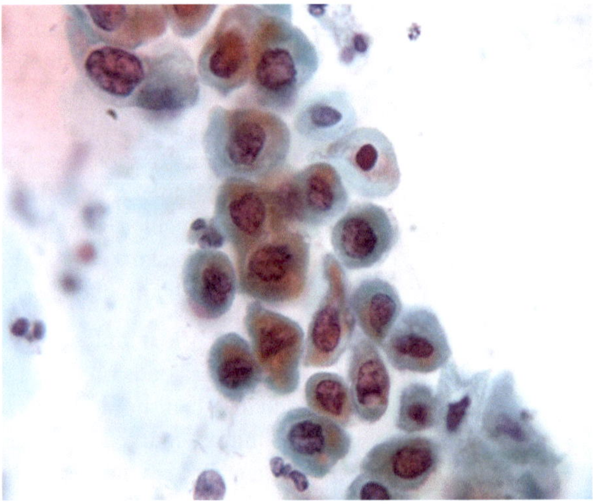

Fig. 7.2 Immature cells (para-basal)

High-grade squamous intraepithelial lesion (HSIL) This represents changes in the smallest squamous, immature cells (para-basal) whose main feature is the loss of the nucleus/cytoplasm ratio (Fig. 7.2). An HSIL diagnosis in cytology includes NIC2, NIC3, and in situ carcinoma in the histological section. Most of the patients diagnosed with HSIL have an NIC2 or NIC3 biopsy. The suggested management for women older than 25 years is colposcopy with an excisional procedure (cone), if the lesion is identified; however, if the high-grade intraepithelial lesion is not confirmed by biopsy, the recommendation is to perform a revision of the cytology and histological material, with an additional immunohistochemical analysis to assess p16 [3, 6].

Squamous cell carcinoma This term refers to an epithelial invasive tumor composed of squamous cells of distinct differentiation degrees. The Bethesda system does not subdivide squamous cell carcinoma similar to the World Health Organization

(WHO) classification: keratinizing, non-keratinizing, papillary, basaloid, warty, squamo-transitional, and lympho-epithelial. This is because the morphological characteristics are not clearly distinguishable using the cytology results [3].

Glandular cell alterations: it is important to consider that cytology primarily detects lesions in the flat epithelium, and it does not detect glandular lesions; given the scarce frequency of the latter and low sensitivity, errors in sampling and the interpretation of results [3].

7.1.2.1 Glandular Epithelium Lesions

Atypical glandular cells (AHCs) This term refers to alterations in the glandular epithelium beyond reactive changes but insufficient to categorize them as adenocarcinoma. The morphological entities that suggest this diagnosis can be benign or malignant: the benign conditions include endocervical and endometrial polyps, endometriosis, endocervical microcystic hyperplasia, adenosis, energetic and lower uterine segment brushings, tubal metaplasia, and Arias-Stella phenomenon; the malignant conditions include high-grade intraepithelial lesions with glandular penetration in situ adenocarcinoma and invasive adenocarcinoma [3].

The Bethesda system subdivides these results as follows:

(a) Atypical endocervical cells (unspecified, NOS)
(b) Atypical endometrial cells (unspecified, NOS)
(c) Atypical glandular cells (unspecified, NOS)
(d) Atypical endocervical cells (favors neoplasia)
(e) Atypical glandular cells (favors neoplasia)

As discussed in the previous paragraph, the Bethesda system categorizes glandular cells according to their site of origin whenever possible because the clinical follow-up and management vary depending on the cell type; however, on several occasions, it is impossible to determine the cells' origin. This is why the term "atypical glandular cells" (AGCs) is more pervasively used in cytology [3].

The 5-year risk of a high-grade intraepithelial lesion after an AGC diagnosis is 10–40%; this seems paradoxical because a high-grade squamous intraepithelial lesion is frequently extended to glandular endocervical spaces, replacing them to such an extent that the smear gives the appearance of a lesion in the glandular epithelium. This is a context in which the cells characteristic of a high-grade lesion are not present in the rest of the smear; based on this, it is the pathologist's or cytopathologist's duty to place a note specifying the probable nature of the lesion to guide the gynecologist. With the AGC diagnosis and a negative HPV molecular test, the risk is 0.09%; however, with an AGC with a positive molecular HPV test, the risk of a high-grade lesion in the squamous epithelium increases to 33% [3, 6].

In situ endocervical adenocarcinoma (IEA) It refers to a high-grade glandular endocervical noninvasive lesion. This cytological interpretation is highly difficult, even for the most experienced cytopthologists, explaining why the "atypical endocervical cells, promotes neoplasia" interpretation is justified. The coexistence of a squamous and a glandular lesion in the cervix must always be considered when an in situ endocervical adenocarcinoma is interpreted. More than half of IEAs frequently have an intraepithelial squamous lesion. According to the ASCCP, the initial management includes colposcopy and endocervical curettage. HPV detection tests are not recommended because they can yield negative results [3].

Adenocarcinoma An adenocarcinoma diagnosis, either endocervical or endometrial, must be given when the following cytologic criteria are observed: tumoral diathesis, hemorrhagic background, abnormal glandular cells with the presence of macronuclei and architectural atypia. Additionally, because cellular morphology can be difficult to interpret, the cytological classification of morphological variants is discouraged because it is poorly reproducible, especially in extrauterine-originated adenocarcinomas, where the clinical correlation is crucial. Patient management depends on the clinical stage [3].

7.1.3 Liquid-Based Cytology and Molecular Biology Studies

In 1996, the FDA approved the first commercial brand of a liquid-based screening method. In this test, the cervical-vaginal specimen collected is placed in a vial with preserving liquid; then, in an automated processing machine, it is spread apart, collected, and transferred to a slide to be stained and microscopically evaluated. The cytomorphologic characteristics of the liquid-based cytology are different from those observed in conventional cytology; consequently, the cells develop dyscohesion, decreased size, a loss of the pattern in which they are arranged, and a lack the inflammatory, hematic, and necrotic background in which they are located [7].

Scientific evidence has been found both in favor and against the use of liquid-based cytology in the detection of precursor lesions and to decrease the incidence of inadequate samples. This has prompted some developed countries to completely substitute the conventional smear, whereas others have maintained the conventional cytology because the high cost of the liquid-based method is considered to be unjustified [8, 9].

In liquid-based samples, it is possible to perform complementary tests, such as the detection of HPV DNA and immunocytochemistry for the specific detection of p16, among others [10]. Currently, it is an acceptable strategy to simultaneously perform cytology and HPV DNA test as a screening method and as a post-treatment follow-up because performing both tests together has shown greater sensitivity and specificity than using them separately. In 2004, the FDA approved the use of HPV detection tests as a screening tool and guide for patient management; the aim of HPV detection is not the detection of all virus genotypes but of the high risk-associated genotypes either through the hybrid capture assay or using PCR (polymerase chain reaction). In 2014, the FDA approved the co-test, i.e., performing the cytologic evaluation along with the collection of a sample for the molecular test at the same time as the screening [4, 10].

7.2 Pathology of Cervical Cancer

7.2.1 Squamous Intraepithelial Lesions

They are defined as "Alterations in the squamous epithelium in the cervix transformation zone, which are induced by HPV infection". Morphologically, they are characterized by maturation anomalies and nuclear anomalies. The first description was published in 1888 by Sir John Williams. Subsequently, the concept of in situ carcinoma (ISC) was defined, and lesions with abnormal characteristics that did not comply with ISC criteria were identified. From the 1950s, some confusing and imprecise terms were coined to refer to these lesions, such as "anaplasia" and "basal cell hyperplasia". In 1952, Reagan and Hicks introduced the term "atypical hyperplasia" for cervical lesions with a higher differentiation grade than ISC but a lower risk of developing invasive carcinoma. Shortly thereafter, it was replaced by "dysplasia", which was stratified as follows: mild, moderate, and severe. In 1956, Koss and Durfee described koilocytes, noting similarities to Reagan's description of mild dysplasia. In 1976, Meisels and Fortin observed an association between these changes and HPV infection. In 1969, Richart proposed that cervical carcinogenesis comprised a spectrum that went from mild dysplasia to carcinoma and introduced the term "*Cervical Intraepithelial Neoplasia*" (CIN) to emphasize the role of these lesions as cancer precursors. In 1975, the WHO proposed the terminology unification and, soon after, the International Society of Gynecological Pathologists (ISGYP) replaced the term "dysplasia" with "Cervical Intraepithelial Neoplasia" (CIN). According to the epithelial thickness or affected strata, mild dysplasia corresponds to CIN-I, moderate dysplasia to CIN-II, and severe dysplasia to CIN-III/ISC [11, 12].

Towards the end of the 1980s, our knowledge of the biology and oncogenic mechanisms of HPV increased as the subjectivity in the distinction between CIN 2 and CIN 3 became apparent. Currently, the WHO recommends the use of a two-grade nomenclature (low grade and high grade) based on the Bethesda System because it is more reproducible and more biologically relevant [13].

Low-grade squamous intraepithelial lesions (LSILs) These are considered the clinical and morphologic manifestations of a productive HPV infection, characterized by basal or parabasal-like cell proliferation that does not occupy more than one-third of the epithelium thickness. Non-atypical mitoses can be observed in the same zone. Maturation exists in the rest of the epithelium, although with an increase in nuclear size and occasionally binucleation. Additionally, viral cytopathic effects can be observed, characterized by hyperchromasia and nuclear outline irregularity, in addition to the presence of a vacuole or perinuclear halo. In superficial stratum cells, parakeratosis or hyperkeratosis can be observed.

Although most LSIL cases are related to high-risk HPV types, infected cells are generally euploid or polyploid.

LSIL patients have a favorable prognosis because many of them present regression within the next 12 months. The risk of progression is related to HPV 16 infection, advanced age, immunosuppression, and tobacco consumption. Currently, there are no biomarkers to predict persistence, progression, or regression in these lesions.

High-grade squamous intraepithelial lesions (HSILs) They are defined as intraepithelial lesions that bear a significant risk of developing invasive carcinoma if left untreated. They are associated with high-risk HPV infection and tend to occur in a more advanced age group than LSILs, but earlier in life than invasive carcinoma, showing an incidence peak between 35 and 39 years. They predominantly localize to the transformation zone and are microscopically characterized by the proliferation of squamous cells with a lower differentiation than those observed in LSIL. Such cells have hyperchromatic nuclei with an irregular outline, and nucleoli are rarely observed. These alterations extend up to the middle or superficial third of the epithelium. Mitoses are more frequent and can be observed in the outermost strata (Fig. 7.3). Some morphologic variants have been described as follows:

(a) "Thin" LSILs. They present histological characteristics of LSILs but have a thickness of less than 10 cells.
(b) Keratinizing LSILs. There is keratinization on the epithelium surface. Dyskeratosis and nuclear pleomorphism are characteristically observed. They are most commonly found in the exocervix.
(c) Condylomatous. These are lesions with the clinical appearance of a condyloma that present changes to LSIL. Such changes can be focal.
(d) Epidermoid papillary in situ carcinoma ("squamo-transitional papillary noninvasive carcinoma"). This consists of a papillary lesion with a thin projections covered by epithelium with HSIL (High-grade squamous intraepithelial lesions) features, morphologically similar to urothelial neoplasms.

Most of these are monoclonal and are more frequently aneuploid than polyploid. In contrast to LSIL (Low-grade squamous intraepithelial lesions), it is more frequent to find DNA integration of HPV.

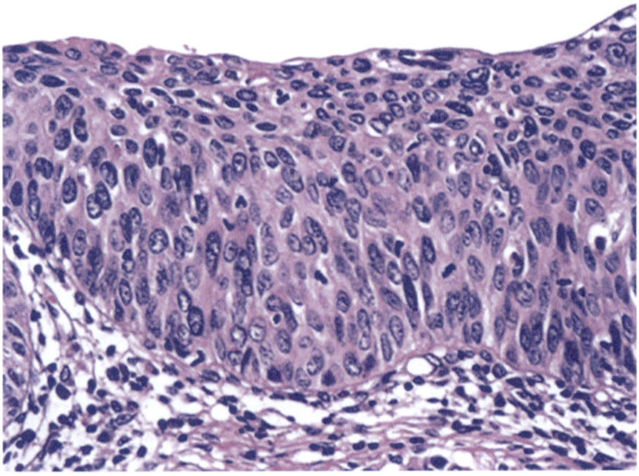

Fig. 7.3 Mitoses are more frequent observed

The main recurrence prognostically identified factors are the size of the lesion and reaction margin state. It has recently been shown that the evaluation of HPV DNA presence at 12 months after treatment is the best predictor of residual or recurrent disease [13].

7.2.2 Epidermoid Microinvasive Carcinoma

The FIGO (International Federation of Gynecology and Obstetrics) defines it as an invasive epidermoid carcinoma diagnosed exclusively by microscopic evaluation and classifies it at clinical stage IAI.

Clinical stage IAI: epidermoid carcinomas with stromal invasion of less than 3 mm in depth and up to 7 mm in horizontal extension.

Clinical stage IA2: epidermoid carcinomas with stromal invasion of more than 3 mm, but less than 5 mm in depth and up to 7 mm in horizontal extension.

The presence of lymphovascular invasion does not affect staging.

The SGO (Society of Gynecological Oncologists) defines microinvasive epidermoid carcinomas as neoplastic epithelia (in situ carcinomas) that invade the stroma in one or more spots with a maximum depth of 3 mm measured from the basal membrane of the epithelium (Fig. 7.4). There must not be the presence of lymphovascular invasion [14].

7.2.3 Epidermoid Carcinoma

It is the second most common neoplasia among women, with a mean presentation age of 55 years. Macroscopically, it presents as an exophytic lesion of papillary or polyploid aspect. The endophytic pattern can also be observed sometimes covered by epithelium

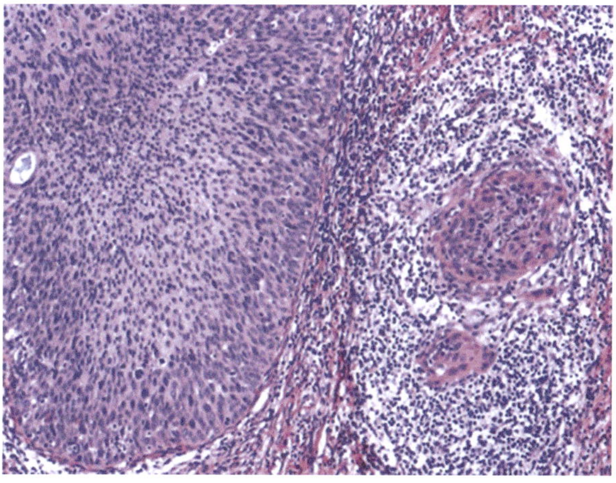

Fig. 7.4 Microinvasive epidermoid carcinomas as neoplastic epithelia (in situ carcinomas)

with normal characteristics. Tumors originated in the canal are poorly visible and difficult for biopsy collection. In advanced stages, tumors can look ulcerated and friable in appearance; palpation shows induration of the cervix and parametrial region [11, 12].

The histologic grade is based on nuclear pleomorphism, nucleolus size, mitotic activity, and necrosis. Epidermoid carcinomas are classified from well to poorly differentiated. The epidermoid carcinoma of the usual type can be keratinizing or non-keratinizing. The latter is constituted by progenitor polygonal cells arranged in mantles or nests, with the presence of intercellular bridges (Fig. 7.5). Individual keratinization can be observed but not the formation of corneal beads (Fig. 7.6). The cytoplasms are eosinophilic and dense because of keratinization. Abundant keratohyalin granules can be observed [13, 15, 16].

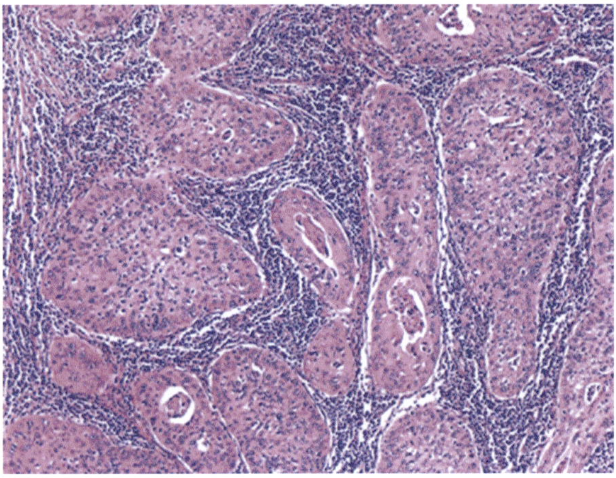

Fig. 7.5 Polygonal cells arranged in mantles or nests, with the presence of intercellular bridges

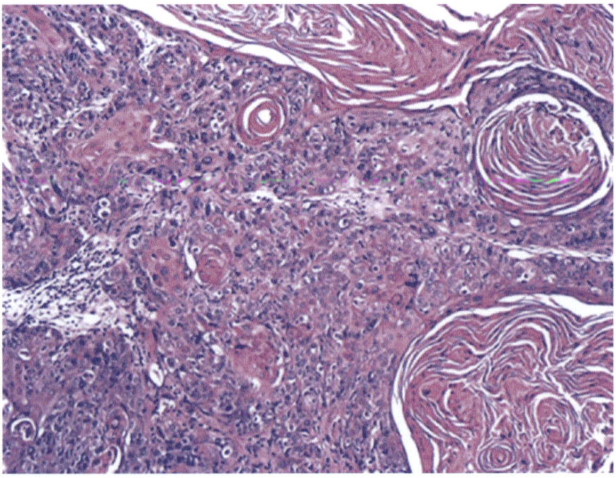

Fig. 7.6 Individual keratinization can be observed but not the formation of corneal beads

7.3 Epidermoid Carcinoma Histologic Subtypes

Basaloid epidermoid carcinoma This is an aggressive variant. It is comprised of nests of basal squamous cells with an immature aspect, similar to those found in cervical in situ carcinoma. Individual keratinization can be observed, but the formation of corneal beads is rare. There is nuclear pleomorphism, marked mitotic activity, geographical aspect necrosis, and comedonecrosis. It is associated with high-risk HPVI (Human Papiloma Virus Infection). It is presented in advanced clinical stages and has a poor prognosis, unlike basal cell epithelioma, an entity with which a differential diagnosis must be performed [17].

Squamous cell verrucous carcinoma This is a very well differentiated squamous cell carcinoma, characterized by an undulating hyperkeratosis, warty surface, and a pushing "infiltrative", bulbous aspect edge. The cytoplasm of neoplastic cells is abundant, and nuclear atypia is minimal. Cytopathologic changes associated with HPVI are not identified. It is a mildly aggressive neoplasia that can recur but does not present metastasis. Unlike condyloma acuminatum, its papillary projections are wide without fibrovascular septa, and koilocytes are not identified [13].

Condylomatous epidermoid carcinoma This is a carcinoma with a condylomatous aspect at low magnification. It presents an architecture similar to that of condyloma acuminatum or to that of Bowenoid lesions of the vulva. The outline is infiltrative, and the presence of koilocytic atypia is characteristic of this variety [18].

Epidermoid carcinoma with papillary pattern This is an epidermoid carcinoma characterized by the formation of thick or thin papillae with fibroconnective tissue septa, covered by an epithelium with similar characteristics to those of ISC (In Situ Carcinoma). Unlike condylomatous carcinoma, it lacks koilocytic atypia and Bowenoid aspect. Given its growth pattern in superficial biopsies, it is frequently impossible to determine the presence of invasion [19].

Epidermoid squamotransitional carcinoma It is a low-frequency variety of cervical carcinoma, occurring in atrophic women; from a histological standpoint, it is indistinguishable from urothelial bladder carcinoma. It can be found in a pure form or with squamous differentiation areas. It is characterized by a papillary growth pattern with fibrovascular septa covered by an atypical stratified epithelium with a urothelial or squamous aspect. Transitional metaplasia has not been proven to be a precursor lesion [20].

Lymphoepithelioma-like epidermoid carcinoma Similar to its counterpart of the head and neck region, this subtype comprises squamous cell nests or trabeculae that are poorly differentiated and surrounded by lymphoplasmacytic inflammatory infiltrate rich in eosinophils. Neoplastic cells are polygonal, with a vesicular prominent nucleus and eosinophilic cytoplasm with poorly defined edges. This explains why the diagnosis by biopsy is discouraged. The prognosis is favorable, with metastatic lymphatic node metastasis lower than that of other epidermoid carcinoma varieties [21].

7.3.1 Glandular Lesion Precursors

In situ adenocarcinoma/high-risk intraepithelial glandular cervical neoplasia (ISA/HIGCN) This is defined as an intraepithelial lesion that contains a malignant aspect glandular epithelium and bears a significant risk of developing invasive adenocarcinoma if left untreated. The most common presentation is through a cytological finding of endocervical atypical glandular cells, frequently associated with HSILs [22].

It is associated with high-risk HPV types, mainly 16 and 18. Morphologically, it is characterized by the presence of atypical epithelial cells that replace the normal endocervical gland cover. Neoplastic cells are columnar, they are arranged in a pseudostratified arrangement, and depletion of the mucous content of the cytoplasm is frequently found. The lobular pattern is conserved because abnormal cells are distributed along the pre-existent glandular outlines (Fig. 7.7). "*Usual*" endocervical-type ISA is the most common form. It presents enlarged hyperchromatic nuclei with thick chromatin and, sometimes, a prominent nucleus. Intestinal differentiation with calciform cells can be observed, or "endometrioid" morphology, characterized by the presence of smaller nuclei and scarce mucus vacuoles in the apical edge of the cytoplasm. It is sometimes possible to identify neuroendocrine or Paneth cells. It is important to recognize intestinal differentiation zones in endocervical glands because their presence almost always indicates a premalignant or malignant lesion, even when cellular atypia is mild.

A morphological variant named "Stratified Mucinous Intraepithelial Lesion" (SMILE) has been described. It consists of a stratified epithelium consistent of atypical nucleus cells that contain small vacuoles with mucin or clear cytoplasm in all of its layers. Additionally, numerous mitoses and apoptotic bodies are observed, as well as a high proliferation index. SMILEs are usually associated with HSILs and/or ISA.

There are lesions with cytologic atypia previously referred to as "*Endocervical Glandular Dysplasia*" (EGD) or "*Low Grade Glandular Cervical Intraepithelial Neoplasia*" (LCIN) with cytological changes with atypia that do not comply with

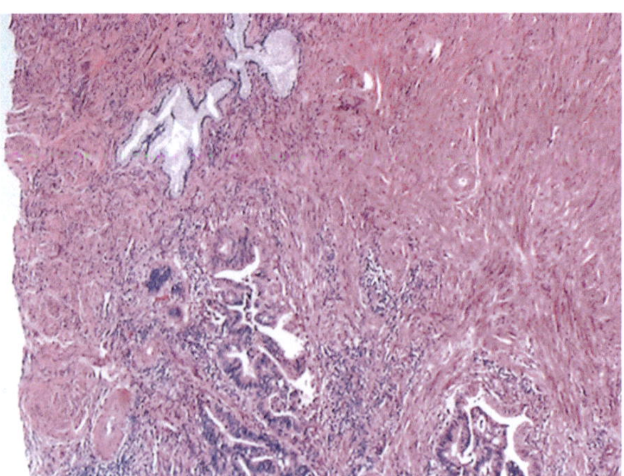

Fig. 7.7 The lobular pattern is conserved because abnormal cells are distributed along the pre-existent glandular outlines

ISA/HCIN. However, the criteria are not well defined, and reproducibility is very low; therefore, it is not considered a specific entity [22].

7.3.2 *Early Adenocarcinoma*

Unlike squamous neoplasias and glandular neoplasias, there is no consensus to determine microinvasive adenocarcinomas. The SGO (Society of Gynecological Oncologists) applies this term to adenocarcinomas that infiltrate the stroma in one or more spots with a depth less than 3 mm from the base of the epithelium and in the absence of lymphovascular permeation. The FIGO (International Federation of Gynecology and Obstetrics) defines them as invasive adenocarcinomas diagnosed by only microscopic evaluation and classified as clinical stage IA.

The clinical stage IAI corresponds to an adenocarcinoma with invasion to the minor stroma of less than 3 mm in depth and up to 7 mm in horizontal extension.

Clinical stage IA2 corresponds to an adenocarcinoma with invasion to the stroma of more than 3 mm, but less than 5 mm and up to 7 mm in horizontal extension.

The presence of lymphovascular invasion does not affect staging. Because there is no consensus, it is recommended, in invasive neoplasias, to determine the depth of the invasion without using the term “microinvasion”. Notably, in adenocarcinomas with an invasion less than 3 mm, the incidence of positive lymphatic nodes is less than 1% [14].

7.3.3 *Adenocarcinoma*

Endocervical adenocarcinoma corresponds to 10–25% of cervical carcinomas. Their increase corresponds to improvements in screening methods and better identification of glandular lesions.

Ninety-four percent of endocervical adenocarcinomas are associated with high-risk HPV infection; the most common are isotypes 18, 16, and 45. Their clinical manifestations include transvaginal bleeding and cervical tumor of the exophytic aspect, with ulceration foci or an infiltrative pattern.

7.4 Adenocarcinoma Histologic Subtypes

Endocervical adenocarcinoma of the usual type It is the most frequent and corresponds to 90% of all uterine cervical adenocarcinomas. Macroscopically, most have an exophytic aspect. Histologically, they present a complex architectural pattern constituted by glands arranged in cribiform or papillary structures with the presence of mucoproduction. Neoplastic cells show stratification, mitotic activity, nuclear enlargement and hyperchromatism, as well as prominent nuclei. Cytoplasms can be eosinophilic (Fig. 7.8) or clear [22].

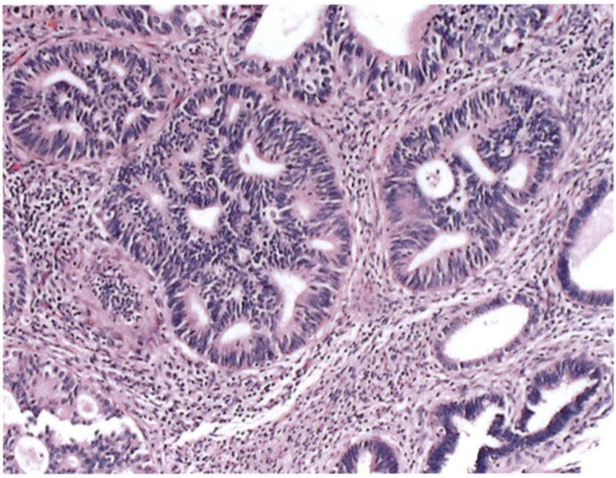

Fig. 7.8 Cytoplasms can be eosinophilic or clear [22]

Mucinous adenocarcinoma This is classified into four variants: usual type, gastric type (minimal deviation adenocarcinoma), intestinal type, and signet ring cells.

Usual type mucinous adenocarcinoma corresponds to a mucoproductor adenocarcinoma that cannot be classified in any other specific variant.

Gastric type adenocarcinoma (minimal deviation adenocarcinoma) corresponds to 1% of cervical adenocarcinomas and, in most cases, are not related to HPVI. An association with the Peutz-Jeghers syndrome has been reported. Histologically, it corresponds to a very well differentiated adenocarcinoma surrounded by stroma that shows scarce or no desmoplastic reaction in some areas. Cases with gastric differentiation present cells with a clear cytoplasm and sharp outlines, with a large, hyperchromatic nucleus. In immunohistochemical analysis, the cells are positive for MUC6 and HIK1083. Their behavior is more aggressive than conventional adenocarcinomas.

Intestinal type mucinous adenocarcinoma is similar to that originated from the intestinal mucosa, with the presence of calciform, argentaffin, and Paneth cells. It is associated with HPVI.

Signet cell mucinous adenocarcinoma is characterized by the focal or diffuse presence of broad cytoplasm cells, occupied by mucus vacuoles that push the nucleus towards the periphery. It can be associated with or without HPVI [22].

Villoglandular adenocarcinoma This presents in young women (mean age of 35 years), and it is associated with high-risk HPVI. Clinically, these are exophytic tumors. Histologically, they show an exophytic pattern constituted by villous or papillary structures covered by an endocervical type columnar epithelium, with mild or moderate atypia and a decrease in mucoproduction. When it is superficial, its prognosis is excellent. Nonetheless, the prognosis changes if the invasive component is poorly differentiated or if it presents lymphovascular permeation [22].

Endometrioid adenocarcinoma This represents 5% of endocervical adenocarcinomas, and it is associated with high-risk HPVI. Histologically, they are similar to its endometrial cavity-originated counterpart. By immunohistochemistry, they are diffusely positive for p16 and express CEA; unlike endometrial cavity endometrioid adenocarcinomas, they are negative for estrogen receptor and vimentin. Their prognosis is better than the usual type mucinous adneocarcinomas [22].

Clear cell adenocarcinoma This is uncommon in the cervix, and it can present in young women with diethylstilbestrol sporadic exposition history in the uterus. It can be associated with high-risk HPVI. Histologically, they are arranged in a tubular-cystic, papillary or solid pattern. The cells are clear; some have the shape of a tack and a high grade. Hiliary intra- or extracellular globes can be observed. The prognosis is similar to that of conventional endocervical adenocarcinoma [22].

Derous carcinoma This neoplasia is extremely rare in the cervix, and it is similar to that originated in the endometrium, salpingo, or ovary. It is most frequently associated with HPVI in young women. It is arranged in a complex papillary pattern covered by cubic cells with a high nuclear grade. Exfoliation of cells or psammoma bodies can be observed. The behavior is associated with patient age, advanced clinical stage, tumors larger than 2 cm, invasion larger than 1 cm, and the presence of lymphovascular permeation [22].

7.4.1 Other Epithelial Neoplasias

Adenosquamous carcinoma This is a neoplasia constituted by adenocarcinoma and epidermoid carcinoma areas in which both components are histologically recognizable (Fig. 7.9). Epidermoid carcinomas with mucoproduction but with a lack of glandular formation or with a solid pattern and absence of squamous differentiation must not be included.

HPVI subtypes 16 and 18 are the most prevalent, and precursor lesions are in situ epidermoid carcinoma and in situ adenocarcinoma.

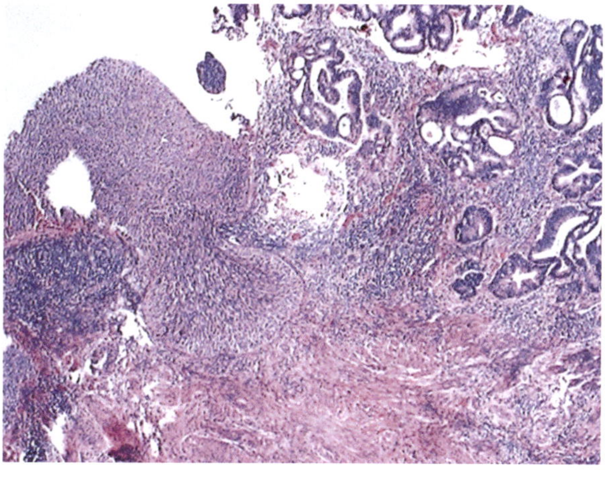

Fig. 7.9 This is a neoplasia constituted by adenocarcinoma and epidermoid carcinoma areas in which both components are histologically recognizable

Although there is some controversy in relation to its prognosis, there is consensus regarding its behavior being similar to that of endocervical adenocarcinoma, stage by stage [23].

Other cervical malignant epithelial neoplasia subtypes include glassy cell carcinoma, adenoid basal carcinoma, adenoid cystic carcinoma, and undifferentiated carcinoma [23].

7.5 Neuroendocrine Tumors

It is recommended to use the terminology of gastric-enteric-pancreatic neuroendocrine tumors for cervical neuroendocrine tumors.

Low-grade neuroendocrine tumor.

Carcinoid tumor
Atypical carcinoid tumor

High-grade neuroendocrine tumor.

Small cell neuroendocrine carcinoma
Large cell neuroendocrine carcinoma

Cervical neuroendocrine neoplasias are associated with HPVI, particularly subtype 18. In immunohistochemistry, they are positive for chromogranin, synaptophysin, and CD65.

Low-grade cervical neuroendocrine neoplasias are rare in this location; they are arranged in an organoid pattern, nests, islets, or trabeculae, constituted by cells with an abundant cytoplasm, nuclei with granular chromatin, and prominent nuclei. The difference between carcinoid tumors and atypical carcinoid tumors is based on the presence of nuclear atypias, mitotic activity, and necrosis foci, which are observed in the latter.

The prognosis for carcinoid tumors is indolent but with metastatic potential. The atypical carcinoid behavior is similar to that of large cell neuroendocrine carcinoma.

Within high-grade neuroendocrine carcinomas, small cell carcinoma is the most frequent, and it is characterized by a monotonous population of small cells with ovoid hyperchromatic nuclei, scarce cytoplasm, and nuclear molding (Fig. 7.10). There are many mitoses, apoptosis, extended necrosis, perineural invasion, and lymphovascular permeation. Large cell neuroendocrine carcinoma is arranged in a diffuse, organoid, trabecular pattern, or similar to laces, constituted by cells with abundant cytoplasm, large nuclei, prominent nuclei, and a high mitotic index. Focal glandular differentiation can be observed.

High-grade neuroendocrine carcinomas are extremely aggressive and are detected in advanced clinical stages. The 5-year survival is 14–39% for large cell neuroendocrine carcinoma in any clinical stage [24].

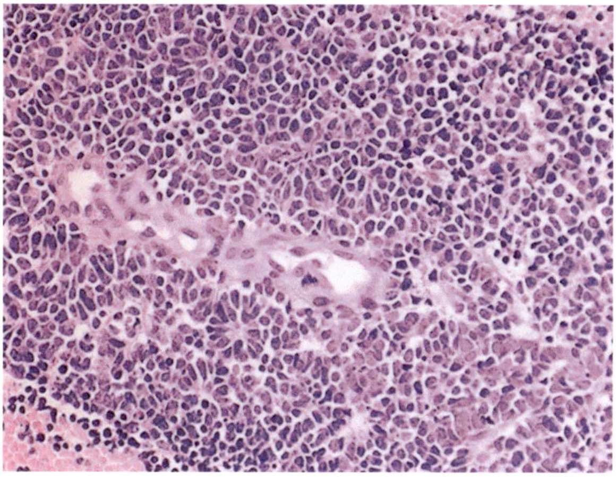

Fig. 7.10 Within high-grade neuroendocrine carcinomas, small cell carcinoma is the most frequent, and it is characterized by a monotonous population of small cells with ovoid hyperchromatic nuclei, scarce cytoplasm, and nuclear molding

References

1. Lazcano-Ponce EC et al. Cáncer de Cuello Uterino. Una Perspectiva Histórica Ginecología y Obstetricia de México. 1994;62:40–7.
2. Lazcano-Ponce EC et al. Quality control study on negative gynecological cytology in Mexico. Diagn Pathol. 1994;10:10–4.
3. Nayar R, Wilbur DC. The Bethesda System for reporting cervical cytology. 3rd ed. New York: Springer; 2015.
4. Massad LS, Einstein MH, Huh WK, Katki HA, Kinney WK, Schiffman M, Solomon D, et al. Update consensus guidelines for the management of abnormal cervical cancer screening tests and cancer precursors. J Low Genit Tract Dis. 2012;17:S1–S17.
5. Katki HA, Schiffman M, Castle PE, Fetterman B, Poitras NE, Loyer T, et al. Five –year risk on CIN3+ and cervical cancer for women with HPV-positive and HPV- negative high-grade pap results. J Low Genit Tract Dis. 2013;17:S50–5.
6. Katki HA, Schiffman M, Castle PE, Fetterman B, Poitras NE, Loyer T, et al. Five –year risk on CIN3+ and cervical cancer for women with HPV testing of ASC-US pap results. J Low Genit Tract Dis. 2013;17:S36–42.
7. Hoda R, Loukeris K, Abdul-Karim F. Gynecologic cytology on conventional and liquid-based preparations: a comprehensive review of similarities and differences. Cancer Cytopathol. 2012;41:257–78.
8. Bernstein S, Sánchez-Ramos L, Ndubisi B. Liquid-based cervical cytologic smear study and conventional Papanicolaou smears: a meta-analysis of prospective studies comparing cytologic diagnosis and sample adequacy. Am J Obstet Gynecol. 2001;185(2):308–17.
9. Davey E, Barratt A, Irwing L, Chan S, et al. Effect of study design and quality on unsatisfactory rates, cytology classifications, and accuracy in liquid-based versus conventional cervical cytology: a systematic review. Lancet. 2006;367:22–132.
10. Cheung A, Szeto E, Leung B, Khoo U, et al. Liquid-based cytology and conventional cervical smears. A comparison study in an Asian screening population. Cancer Cytopathol. 2003;99:331–5.
11. Arends MJ, Buckley CH, Wells M. Aetiology, pathogenersis and pathology of cervical neoplasia. J Clin Pathol. 1998;51:96–103.
12. Darragh TM, Colgan TJ, Cox T, et al. The lower anogenital squamous terminology standardization project for HPV-associated lesions: background and consensus recommendations from

the College of American Pathologists and the American Society for Colposcopy and Cervical Pathology. J Low Gen Tract Dis. 2012;16(3):205–42.
13. Stoler M, Bergeron C, Cogan TJ, Ferenczy AS, et al. Squamous cell tumours and precursors. In: Kurman RJ, Carcangiu ML, Harrington CS, Young RH, editors. WHO classification of tumours of female reproductive organs. 4th ed. Lyon: IARC; 2014.
14. Malpica A, Deavers MT, Euscher E. Squamous lesions of uterine cervix. In:Biopsy interpretation of the uterine cervix and corpus. Philadelphia: Lippincott Williams & Wilkins; 2010.
15. Kurman RJ, Ronett BM, Sherman ME, Wilkison EJ. Tumor of cérvix, vagina and vulva. 3rd series, Fascicle 4. Washington, DC: American Registry of Pathology in collaboration with de Armen Forces Institute of Pathology; 2010. p. 431.
16. Stoler MH. The pathology of cervical neoplasia. In: Rohan TE, Shan KV, editors. Cervical cancer: from etiology to prevention. New York: Kluwer Academic Publishers; 2004.
17. Grayson W, Cooper K. A reappraisal of "basaloid carcinoma" of the cervix, ans differential diagnosis basaloid cervical neoplasms. Adv Anat Pathol. 2002;9:290–300.
18. Kurman RJ, Toki SMH. Basaloid and warty carcinoma of the vulva. Distinctive types of squamous cell carcinoma frequently associated with human papillomaviruses. Am J Surg Pathol. 1993;17:133–45.
19. Brinck U, Jacob C, Bau O, Fuzesi L. Papillary squamous cell carcinoma of the uterine cérvix: report of three cases and a review of its classification. Int J Gynecol Pathol. 2000;19:231–5.
20. Albores Saavedra J, Young RH. Transitional cell neoplasms (carcinomas and inverted papillomas) of the uterine cervix. A report of five cases. Am J Surg Pathol. 1995;19:1138–45.
21. Martorell MA, Julian JM, Calabuig C, Garcia-Garcia JA, Perez-Valles A. Lymphoepithelioma-like carcinoma of the uterine cervix. Arch Pathol Lab Med. 2002;126:1501–5.
22. Wilbur DC, Colgan TJ, Ferenczy AS, Hirschowitz L, et al. Glandular tumors and precursors. In: Kurman RJ, Carcangiu ML, Harrington CS, Young RH, editors. WHO classification of tumours of female reproductive organs. 4th ed. Lyon: IARC; 2014.
23. Colgan TJ, Kim KR, Hirschowitz L, WG MC. Other epithelial tumours. In: Kurman RJ, Carcangiu ML, Harrington CS, Young RH, editors. WHO classification of tumours of female reproductive organs. 4th ed. Lyon: IARC; 2014.
24. Colgan TJ, Kim KR, Hirschowitz L, WG MC. Neuroendocrine tumours. In: Kurman RJ, Carcangiu ML, Harrington CS, Young RH, editors. WHO classification of tumours of female reproductive organs. 4th ed. Lyon: IARC; 2014.

Chapter 8
Cervical Cancer Staging

Alhely López-Arias, David Isla-Ortiz, Salim Barquet-Muñoz, and David F. Cantú-de-León

Abstract Cervical cancer (CC) is an important cause of morbidity and mortality worldwide in female populations. Because the prognosis and management of these patients depends on proper staging, emphasis must be placed on ensuring that health care professionals are perfectly familiar with current standards. Cervical Cancer staging is still achieved clinically. In some cases, it relies on surgical staging and diagnostic imaging tools that have widely progressed to improve their ability to detect tumor foci and distant site extensions. A section about preinvasive lesions is included in this chapter as a preamble to invasive lesions, which are the topic of the present text.

Keywords Cervical cancer • Staging • Clinical profile • Prognosis • TNM • FIGO • Physical examination

A. López-Arias, MD
Clinical Research, Instituto Nacional de Cancerología-México, Mexico City, Mexico

D. Isla-Ortiz, MD • S. Barquet-Muñoz, MD
Department of Gynecologic Oncology, Instituto Nacional de Cancerología-México, Av. San Fernando No 22, Col. Sección XVI, Mexico City, Mexico, 14080

D.F. Cantú-de-León, MD, MSc, PhD (✉)
Department of Gynecologic Oncology, Instituto Nacional de Cancerología-México, Av. San Fernando No 22, Col. Sección XVI, Mexico City, Mexico, 14080

Division of Research, Instituto Nacional de Cancerología-México, Mexico City, Mexico
e-mail: dcantude@gmail.com

J.G. de la Garza-Salazar et al. (eds.), *Cervical Cancer*,
DOI 10.1007/978-3-319-45231-9_8

8.1 Uterine Cervix Preinvasive Lesions

HPV infection precedes the CC carcinogenic process (as discussed in a previous chapter). Most invasive lesions are preceded by an intraepithelial lesion or a Cervical Intraepithelial Neoplasia (CIN). Most CIN develop in the cervix transformation zone, which is located in the squamo-columnar junction between the endocervix columnar epithelium and the ectocervix squamous epithelium. This area is called the transformation zone because it undergoes a columnar epithelial metaplasia process toward the external cervical orifice in response to different factors, including pH and hormonal changes, throughout a woman's life. CIN's form a spectrum comprising a neoplastic cell continuum according to observed changes in the cytoplasm, the loss of nuclear polarity, pleomorphism, and mitosis. They are divided into CIN 1, in which only the inferior one-third of the epithelium is affected; CIN 2, in which the lesion extends up to the middle one-third of the epithelium, and CIN 3, in which the lesion has extended through the entire thickness of the epithelium [1].

The mean time to a CIN 3 or in situ carcinoma development from the moment of an initial HPV16 infection is between 7 and 12 years, whereas in a high risk HPV-positive CIN 1, the development time is 6 years [2].

The most widely used CC screening study is still cervical-vaginal cytology. It is important to disclaim the notion that colposcopy is not a screening method because it requires an extensive amount of resources and preparation to be adequately performed. However, all cytological abnormalities must be further analyzed by colposcopy. The goal is to reveal aberrations that can guide biopsy collection with the aim of ruling out invasive cancer [3].

8.2 Treatment of Premalignant Lesions

Low grade squamous intraepithelial lesions (LG-SILs) and atypical squamous epithelium of undetermined significance (ASE-US).

Because LG-SILs can spontaneously resolve within less than 24 months, women diagnosed with LG-SIL may be kept under surveillance, with periodic cytological exams every 6 months [4]. Recent recommendations include the use of a "co-assay", in which the results of a high-risk HPV detection test are combined with (e.g.: hybrid capture) a cytological test because the combination results in sensitivity that reaches 90–100% [5] and better predicts the development of high grade lesions or cancer.

In the case of a negative high-risk HPV test but a LG-SIL-coherent cytology, it is recommended that the test be repeated after 1 year. If at that time the cytology shows AS-EUS, a larger lesion, or the presence of a high-risk HPV virus, a colposcopy and guided biopsy are performed. Conversely, if both tests yield negative results, no cytological propagation is observed, and the high risk-HPV virus test is also negative, both tests can be repeated in 3 years [6].

In contrast, in postmenopausal women, LG-SIL cases can be assessed by performing a co-assay within 6 months or directly proceeding to perform a colposcopy and a biopsy. If the HPV test yields negative results for the presence of high-risk viruses or no lesions are identified in colposcopy, the co-assay is performed 1 year later. If the result is AS-EUS or higher, colposcopy is performed, otherwise, routine screens are performed [7].

In patients with CIN1 according to biopsy results in which this finding is preceded by a cytological determination of LG-SIL or AS-EUS, the co-assay must be performed after 1 year. If both are negative, routine screens are performed. If CIN 1 persists for 2 years, it is acceptable to either continue with surveillance or treat the lesion. Both ablation and scission can be used, but the former treatment implies a satisfactory colposcopy. In cases in which the second assessment shows CIN 2 or higher, the lesion must be treated.

In patients with CIN 2 preceded by LG-SIL or AS-EUS, the follow-up protocol is more intense. It includes a diagnostic scission procedure, and during follow-up, the co-assay is performed once every 1 or 2 years. If patients show normal results in successive assays, they return to 3 year follow-up [8].

Current recommendations suggest performing a colposcopy when the examination shows an ASC-US, LG-SIL, H-ASC and Atypical Glandular Cells (AGC) and when there is a positive HPV test. After LG-SIL cytology and an inadequate colposcopy or positive endocervical curettage, an excisional procedure is recommended to achieve a more accurate diagnosis and treatment protocol. Any CIN 2 or CIN 3 histological diagnosis based on a cervical biopsy must be followed by excision of the transformation zone unless the patient is pregnant [7].

In cases in which a malignant macroscopic lesion is identified in the cervix uteri, it is necessary to perform a staging procedure, that corresponds to the magnitude of the disease. It is also important to know the signs and symptoms that are presented in invasive disease.

8.3 Clinical Profile and Physical Examination

All women with precursor lesions or in situ carcinoma are asymptomatic, although there may be clinical manifestations that are associated with the disease because of the presence of concomitant infections. In invasive cancer cases, as dissemination progresses, signs and symptoms begin to appear. The most frequent sign is transvaginal hemorrhage, which is most often post-coital, intermenstrual, or postmenopausal. Moreover, tumor necrosis produces serosanguinous smelly fluid.

These types of symptoms appear early in exofitic tumors of the ectocervix. However, in endocervical tumors, the manifestations are subtle, even in advanced disease. This underscores the importance of perfect endocervical canal sampling, during which the sample is obtained prior to the cytology [9].

In locally advanced and metastatic stages, the patient may lose weight and have inguinal and/or supraclavicular lymph node enlargement. A bad smell can also be perceived as a result of postcoital bleeding. Bladder or rectal invasion result in the appearance of fistulae, hematuria and hematochezia, pelvic pain, sciatic nerve region pain, leg edema, lumbar pain, and, in the presence of extension to the contiguous viscera, sacral plexus affection and lymphatic, vascular or uretral obstruction.

It is worth mentioning that exploration is more difficult in postmenopausal women because lesions are frequently located in an endocervical location and the uterine cervix is atrophic and not easy to visualize. Furthermore, vaginal examinations are more difficult in these patients because of atrophia, the loss of elasticity, and a reduction in patient complaint.

After an inspection, a bimanual exploration is performed to evaluate the shape, dimensions, and mobility of the uterus, including the uterine cervix and parametria. The uterus may be enlarged because of endometrial infiltration, uterine collection, or the presence of concomitant miomatosis and the possible coexistence of anexial involvement. If the uterus is fixed, it is certain to be because of tumor infiltration towards the pelvic wall. To evaluate its extension towards the parametria, bladder, and rectum, it is necessary to perform a careful rectovaginal exploration: the right side of the pelvis (parametrium) is palpated with the right hand, and the left side is palpated with the left hand (introducing the middle finger through the rectum and the index finger through the vagina [9]). When a parametrium is involved, it is usually irregular, nodular and painful at touch.

During the physical examination, it is important to explore the lympho-porting areas. If, during the exploration of the supraclavicular or inguinal region, any suspicious increase in the volume of lymph nodes is noticed, fine needle aspiration biopsy can reasonably rule out metastatic disease.

Additional analyses can be useful for accurate staging, and, in some cases, laboratory results can be prognostic (e.g., hemoglobin). It is important to keep in mind that these tools provide only more precise information that is difficult to obtain through physical examination.

A very important prognostic factor that can differ across clinicians during exploration is tumor size. Hence, confirmation by a qualified expert is crucial, mainly during the early stages of the disease, because tumor size, depth of invasion, and stromal involvement are correlated with each other [9].

In clinical stages II, III, and IV, poor prognostic indicators include the presence of the disease in the pelvic nodes, a growth in the size of the primary tumor, low hemoglobin levels, and functional status.

8.4 Clinical Staging

In cervical cancer, stage assigning is based on clinical data. Experience is required for staging to be reproducible and reliable. Thus, CC clinical staging rules are based on gynecological clinical explorations that are performed by an expert, preferably while the patient is under anesthesia (although this depends on the health center). The initially assigned clinical stage should be maintained and remain unchanged despite subsequent new discoveries even in cases of recurrence [10].

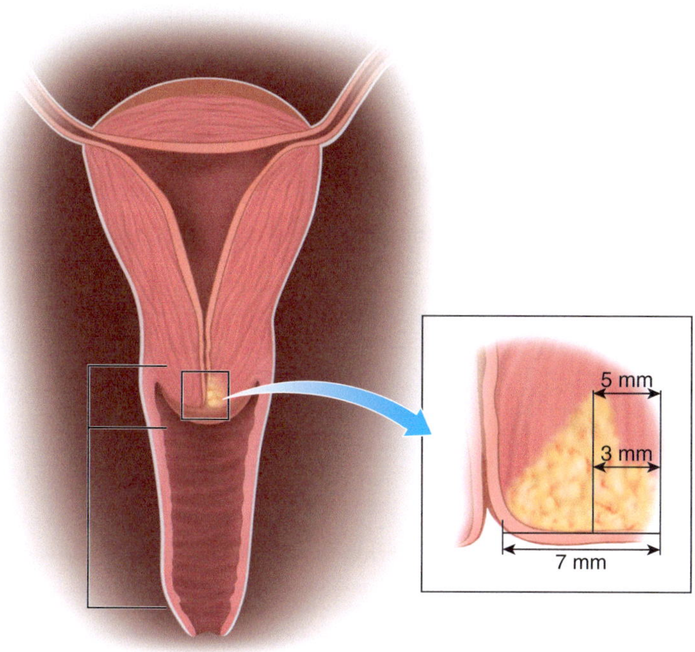

Fig. 8.1 Stage Ia1: There is a cancerous area of 3 millimeters (mm) or smaller in depth, and 7 mm or smaller in length. Stage Ia2:There is a cancerous area larger than 3 mm but not larger than 5 mm in depth, and 7 mm or smaller in length

The currently used staging system is the one that was adopted by the International Federation of Gynecology and Obstetrics (FIGO). It should be taken into consideration that the staging system is useful only for comparative purposes and must not be taken as an indication of norms. Each clinical case must be individually considered and supported by imaging methods before proposing the best treatment plan. According to the FIGO, clinical exploration is the gold standard for CC staging. Tumor diameter, vaginal infiltration, and tumor extension to parameters and septi (e.g., the vesicovaginal septum and rectovaginal septum) represent the morphological parameters that should be considered during CC staging, as follows:

In 2009, FIGO revisited CC staging and established the following [11]:

Stage 0: In situ carcinoma, intraepithelial carcinoma.
Stage I: Carcinoma strictly limited to the cervix (Fig. 8.1).

Stage Ia: Invasive cancer identified only in microscopy, stromal invasion is no more than 5 mm deep and 7 mm wide.
Stage Ia1: Stromal invasion <3 mm deep and <7 mm in extension or width.
The incidence of lymphatic nodal metastasis in stage IaI is 0.1–2.6%, in most cases, it is less than 1% [12].

Stage Ia2: Stromal invasion >3 mm but <5 mm in depth and <7 mm in extension. In this stage, the risk of metastasis to pelvic and para-aortic lymph nodes ranges from 0 to 9.7% [13].

The depth of the invasion must not be more than 5 mm from the base of the epithelium and the surface of the glands from which they originate. The involvement of the vascular, venous of lymphatic space must not alter staging.

Stage Ib: Lesions clinically confined to the cervix or preclinical lesions larger than stage Ia2.

Stage Ib1: Lesions clinically visible but no larger than 4 cm.

The risk of nodal pelvic or para-aortic metastasis in stage Ib1 ranges from 10% to 22% [14].

Stage Ib2: Clinically visible lesions are larger than 4 cm (Fig. 8.2).

Stage II: The Carcinoma has extended further than the uterus but not to the pelvic wall or the inferior one-third of the vagina.

Stage IIa: Engagement of two thirds of the superior part of the vagina without affecting the parametrium.

Stage IIa1: Clinically visible lesion <4 cm in its largest dimension.

Stage IIa2: Clinically visible lesion >4 cm in its largest dimension (Fig. 8.3).

Stage IIb: Parametrium infiltration without affecting the pelvic wall.

Pelvic lymph node metastasis is generally 10–27% in stage II, and para-aortic lymph node involvement occurs in 7–25% of stage II cases [12]. Other authors claim that in stage IIb, the incidence of para-aortic node involvement is 19.8% [15] (Fig. 8.4).

Stage III: Involvement of the inferior third of the vagina or extension to the pelvic wall. In a rectal examination, no cancer-free space is observed between the tumor and the pelvic wall. All hydronephrosis and non-functioning kidney are included unless they can be attributed to other causes.

Stage IIIa: Involvement of the inferior third of the vagina but extension no to the pelvic wall.

Stage IIIb: Extension towards the pelvic wall and hydronephrosis or a non-functioning kidney (Fig. 8.5).

Nodal involvement in this stage extends to the pelvic nodes in as many as 43% and to the para-aortic nodes in 7–25% of cases [12]. Other authors argue that in stage III, nodal affection is usually up to 27.5% [15].

Stage IV: Extension out of the pelvis or a clinically invasion of bladder mucosa or rectum.

Stage IVa: Tumor involves bladder or rectal mucosa.

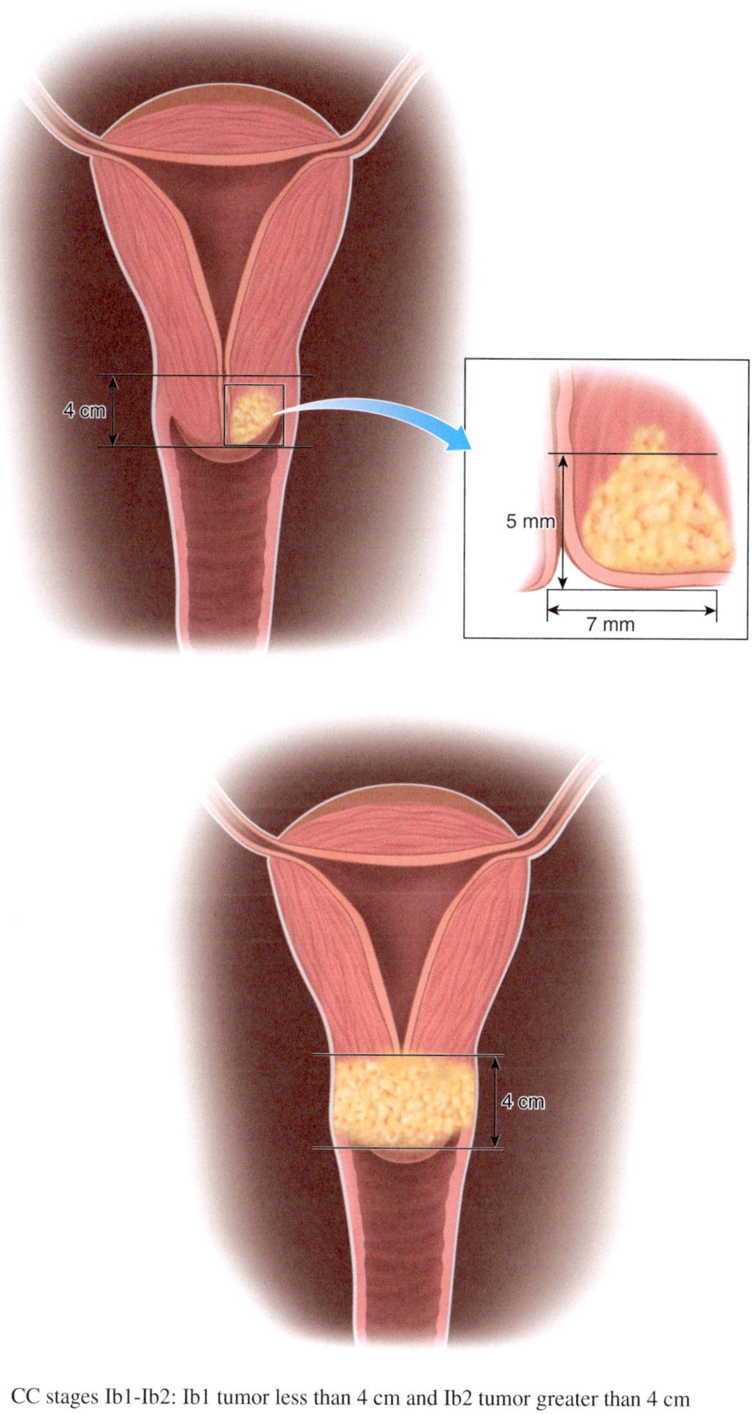

Fig. 8.2 CC stages Ib1-Ib2: Ib1 tumor less than 4 cm and Ib2 tumor greater than 4 cm

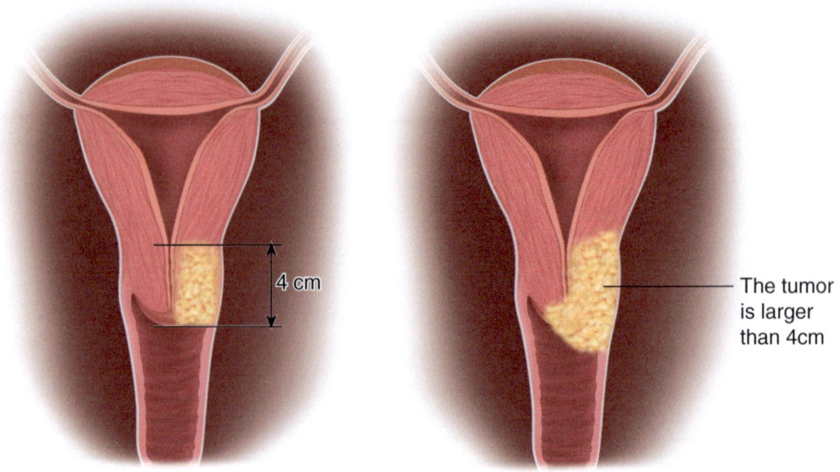

Fig. 8.3 Stages IIa1-IIa2. The tumor has not spread to the tissue next to the cervix, also called the parametrial area.

Fig. 8.4 CC stages IIb. The tumor has spread to the parametrial (tissue surrounding the uterus) area.

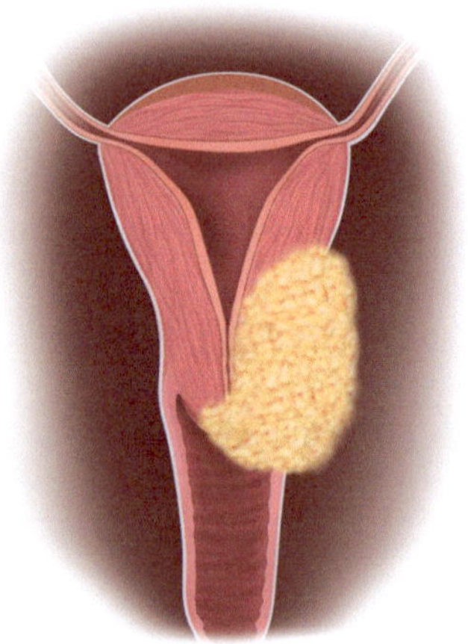

Stage IVb: Distant metastasis or disease outside the true pelvis (Fig. 8.6).

Nearly 5–35% of CC patients will develop metastasis to the lungs. Some other common metastasis sites are the bones (16%), liver (3%) and intestines. Bone affection happens via hematic dissemination, and small intestine affection can occur as a result of the direct extension of the para-aortic nodes or via peritoneal dissemination [16].

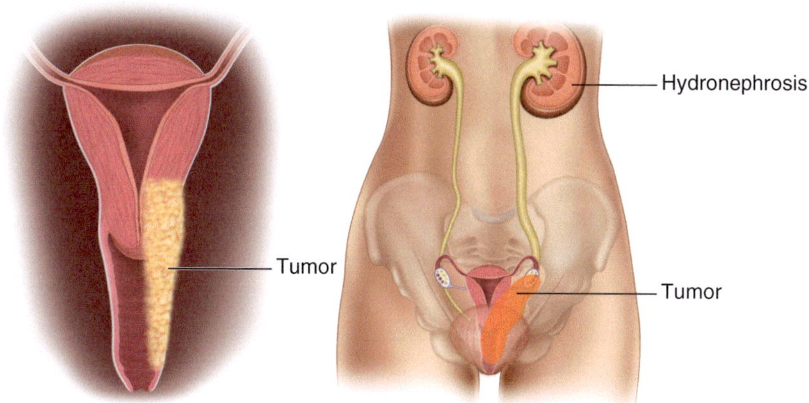

Fig. 8.5 CC stages IIIa. The tumor involves the lower third of the vagina, but it has not grown into the pelvic wall. IIIb. The tumor has grown into the pelvic wall and/or causes hydronephrosis or nonfunctioning kidneys.

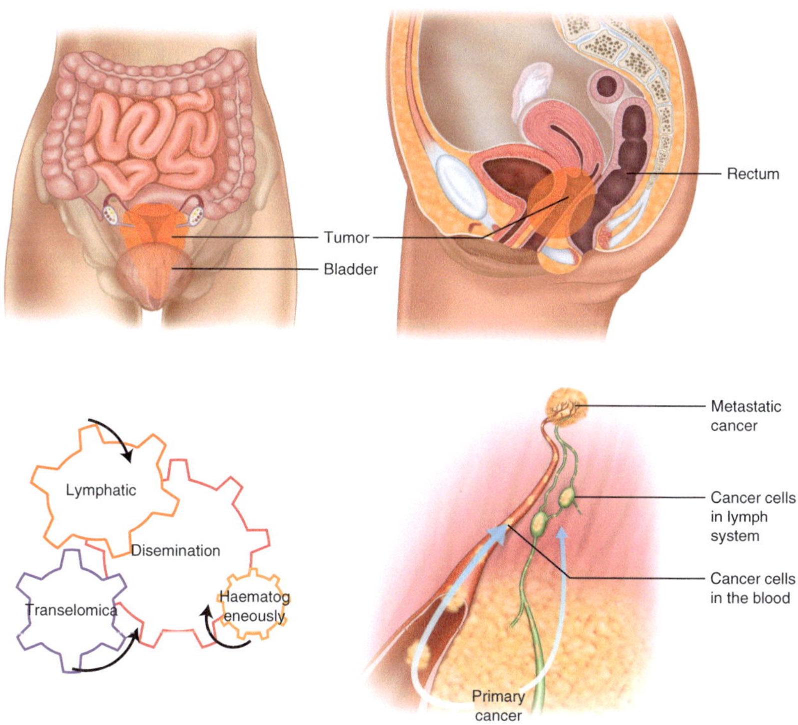

Fig. 8.6 CC stages IVa and Ivb. The tumor has spread to the mucosa (lining) of the bladder or rectum and grown beyond the pelvis.

8.5 Surgical Staging

When performing surgical treatment, histopathological findings can affect CC staging. Thus, the TNM nomenclature, which was approved by the American Joint Committee on Cancer (AJCC) and is in its 7th edition, is generally used.

The cases must be classified as CC if the primary site of origin is the cervix. All histologic types are included. The grade is determined according to the widely used methods, but the grade does not affect staging.

The nomenclature includes the following:

Tx = The primary tumor cannot be assessed.
T0 = No evidence of a primary tumor.
Tis = In situ carcinoma.

- T1 = Cervical carcinoma confined to the uterus.
  - T1a = Invasive carcinoma diagnosed by microscopy only.
  - T1a1 = Stromal invasion of 3 mm or less in depth and 7 mm or less in horizontal extension.
  - T1a2 = Stromal invasion of more than 3 mm but less than 5 mm with a horizontal extension of 7 mm or less.
  - T1b = Clinically visible lesion confined to the cervix or microscopically visible but larger than T1a/Ia2.
  - T1b2 = Clinically visible lesion of 4 cm or less at its largest part.
- T2 = Cervical carcinoma that invades further than the uterus but not towards the pelvic wall or the inferior one-third of the vagina.
  - T2a = Tumor without invasion to the parametria.
    - T2a1 = Clinically visible lesion of 4 cm or less in its largest part.
    - T2a2 = Clinically visible lesion of more than 4 cm in its largest part.
  - T2b = Tumor with invasion into the parametria.
- T3 = Tumor is extended to the pelvic wall or involves the inferior one-third of the vagina, and/or causes hydronephrosis or a dysfunctional kidney.
  - T3a: The tumor involves the inferior one-third of the vagina without extending to the pelvic wall.
  - T3b: Tumor has extended to the pelvic wall and/or causes hydronephrosis or a non-functioning kidney.
- T4 = The tumor invades the bladder or rectum mucosa or it extends further than the true pelvis.

  Nx = Regional lymphatic nodes cannot be evaluated.
  N0 = There is no metastasis to regional lymphatic nodes.
  N1 = Metastasis to regional lymphatic nodes.

M0 = No distant metastasis.

M1 = Distant metastasis (including peritoneal extension, the supraclavicular, mediastinal, or para-aortic nodes, and the lungs, liver, or bones).

In most clinical scenarios, the first treatment is defined by the clinical stage, while the pathological stage is useful for direct adjuvant therapy, whether it includes radiotherapy or chemotherapy.

The pathologic classification of TNM does not replace the TNM clinical classification but instead provides additional information mostly related to local and distant recurrence and reveals the presence of hidden residual disease or micrometastases, at the beginning of presentation [17].

Cervical cancer is disseminated through the lymphatic system. Hence, the first place where metastases appear is the pelvic lymph nodes, followed by the para-aortic nodes. Laparotomy and laparoscopy are the most widely used methods for nodal evaluation in CC, given that they have similar sensitivities. The most important survival prognosis factor is a nodal status [18].

8.6 Imaging Studies

Although the FIGO staging system does not include imaging to stage CC, committees promote the use of these imaging techniques to allow for the determination of prognostic factors, such as tumor size, parametrial involvement or pelvic wall involvement, and adjacent organ invasion or lymphatic node metastasis [19]. These are valuable for determining a treatment plan, but must not be used to modify the initial clinical stage of the patient.

In has been shown that transrectal ultrasound is superior to MRI for detecting tumor after biopsies because it calculates volume with a higher precision and evaluates parametrial invasion. The role of the ultrasound has improved as a result of the advent of novel technologies and the implementation of high frequency transducers that allow a higher quality image to be obtained. The advantages of ultrasound over MRI are that the former has a lower cost, is less invasive and faster to be performed, more availability, and does not require contrast, unlike MRI. However, ultrasound is operator-dependent, and interpretation of ultrasound data is therefore variable [20].

CT- scan (Computed Axial Tomography) has a sensitivity of 32–80% in the evaluation of CC and a parametrial invasion sensitivity of 17–100% with a mean of 64% in CC. Specificity is 50–100%, with a mean of 81%. The VPP to evaluate nodal involvement is 51–65%, with a VPN of 86–96% and a sensitivity of 31–65% [21]. However, Innocenti et al. reported that transvaginal ultrasound had a higher sensitivity for detecting parametrial infiltration than surgical staging (78% vs 50%, $p = 0.06$) [22, 23].

Excretory urography is the only imaging tool that is recommended for diagnosing ureteral obstruction according to the FIGO. It is mandatory for all patients except those in early stages IA1 to IB1. Its use requires intestinal preparation, proper renal function, and the use of contrast agents, and it is thus a very expensive method that is more time-consuming and takes a longer time to yield results than other methods. Nonetheless, no recent studies have supported the use of the ultrasound as an alternative imaging tool for detecting ureteral obstructions or hydronephrosis [24].

The advantages of the pyelogram are that it allows for an intermediate visualization of the whole urinary system, the urinary tract and the parenchyma, and presents the possibility of allowing the identification of interrelationships, such as those between the cup and the renal papilla, ureter alterations or those in the ureteric mucosa, and the presence of fistulae [25]. Its disadvantages include the following: it uses ionizing radiation and contrast, it is more expensive than ultrasound, its precision depends on renal function, it has a low definition for observing minimal lesions, and it provides a poor characterization of renal masses. Generally, this imaging method is not indicated for CC patients because ultrasound, CT-scan and MRI provide a better evaluation and higher precision [25].

Chest X-ray is used to evaluate pleural effusions and metastatic disease to the lung parenchyma in stage IVB patients. Although it does not have the specificity of chest CT-scan, it has a lower cost and is available in more hospital units [21].

In 2015, Devine proposed a CC staging system that was based on MRI findings, as follows [26]:

Stage I: Tumors in microinvasive stage IA are not observed in MRI, although they can be detected as early reinforcement foci in dynamic contrast images.

Stage II: Tumor invasion towards the vagina can be observed as T2 hyperintensity. It interrupts the vaginal walls, which are normally hypointense. It is important to keep in mind that physical exploration is more precise than MRI for observing vaginal fornices, and MRI is superior to gynecological exploration for detecting parametrial invasion (sensitivity, 69% and specificity, 93%). The precision of physical exploration is 50%.

Stage III: The internal obturator, the levator ani, and the piriform muscles show hyperintense infiltration when a tumor is involved.

Stage IV: When there is invasion into adjacent organs, a separation plane loss can be observed in the fat between the cervix and the bladder or the rectum. The abnormally high signal intensity in the vesical wall is an indicator of tumor involvement, but is confirmed with cystoscopy as a bullous edema.

When extrapelvic retroperitoneal lymph node enlargements are identified using CT or MRI, a guided biopsy is recommended to confirm the findings and better planning the treatment regimen.

The sensitivity (66.6%) and specificity (98%) of MRI are higher than the rates for gynecological exploration for local disease, also has a 50% sensitivity and 96.8% specificity to detect metastasis to the pelvic nodes, and 66.6% sensitivity and 100% specificity for paraortic nodes [27]. Detecting metastasis to lymph nodes using MRI is based upon size, including a 1 cm or larger axis diameter. Larger nodes are generally reactive, while smaller ones can contain neoplastic activity microscopic foci.

PET and PET/CT are the most accurate diagnostic methods that can be used to evaluate exptrapelvic disease in locally advanced CC. Their high rate of true-positive results suggests that surgical staging is unnecessary when using PET-CT, when there is high uptake in the para-aortic nodes. The para-aortic node involvement false positive rate is 12%, and these cases are mainly attributed to nodal disease of 5 mm or less. If we only consider the patients with pelvic uptake, the para-aortic node false negative rate is 22% [28] However, when evaluating hepatic metastasis, there is a higher sensitivity and specificity in PET/MRI or even MRI over PET/CT [29]. In spite of its actual importance, surgical staging of the retroperitoneal nodes is highly relevant because it allows us to more accurately detect pelvic or para-aortic metastases , improving survival rates when more radical treatment is advised.

In 2004, 531 new cases of invasive cancer were registered in the INCan's records. The resulting clinical stage distribution was as follows: CSI: 19%, CSII: 40%, III: 24%, IV: 5%, and 11%. Patients were not classified according to any previous treatment. These results show that there is a tendency to diagnose in less advanced stages, thanks to screening and prevention methods that have recently gained recognition.

8.7 Conclusions

Cervical Cancer staging is performed in a clinical setting because it requires basic tools that can be used in any hospital clinic throughout the world. Proposing a universal classification system would allow the establishment of a common language for the international medical community. However, histopathological staging is necessary to widen the available sources of information and to assess patient prognoses. Imaging methods are mainly helpful in patients in advanced disease stages or patients who are recurrent. Hence, it is important to plan more accurate therapeutic strategies as a function of each patient's stage.

References

1. Galgano MT, Castle PE, Atkins KA, Brix WK, Nassau SR, Stoler MH. Using biomarkers as objective standards in the diagnosis of cervical biopsies. Am J Surg Pathol. 2010;34(8):1077–87. doi:10.1097/PAS.0b013e3181e8b2c4.
2. Schlecht NF, Platt RW, Duarte-Franco E, Costa MC, Sobrinho JP, Prado JCM, Ferenczy A, Rohan TE, Villa LL, Franco EL. Human papillomavirus infection and time to progression and regression of cervical intraepithelial neoplasia. J Natl Cancer Inst. 2003;95(17):1336–43. doi:10.1093/jnci/djg037.
3. De Palo G. Colposcopía y patología del tracto genital inferior. 2nd ed. Buenos Aires: Panamericana; 1997.

4. Massad LS, Einstein MH, Huh WK, Katki HA, Kinney WK, Schiffman M, Solomon D, Wentzensen N, Lawson HW. ASCCP consensus guidelines conference (2013) 2012 updated consensus guidelines for the management of abnormal cervical cancer screening tests and cancer precursors. J Low Genit Tract Dis. 2012;17(5 Suppl 1):S1–S27. doi:10.1097/LGT.0b013e318287d329.
5. Cox JT. Human papillomavirus testing in primary cervical screening and abnormal Papanicolaou management. Obstet Gynecol Surv. 2006;61(6 Suppl 1):S15–25. doi:10.1097/01.ogx.0000221011.01750.25.
6. Lörincz AT, Richart RM. Human papillomavirus DNA testing an adjunct to cytology in cervical screening programs. Arch Pathol Lab Med. 2003;127(8):959–68. doi:10.1043/1543-2165.
7. Bornstein J, Bentley J, Bösze P, Girardi F, Haefner H, Menton M, Perrotta M, Prendiville W, Russell P, Sideri M, Strander B, Tatti S, Torne A, Walker P. 2011 colposcopic terminology of the International Federation for Cervical Pathology and Colposcopy. Obstet Gynecol. 2012;120(1):166–72. doi:10.1097/AOG.0b013e318254f90c.
8. Centers for Disease Control and Prevention (CDC). Recommendations on the use of quadrivalent human papillomavirus vaccine in males – Advisory Committee on Immunization Practices (ACIP) 2011. MMWR Morb Mortal Wkly Rep. 2011;60(50):1705–8.
9. Di Saia P, Creasman WT. Clinical gynecologic oncology. 8th ed. Philadelphia: Elsevier; 2012.
10. Wiebe E, Denny L, Thomas G. Cancer of the cervix uteri. Int J Gynecol Obstet. 2012;119(S2):S100–9. doi:10.1016/S0020-7292(12)60023-X.
11. Pecorelli S, Zigliani L, Odicino F. Revised FIGO staging for carcinoma of the cervix. Int J Gynaecol Obstet. 2009;105(2):107–8. doi:10.1016/j.ijgo.2009.02.009.
12. Tse KY, Ngan HY. The role of laparoscopy in staging of different gynaecological cancers. Best Pract Res Clin Obstet Gynaecol. 2015;29(6):884–95. doi:10.1016/j.bpobgyn.2015.01.007.
13. Van Meurs H, Visser O, Buist MR, Ten Kate FJ, van der Velden J. Frequency of pelvic lymph node metastases and parametrial involvement in stage IA2 cervical cancer: a population-based study and literature review. Int J Gynecol Cancer. 2009;19(1):21–6. doi:10.1111/IGC.0b013e318197f3ef.
14. Landoni F, Maneo A, Colombo A, Placa F, Milani R, Perego P, Favini G, Ferri L, Mangion C. Randomised study of radical surgery versus radiotherapy for stage Ib-IIa cervical cancer. Lancet. 1997;350:535–40. doi:10.1016/s0140-6736(97)02250-2.
15. Chu KK, Chang SD, Chen FP, Soong YK. Laparoscopic surgical staging in cervical cancer--preliminary experience among Chinese. Gynecol Oncol. 1997;64(1):49–53. doi:10.1006/gyno.1996.4527.
16. Gallup DG (2008) The spread and staging of cervical cancer. Glob Libr Women's Med. ISSN 1756–2228. doi:10.3843/GLOWM.10231. http://www.glowm.com/section_view/heading/The%20Spread%20and%20Staging%20of%20Cervical%20Cancer/item/231
17. Gospodarowicz M, Brierley J, O'Sullivan B. Principles of cancer staging for clinical obstetrics and gynecology. Best Pract Res Clin Obstet Gynaecol. 2015;29(6):767–75. doi:10.1016/j.bpobgyn.2015.05.003.
18. Somashekhar SP. Does debulking of enlarged positive lymph nodes improve survival in different gynaecological cancers? Best Pract Res Clin Obstet Gynaecol. 2015;29(6):870–83. doi:10.1016/j.bpobgyn.2015.04.010.
19. Balleyguier C, Sala E, Da Cunha T, Bergman A, Brkljacic B, Danza F, Forstner R, Hamm B, Kubik-Huch R, Lopez C, Manfredi R, McHugo J, Oleaga L, Togashi K, Kinkel K. Staging of uterine cervical cancer with MRI: guidelines of the European Society of Urogenital Radiology. Eur Radiol. 2011;21(5):1102–10. doi:10.1007/s00330-010-1998-x.
20. Moloney F, Ryan D, Twomey M, Hewitt M, Barry J. Comparison of MRI and high-resolution transvaginal sonography for the local staging of cervical cancer. J Clin Ultrasound. 2015; doi:10.1002/jcu.22288.
21. Siegel CL, Andreotti RF, Cardenes HR, Brown DL, Gaffney DK, Horowitz NS, Javitt MC, Lee SI, Mitchell DG, Moore DH, Rao GG, Royal HD, Small Jr W, Varia MA, Yashar CM, American

College of Radiology. ACR appropriateness criteria pretreatment planning of invasive cancer of the cervix. J Am Coll Radiol. 2012;9(6):395–402. doi:10.1016/j.jacr.2012.02.021.
22. Alcázar JL, Arribas S, Mínguez JA, Jurado M. The role of ultrasound in the assessment of uterine cervical cancer. J Obstet Gynecol India. 2014;64(5):311–6. doi:10.1007/s13224-014-0622-4.
23. Innocenti P, Pulli F, Savino L, Nicolucci A, Pandimiglio A, Menchi I, Massi G. Staging of cervical cancer: reliability of transrectal US. Radiology. 1992;185(1):201–5.
24. Vanderpuye V. Renal sonography in the diagnosis of renal obstruction or hydronephrosis in patients with cervical cancer. J Clin Ultrasound. 2002;30(7):424–7. doi:10.1002/jcu.10092.
25. Dalla Palma L. What is left of i.v. urography? Eur Radiol. 2001;11(6):931–9. doi:10.1007/s003300000080126.
26. Devine C, Gardner C, Sagebiel T, Bhosale P. Magnetic resonance imaging in the diagnosis, staging, and surveillance of cervical carcinoma. Semin Ultrasound CT MR. 2015;36(4):361–8. doi:10.1053/j.sult.2015.05.004.
27. Bourgioti C, Chatoupis K, Rodolakis A, Antoniou A, Tzavara C, Koutoulidis V, Moulopoulos LA. Incremental prognostic value of MRI in the staging of early cervical cancer: a prospective study and review of the literature. Clin Imaging. 2015;40(1):72–8. doi:10.1016/j.clinimag.2015.09.012.
28. Gouy S, Morice P, Narducci F, Uzan C, Gilmore J, Kolesnikov-Gauthier H, Querleu D, Haie-Meder C, Leblanc E. Nodal-staging surgery for locally advanced cervical cancer in the era of PET. Lancet Oncol. 2012;13(5):e212–20. doi:10.1016/S1470-2045(12)70011-6.
29. Queiroz MA, Kubik-Huch RA, Hauser N, Freiwald-Chilla B, von Schulthess G, Froehlich JM, Veit-Haibach P. PET/MRI and PET/CT in advanced gynaecological tumours: initial experience and comparison. Eur Radiol. 2015;25(8):2222–30. doi:10.1007/s00330-015-3657-8.

Chapter 9
Imaging in Cervical Cancer

Yolanda Villaseñor-Navarro, Irlanda Pacheco-Bravo, Juan Armando Reyes-Pérez, Guinevere Virginia López-Tecamachaltzi, Francisco Osvaldo García-Pérez, Roberto Alejandro Cruz-Morales, and Carlos Martín Galindo-Sarco

Abstract Cervical cancer (CC) is diagnosis based on histopathological analysis. Although cancer staging is performed clinically, using the International Federation of Gynecology and Obstetrics (FIGO) criteria, cancer staging systems have been shown to be deficient for the examination of prognostic factors of CC, including tumor size and infiltration of the parametria or pelvic wall, as well as for the evaluation of nodal metastases. In this regard, imaging methods are considered crucial in the assessment of CC, as imaging data complement the information obtained from a clinical examination.

Ultrasound has a limited role in CC staging; it is inadequate for assessing nodal status or pelvic wall involvement. Tomography is used to evaluate adenopathies, define the extent of disease progression, assess metastasis, plan radiotherapy, and guide percutaneous biopsy. Magnetic resonance imaging (MRI) has been established to be superior for the characterization of lesions and local extension of disease. The main indications for 18F-FDG positron emission tomography-computed tomography (PET-CT) are initial staging (determination of locoregional nodal involvement and extrapelvic extension), evaluation of the response to therapy and detection of recurrence.

Keywords FIGO • Staging • Recurrence • Tomography • Magnetic resonance imaging • PET-CT

Y. Villaseñor-Navarro, MD • I. Pacheco-Bravo, MD (✉)
J.A. Reyes-Pérez, MD • G.V. López-Tecamachaltzi, MD
F.O. García-Pérez, MD • R.A. Cruz-Morales, MD
C. Galindo-Sarco, MD
Department of Radiology, Instituto Nacional de Cancerología-México,
Av. San Fernando No 22, Col. Sección XVI, Mexico City, Mexico, 14080
e-mail: drairlandapacheco@hotmail.com

J.G. de la Garza-Salazar et al. (eds.), *Cervical Cancer*,
DOI 10.1007/978-3-319-45231-9_9

9.1 Introduction

Given its epidemiological features, cervix cancer is still diagnosis based on a clinical examination, despite an error rate of up to 32% in stage IB patients and up to 65% in stage III patients according to the International Federation of Gynecology and Obstetrics (FIGO). Clinical staging has been shown to be unsuitable for the evaluation of prognostic factors, such as invasion of the parametria and pelvic wall, tumor size, and locoregional and distant nodal metastases [1].

Cervical Cancer (CC) staging is fundamental for treatment planning, and this process implies a reliable, practical and reproducible staging method that facilitates the assessment of the treatment response, prediction of prognosis, and exchange of information among different oncological treatment centers. Magnetic resonance imaging (MRI) is an imaging modality that plays a predominant role in the evaluation of disease extension and spread [2].

Recent studies have reported discrepancies between clinical evaluation results and MRI data; for instance, the characteristics endocervical lesions are often conflicting, with an underestimation of the tumor size based on the clinical examination compared to the tumor size based on MRI. In general, the accuracy of MRI in estimating the tumor size is 93%, while the accuracy of clinical staging is less than 60% [3].

The revised FIGO staging guidelines recommend performing computed tomography (CT) or MRI whenever such an imaging method is available. The use of CT is unsuited for local staging but is highly useful for detecting extrauterine affection, including nodal affection, fistula, or distant disease. Conversely, MRI provides high-contrast resolution of soft tissue and enables the clear definition of the local extension of the primary tumor and metastatic lesions [4].

Currently, MRI has no defined indication in stage IA patients, as stage IA cancer is by definition a microscopic disease that is undetectable on MRI. Thorax radiography (TR) and PET are considered for patients with distant disease. Early stage (IIA1 and IB1) CC patient treatment includes surgery; thus, it is crucial to identify tumor extension beyond cervix in order to plan the course chemotherapy and radiotherapy for these patients.

9.2 Technical Recommendations Concerning Cervical Cancer Assessment Using Different Diagnostic Tools

9.2.1 Ultrasound

This method is affordable, non-invasive, and widely used in different studies and treatment centers. Hence, ultrasound has gained popularity for CC analysis during the last two decades. Reports by Fisherova and Testa have described its high

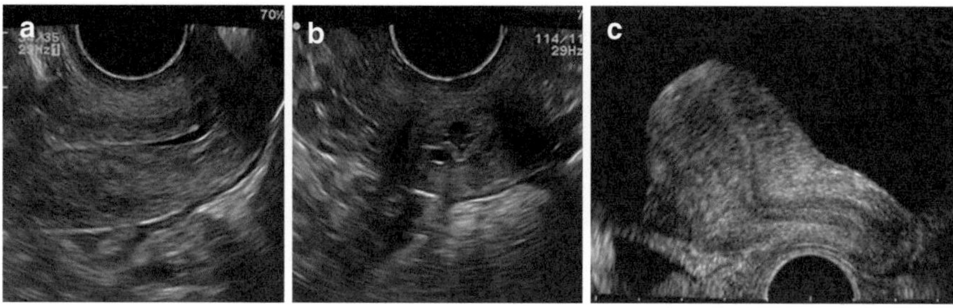

Fig. 9.1 Normal appearance of cervix by transvaginal ultrasound, sagittal axis (**a**) and axial axis (**b**), transrectal ultrasound of the uterus and cervix (**c**)

sensitivity and specificity in the detection of primary lesions as well as locoregional extension [5, 6].

In the study of this type of neoplasia, tone must combine abdominal and pelvic suprapubic ultrasound to search for adenopathies. Additionally, transvaginal ultrasound and transrectal ultrasound are needed to evaluate local extension and Doppler color ultrasound is applied to assess, tumor angiogenesis in vivo in a non-invasive manner [7].

To achieve high accuracy using ultrasound, it is recommended to consider three variables: the operator, who needs some degree of experience; a high-resolution ultrasound system equipped with multifrequency convex and endocavitary transducers that is capable of color, spectral and power Doppler imaging. Additionally, the ultrasound data must be stored as static images or video for post-procedural analysis. Finally, during each evaluation, the patient's habitus and general conditions must be considered to perform a complete assessment [8].

Transvaginal exploration is the optimal approach to the study of the uterus, as this approach adequately locates the anatomy, the annexes, and the pelvic peritoneum [8]. Cervix-dependent lesions are identified as non-compressible lesions that can vary in morphology in relation to their growth pattern (exophytic or endophytic). A color Doppler system enables the identification of cervix-dependent lesions based on a notable increase in their vascularity [9].

After detection and measurement of the orthogonal diameters of a tumor, stromal infiltration is evaluated (classified as one-third, two-thirds, or complete invasion), and tumor extension to anterior, lateral, or posterior parametria is explored. Parametrial invasion is detecting using color Doppler imaging, which facilitates the discrimination of vascular structures from tumoral tisssue [9].

The transrectal approach is beneficial to patients with an intact hymen, with stenotic vagina, with previous brachytherapy; the main indication of this approach in patients with CC is the evaluation of advanced disease extending to the parametrium, rectum, and vagina (Fig. 9.1) [8].

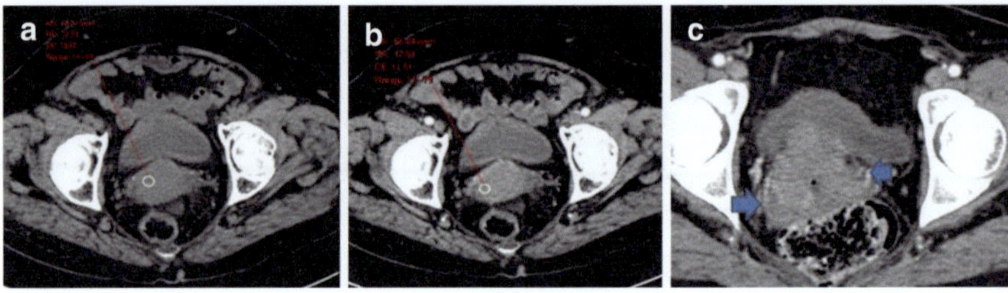

Fig. 9.2 Axial images in CT in single phase (**a**) and contrast phase (**b**) in the same patient, the cervix is enlarged whithout enhancement; other patient (**c**) with a tumor larger and with heterogeneous enhancement, the arrows point the tumor with parametrial extension

9.2.2 Computed Tomography

Among its different methods, CT is widely available and provides images with high spatial resolution within a short period. However, even after image reconstruction and contrast medium administration, the resolution of soft tissue remains unsatisfactory.

Small primary CC lesions usually appear isodense compared to the cervix, while larger lesions tend to be hypodense, necrotic and heterogeneous [10]. However, even further extended neoplasias may appear only as an unspecific increase in cervical volume (Fig. 9.2).

It is currently necessary for a patient to ingest 750–1000 ml of hydrosoluble contrast solution; oral contrast medium is useful for discriminating intestinal loops from lesions, particularly in patients with recurrence or distant disease. Subsequently, 120 ml of non-ionic contrast material is injected intravenously through an injector at a rate of 3 ml/s. After a 50 s delay, the images are acquired in a caudo-cephalic direction to observe the uterus and the cervix in their greatest relief. Additionally, a collimation of 5 mm, a table speed of 12.5 mm per rotation, and 3–5-mm-thick reconstructions are suggested [10].

The adequate application of contrast medium and table direction during study acquisition allows for discrimination of the uterine body from the cervix, which shows characteristic secondary zonal relief against the different components of the central glandular mucosa, internal fibromuscular stroma, and external fibroglandular stroma, conferring the uterine body with a "target-like" appearance in axial plane images [11].

9.2.3 Magnetic Resonance Imaging

In the authors' experience in CC patient diagnosis and follow-up at their institute, imaging studies are performed using a 3 T Discovery 750 W imager (General Electric) equipped with a 16-channel superficial antenna, although diagnostic images can also be obtained using a 1.5 T magnet.

Patient preparation includes a 4- to 6-h fast, with the aim of diminishing peristalsis during imaging. The creatinine concentration in serous fluid must be known before deciding whether to administer endovenous contrast. To this end, veins in the forearm fold are preferentially chosen; it is also preferable to administer 20 mg (1 ampule) of hyoscine N-butylbromide 30–40 min before the initiation of imaging [3].

The key to adequate staging with MRI images is on the utilization of sequences that use a field of view (FOV) of 16–24 cm, a slice thickness of 3–5 mm, a base sequence for the evaluation of parametrial invasion of T2, and an imaging plane perpendicular to the longitudinal axis of the cervical canal, especially for imaging of the supravaginal cervix; the protocol duration is 30–40 min [3].

The T2 imaging sequences obtained using the below protocol are produced in the sagittal and oblique planes (acquired perpendicularly to the long cervical canal). The slice thickness is 5 mm, with a 1 mm inter-slice interval. The images are acquired with a 24 cm FOV and a 288 × 288 matrix. Optionally, sequences with fat saturation can be obtained to evaluate lesions showing signal that is distinct from that of the stroma and cervical canal and to evaluate tumor extension to the uterus, parametrium, and adjacent organs [3].

T1 sequences in the oblique plane are obtained using a 5 mm slice thickness, a 1 mm inter-slice interval, and a 320 × 320 matrix. Additionally, Diffusion-weighted imaging (DWI) sequences with a B value of 700 s/mm^2 in the sagittal and oblique planes can be employed. Whenever needed, the apparent diffusion coefficient (ADC) is processed in the work module to evaluate the behavior of the lesions that have greater signal than the remainder of the stroma and to perform quantitative measurements of the area of interest; ADCs less than 1.2×10^{-3} mm^2/s are considered positive as hypointense [3]. In some centers, gel is applied to the vagina for adequate evaluation of the vaginal and cervical fornices; this method is useful in patients with exophytic tumor growth. In our institution, this is not routinely performed because most of the patients do not agree to use it.

9.3 Main Diagnostic Aspects to Evaluate in Each Image Method

9.3.1 Imaging Features Considered in the Detection of Cervix Cancer

The imaging modalities used to evaluate CC extension include excretory urography (EU), barium enema, ultrasound, MRI, and PET. An important goal in CC staging is to discriminate early disease (IA and IB stages) that can be treated with surgical resection from more advanced disease requiring radiotherapy and probably chemotherapy.

Recent studies showed a decrease in the use of EU, barium enema, and lymphangiography and an increase in the use of CT. In spite of its proven superiority over

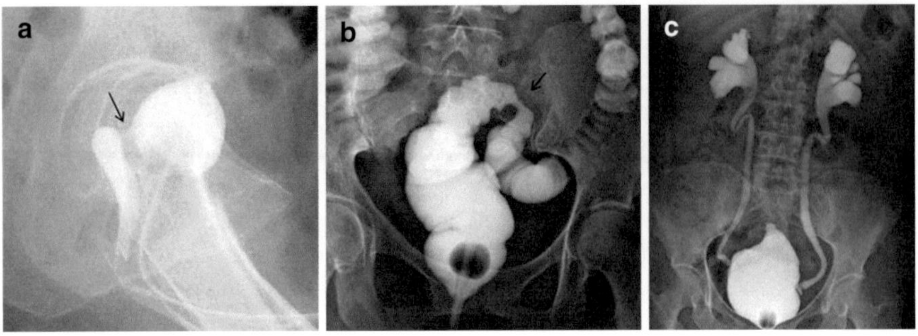

Fig. 9.3 Retrograde Cystogram shows fystula vesico-vaginal (**a**) point with *arrow* in a patient with hysterectomy, in (**b**) barium enema shows a estenosis in the sigmoid post-radiotherapy, retrograde cystogram (**c**) with vesico-ureteral reflux after reinsertion ureteral

other techniques, MRI remains underused in the detection of recurrent disease [5]. Iodine-based and barium-based contrasts are useful in the evaluation of treatment complications, such as fistulae, stenotic zones, vesicoureteral reflux, and ureteral lesion-related hydronephrosis (Fig. 9.3).

9.3.1.1 Ultrasonography

Transvaginal ultrasonography (TVU) has limited utility for cervix cancer tumor evaluation.

Transrectal ultrasonography (TRU) has shown higher accuracy than clinical examination (83% vs. 78%) and, in some studies, even MRI (90% vs. 81%) for the detection of tumors and 99% vs. 95% for the detection of parametrial invasion [5].

TRU has higher accuracy than CT or IRM for the detection of bladder invasion, based upon intact mobility over the uterine neck. However, the main disadvantages of TUR are the inability to evaluate the lateral walls of the pelvis and locoregional nodes [7].

As for the role of echography in the detection of lymphatic nodes in CC, Madsen et al. showed that the sensitivity of this technique is low (23%) but that it has an acceptable positive predictive value (71%) in a series of 109 women.

Fisherova et al. described the ultrasound evaluation technique in women with CC. Detailed evaluation allows for measurement of tumor size to determine the depth of stromal infiltration; the tumor location; parametrial, bladder and rectal involvement; and even the presence of pelvic lymphatic nodes [8].

Doppler Ultrasound in Cervical Cancer

Angiogenesis, the production of new vessels in a specific area, has been demonstrated to be an essential event in tumor growth and progression. In the specific case of CC, angiogenesis has been shown to constitute an independent prognostic factor

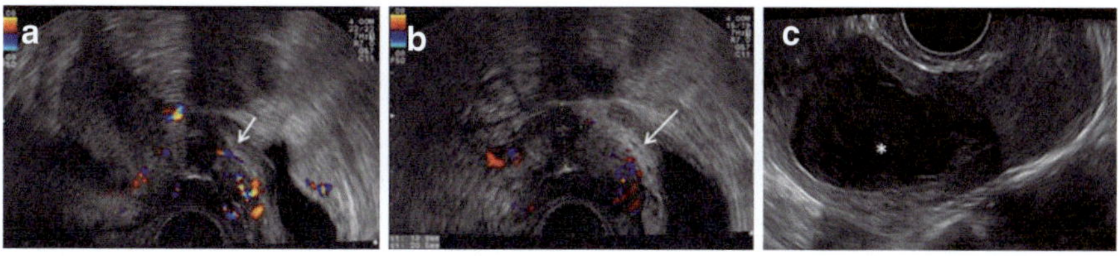

Fig. 9.4 26 years-old women with cervical lesion, sagittal (**a**) and axial (**b**) transrectal ultrasound images show an hypoechoic, solid cervical tumor (*arrow*) with increase in blood flow signals on color Doppler ultrasound, (**c**) sagittal transvaginal ultrasound image, shows a cervical tumor obliterates the endocervix and is present an intrauterine fluid collection, hematometra (*)

and to predict recurrence. The first studies that evaluated blood flow hemodynamics in CC were published in the 90s and were focused on the main cervical supply vessels: the uterine artery and its cervical branches; these studies found that the pulsation index (PI) was lower in healthy women [7].

The first report on an analysis of intratumoral vessels in CC was published by Hsieh et al. in 1995. These authors found that 46.2% of CC patients showed an increase in blood flow signals on color Doppler ultrasound. It was reported that patients with detectable color signals more frequently showed lymphatic node involvement than those who showed no changes on color Doppler imaging (33% vs 5.7%, $p = 0.005$), and detection of color Doppler imaging signals correlated with a higher cell proliferation index. No differences in tumor stage, patient age, clinical staging, histologic type, or the DNA ploidy of the tumor cells were observed (Fig. 9.4) [7].

9.3.1.2 Computed Tomography

CT has an accuracy in CC ranging from 32% to 80%. Its sensitivity and specificity in the detection of parametrial invasion vary from 17% to 100%, with a mean of 64%, and 50% to 100%, with a mean of 81%, respectively. The consensus from the literature is that the value of CT is increased in the most advanced stages of the disease but that CT has limited value (a positive predictive value of 58%) in the evaluation of early parametrial invasion. CT has high accuracy in the detection of advanced disease. However, a recent study by ACRIN® reported that CT has a sensitivity of only 42% for the detection of advanced disease, with ranges of sensitivity and specificity for detecting parametrial invasion of 14–38% and 84–100%, respectively (Fig. 9.5) [10].

The main limitation of CT to local staging is inadequate discrimination between the tumor and normal cervical stromal tissue or parametrial structures (because of tissue isodensity). Thus, CT is chiefly used to evaluate advanced disease and metastasis to lymph nodes. The positive predictive value for nodal affection is between 51% and 65%, with a negative predictive value of 86–96% and a sensitivity range of 31–65%. A finding of tumor size (>1 cm) alone on CT can be a low-sensitivity parameter for malignant adenopathies and can miss microscopic metastases. Other uses of CT are detection of distant metastases, planning of radiotherapy and guidance of intervention procedures (Fig. 9.6) [10, 11].

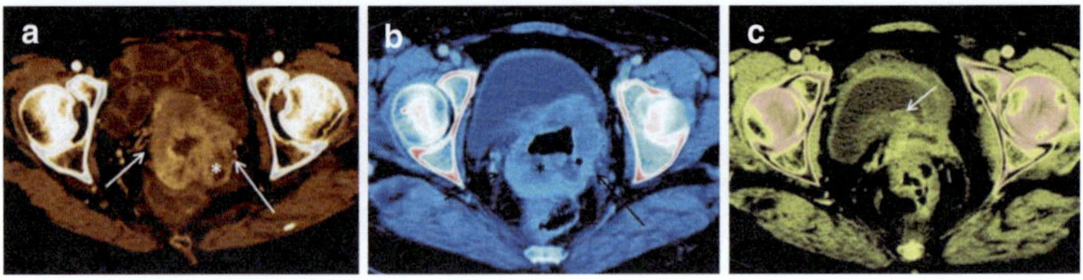

Fig. 9.5 Axial enhanced CT image of the tumors of the 4 cm or more size, in (**a**) women (52 years old), (**b**) and other patient with 46 years old, in both of them: enhancement and hypodense areas and isodensity (*) which represent necrosis and parametrial extension (*arrows*), in the left the enhancement the ligaments uterosacral. In (**c**) shows infiltration to the vesical wall (*) by epidermoid carcinoma in a patient 46 years old and cervical cancer clinical stage IIIB

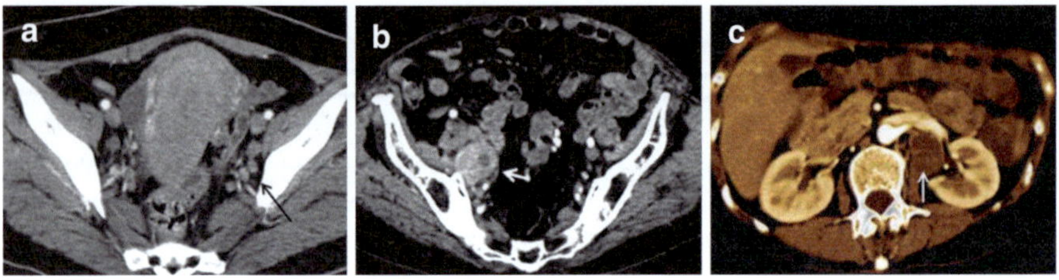

Fig. 9.6 Lymph metastasis (*arrows*) in left ganglionic chain obturator (**a**), right iliac common (**b**) and paraortic chain (**c**), round, with moderate enhancement, in (**b**) and (**c**) we have changes by necrosis

Others have stated that CT has an accuracy of 76–80% for the detection of parametrial invasion, which is identified as eccentric parametrial masses, obliteration of periureteral fat planes and shrinkage of vascular structures. Due to its poor resolution of soft tissue, CT may overestimate parametrial invasion [11].

9.3.1.3 Magnetic Resonance Imaging

MRI offers high-resolution contrast and high-quality contrast in soft tissue, enabling the generation of multiplanar slices and three-dimensional reconstructions with maximum intensity projections. The use of functional MRI parameters, such as flux, temperature, tissue oxygenation, dynamic perfusion, and diffusion, further assist in treatment planning and treatment response evaluation [3].

MRI allows for the determination of the size, location, local extension, and stromal invasion depth of the tumor. Thus, MRI is superior to clinical evaluation, considering that lesions smaller than 5 mm have been found in surgical specimens in 70–94% of the cases.

The accuracy of MRI varies from 75% to 96%; its sensitivity and specificity for parametrial invasion range from 40% to 57% and from 77% to 80%, respectively. In studies comparing MRI with CT in the evaluation of parametrial invasion, MRI was superior; it was also demonstrated that the accuracy of MRI is not improved by the

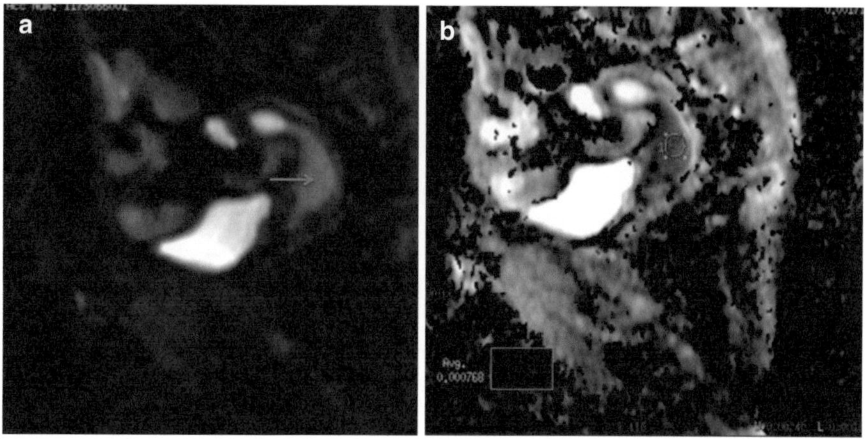

Fig. 9.7 On a sagittal diffusion-weighted MR image (b = 700 sec/mm^2), the tumor (*arrow*) has high signal intensity (**a**) in the apparent diffusion coefficient (ADC) map (**b**) is hypointense with value 0.7×10^{-3} mm/s^2

use of a 3.0-T magnet. The ADC of MRI for CC is inferior to that for normal cervical stroma, providing higher resolution between normal cervical stromal tissue ($1.33–2.0 \times 10^{-3}$ mm^2/s) and cervical tumoral tissue ($0.757–1.11 \times 10^{-3}$ mm^2/s). Applying DWI sequences, which do not require intravenous contrast, adds approximately 2 min to the established protocol (Fig. 9.7) [3].

The addition of DWI examination improves interobserver agreement and is greatly helpful, particularly when T2 sequences are not conclusive or the image acquisition is deficient. Metastatic lymph nodes also show significantly lower ADCs than benign lymph nodes, as observed in abnormal nodes as small as 5 mm. MR spectroscopy with C-choline measurement does not provide any additional benefit. In the evaluation of nodal disease, the sensitivity and specificity ranges of MRI are 30–73% and 93–95%, respectively (similar to those of CT) [3].

9.3.1.4 PET-CT

The prognosis of invasive CC is based on the stage, size, and histologic grade of the primary tumor, as well as on the nodal status; therefore, staging of the disease is essential in treatment determination. PET-CT shows higher sensitivity and specificity than conventional imaging methods for the evaluation of extrapelvic extension and tumor recurrence [12].

The principal indications for 18F-FGD PET-CT are initial staging (the determination of locoregional nodal involvement and extrapelvic extension), evaluation of the response to therapy, and detection of recurrence.

^{18}FGD PET-CT is also useful for tumor margin determination and ureteral obstruction identification, even in the absence of significant dilation. Furthermore, ^{18}FGD PET-CT is useful in the discrimination of residual or recurrent disease from post-radiation fibrosis when tomography findings are inconclusive [13, 14].

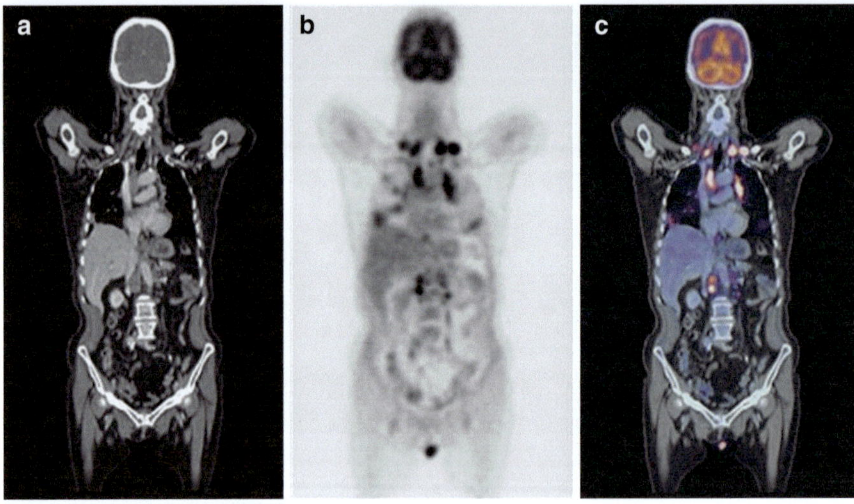

Fig. 9.8. Woman 52 years old. (**a**) CT with contrast, and coronal reconstruction. They identify themselves lymphadenopathies: supraclaviculares, mediastinales and retroperitoneal. (**b**) The hypermetabolism by MIP, shows hypermetabolism in the morphologic study, and additionally is evident the pulmonary alteration. (**c**) Study with fusion of PET/CT with ^{18}FDG

In recent studies, PET-CT showed the highest sensitivity (79–84%) and specificity (95–99%) for nodal staging, compared to 47–50%, and 92–97%, respectively, for tomography, and 56–72% and 90–97%, respectively, for MRI.

Due to its high sensitivity and positive predictive value, PET-CT should be the imaging technique of choice for the evaluation of extrapelvic disease prior to surgical treatment (Fig. 9.8).

PET-CT has been used in some cases to assist in radiotherapy planning because the standard external radiotherapy dose is presumably insufficient to provide locoregional control of advanced disease. Because 18-fluoromisonidazole (F-MISO) labels hypoxic areas, this agent is useful in the planning of intensity-modulated radiotherapy [15, 16].

9.3.2 Imaging Characteristics of Cervix Cancer that Are Useful for Staging

9.3.2.1 Radiological Approach and FIGO Staging

In June 2009, the FIGO staging committee presented a review on CC staging, updating the previous 1998 version. Although the revised FIGO staging system does not include imaging studies in the evaluation of CC, for the first time, the committee recommended imaging techniques, when available, for the assessment of important prognostic factors, such as tumor size, parametrial and/or pelvic lateral wall invasion, adjacent organ invasion, and distant lymph node metastasis. Imaging studies are complementary to clinical evaluation. According to the FIGO, MRI is the optimal option for the assessment of CC of IB1 or higher stage.

On the other hand, young patients bearing small tumors and desiring to preserve fertility may choose a more conservative surgical procedure (trachelectomy). In such cases, MRI is mandatory to determine the tumor size (<2 cm), the cervical length (>2.5 cm), and the distance from the tumor to the internal cervical orifice (>1 cm) [17].

Stage I

The normal cervix has a round shape typically observed in axial oblique images. In enhanced T2 images, three distinct uterine neck images are observed: the mucosa is thin and hyperintense, the stoma is thick and hypointense, and the inner smooth muscle layer shows an intermediate signal. Generally, MRI is not indicated for the evaluation of stage IA CC, as such tumors do not show signal abnormalities.

Stage IB tumors have intermediate to high signal intensity relative to that of the cervical stroma in T2 enhanced images and have variable hyperintensity compared to the stroma on dynamic contrast-enhanced MRI (DCE-MRI). The tumor growth pattern may vary between exophytic, infiltrative, and endocervical [3, 12, 18].

Stage IB tumors are subclassified in IB1 and IB2 based on their size (<4 cm or ≥4 cm, respectively). The tumor size must be measured in two orthogonal directions and in three dimensions. MRI has 90% accuracy in the assessment of tumor size. Accuracy of MRI in tumor size is very important because the clinical examination is not reliable in this regard, especially fir endocervical lesions. The tumor size can also determine the type of treatment; fertility-preserving surgery is possible for tumors smaller than 2 cm, and chemo/radiotherapy may be chosen for tumors larger than 4 cm, even in the absence of parametrial invasion. MRI is helpful in the evaluation of cervical length and of the distance of the tumor from the internal orifice in patients who are candidates for fertility-preserving surgery (Fig. 9.9) [3, 18].

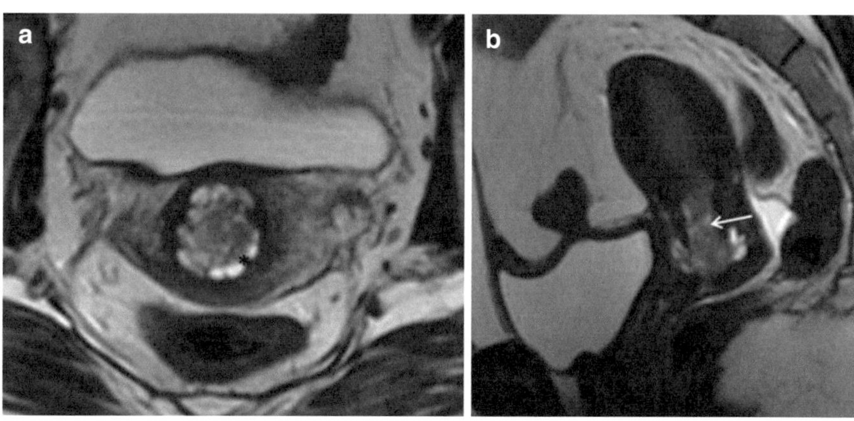

Fig. 9.9 Axial (**a**) and sagittal plane T2-weighted images (**b**). Endocervical lesion in cervix with high and heterogeneous signal in comparison with the cervical stroma; maxim diameter 2 cm (*arrow*). Stage IB1. Naboth cysts (*)

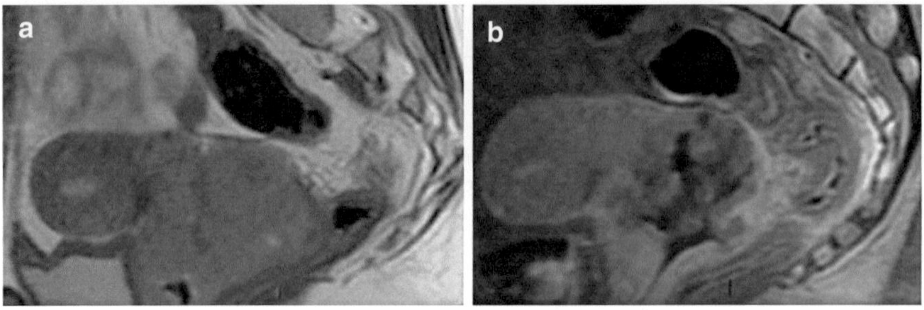

Fig. 9.10 Sagittal plane, T2-weigthed image (**a**) and T1-weigthed imaged after contrast medium administration (**b**) shows an amorphous tumor. The lesion is localized at endocervix with extension at uterus and vagina superior third. Stage IIA2

Stage II

Stage II is defined as the involvement of two thirds of the superior vagina, without parametrial invasion. Vaginal extension is detected as a focal loss of signal towards the vaginal wall in T2-weighted contrast-enhanced sequences. Similarly to stage IB, stage IIA is subclassified into IIA1 and IIA2 based on tumor size (<4 cm and ≥4 cm, respectively). Cervical exophytic tumors can occasionally imitate apparent vaginal extension; however, the hypointense vaginal ring remains intact in such cases.

Invasion to the parametrium may occur in stage IIB CC, and such invasion alters the hypointensity of the cervical stroma without extending to the pelvic lateral wall. The presence of an intact cervical stroma (with a thickness greater than 3 mm) has a very high negative predictive value of 96% for parametrial invasion. Conversely, the positive predictive value of this factor is low (82–86%). Other potential indicators of parametrial invasion include distortion of the uterine neck, lateral displacement of the invaded parametrium, loss of the interphase between the tumor and the parametrium, increased soft tissue signal after gadolinium administration and spread along the uterosacral ligaments (Fig. 9.10) [3, 18].

Mistakes in the interpretation of parametrial invasion can occur in the presence of a previous biopsy with hemorrhage or of peripheral stromal edema, with consequent loss of detectability of the actual tumor margins; other misdiagnosed cases are endometriosis and voluptuous intravaginal tumors. Interruption of the stromal ring in tumors that involve the vaginal portion of the uterine neck together with an intact fornix excludes parametrial invasion.

When the entire thickness of the cervical stroma is interrupted, even in the absence of parametrial invasion, microscopic invasion cannot be excluded. The sensitivity and specificity of IRM for the evaluation of parametrial invasion have been shown to vary from 44% to 100% and from 87% to 93%, respectively [3, 18].

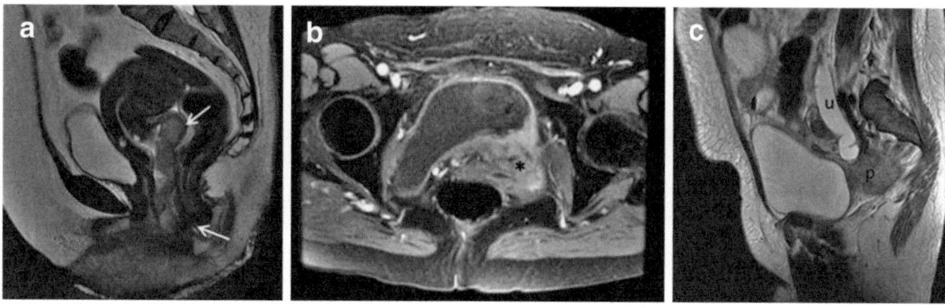

Fig. 9.11 Sagittal plane, T2-weigthed image (**a**), axial plane, T1-weigthed image after contrast medium administration (**b**) and sagittal plane, T2-weigthed image (**c**). Cervical lesion (*) with extension to vagina and left parametrio (*p*) distal ureter (*u*) is expanded

Stage III

Invasion directly to the inferior third of the vagina without extension to the lateral wall of the pelvis is present in stage IIIA CC.

Stage IIIB CC extends through the lateral wall of the pelvis and is defined as the presence of tumor tissue within 3 mm of the lateral pelvic wall muscles. Hydronephrosis caused by obstruction of the ureter and the iliac vessel is also present in stage IIIB disease (Fig. 9.11).

Direct invasion of the bladder or the rectal mucosa is defined as stage IVA CC: interruption of the muscularis propa showing hypointensity and mucosal invasion by a polypoid mass result in high signal intensity along the anterior face of the posterior wall of the bladder. Vesicovaginal or rectovaginal fistula is observed in some cases. Invasion of the bladder is more common than rectal invasion because the area at the back wall of the bladder is exposed and because rectovaginal septum separates the posterior rectal fornix. Bullous edema can mimic bladder invasion but can be distinguished based on the presence of an intact bladder mucosa on DCE-MRI (Fig. 9.13). The sensitivity and specificity of MRI for predicting bladder and/or rectal invasion vary between 83% and 100% and between 88% and 100%, respectively. Stage IVB refers to distant metastases beyond the pelvic lymph nodes to para-aortic and inguinal lymph node, lung, liver and bone tissue (Fig. 9.12) [3, 18, 19].

Another important aspect to evaluate is nodal status. The sensitivity and specificity of MRI for evaluating nodal disease are from 50% to 70% and from 90% to 96%, respectively. MRI using ultra-small paramagnetic iron oxide particles (lymphography) increases the sensitivity and specificity for detecting such metastatic nodes to 90–100% and to 95%, respectively [19].

Corine et al. stated that the DWI sequence is an appropriate tool in MRI for assessing not only primary lesions but also suspicious lymph nodes after chemotherapy. DWI alone has comparable value to PET. Therefore, Corine et al. recommended the use of DWI for evaluation of the pelvis and abdomen.

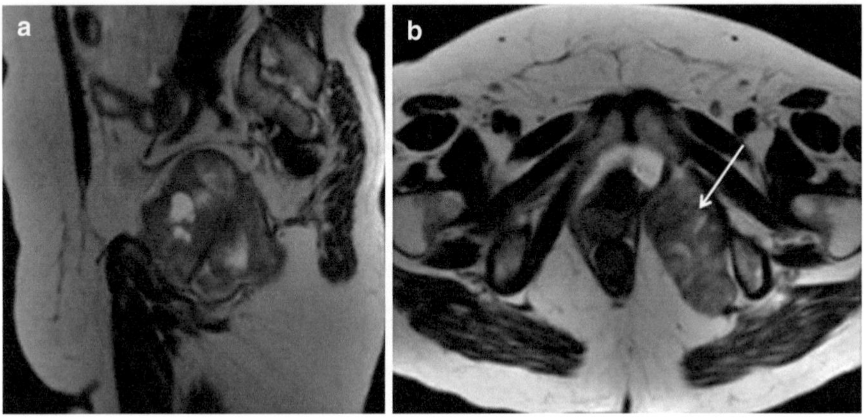

Fig. 9.12 Sagittal (**a**) and (**b**) axial T2-weigthed MR image show heterogeneous lesion with extension to the uterus and left isquiorrectal fossa and internal obturator muscle (*arrow*) and urinary bladder. Stage IV A

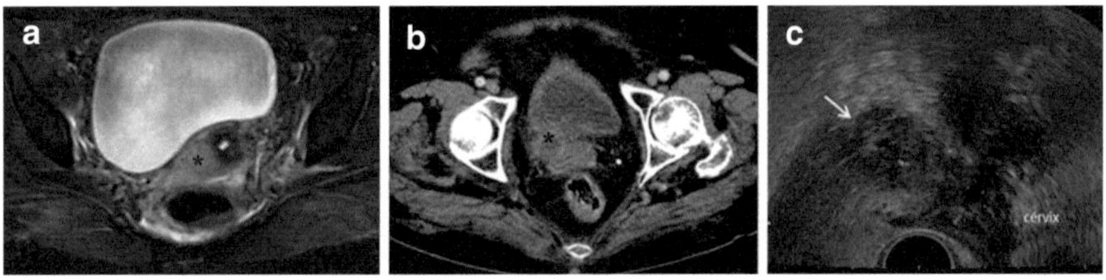

Fig. 9.13 Stage IIIB cervical cancer in 64-years old woman treated with chemotherapy, braquitherapy and teletherapy, shows parametrial recurrence. Axial plane, T2-weighted MR image (a), axial contrast-enhanced CT image (**b**) and trans-rectal ultrasound with biopsy (**c**) (*) *arrow* shows the lesion

The criteria used to diagnose suspicion of lymph node metastasis are a maximum tumor size of the short axis greater than 1 cm (pelvis and abdomen), round shape, irregular margins, signal similar to the primary lesion, and the presence of necrosis [20, 21]. Pannu et al. reported that the maximum dimensions of normal lymph nodes at specific sites are 7 mm in the internal iliac chain, 9 mm in the common iliac chain and 10 mm in the external iliac chain (Fig. 9.6) [22].

Nodal spread is characteristic of CC and commonly occurs in a defined order. The paracervical lymph nodes are the first affected, followed by the parametrial, paraureteral, obturator, hypogastric, external iliac, and common iliac lymph nodes. When the common iliac lymph nodes are affected, further extension to the inguinal, presacral and para-aortic lymph nodes is common. Finally, CC metastasizes to the mediastinal and supraclavicular nodes. When suspicious extrapelvic retroperitoneal lymph nodes are identified, performance of guided biopsy is recommended for confirmation of the histological status and the treatment plan [20, 21].

9.4 Recurrence Evaluation

In 2003, 24,094 new cases of CC were diagnosed in Mexico, of which 38.2% were invasive lesions and 61.7% were in situ carcinomas. In the worldwide literature, 50% of CC patients are diagnosed with stage I disease; the 5-year survival rate for this group is higher than 90%. However, 35% of patients have persistent or recurrent disease after ending their therapy, and 75% of recurrences occur within the 2nd or 3rd year [1, 4, 17].

According to the FIGO, the risk of recurrence depends on the histologic type (e.g., clear cell carcinoma has a worse prognosis than other subtypes), tumor volume, depth of stromal invasion, lympho-vascular invasion, parametrial extension, lymph node involvement at the time of surgery, margin status, and histology.

The vagina and the central pelvis are the most frequent sites of recurrence. Recurrences are asymptomatic in 46–95% of patients. Symptoms include abdominal and pelvic pain, symptoms affecting the legs (pain or lymphedema), vaginal discharge or bleeding, urinary symptoms, cough and weight loss.

The clinical evaluation for CC recurrence includes a complete bimanual and rectovaginal examination of areas that are susceptible to HPV using a mirror (recurrent asymptomatic disease detection rate of 29–75%). Physical examination can detect many cases of recurrent disease in high-risk patients (based on positive pelvic lymph nodes, surgical margins and/or positive parametrium). Exfoliative cytology and physical examination have limitations that, in combination with factors such as obesity and radiotherapy-induced changes, contribute to its low accuracy. Therefore, imaging and laboratory studies are indicated in cases of strong clinical suspicion of recurrence [17].

The imaging modality selected for the evaluation of recurrence should include the entire body to exclude the presence of distant disease. Chest radiography has a detection rate of 20–47%, and its use is recommended in patients who have received radiotherapy.

In pelvic ultrasound studies, the appearance of vaginal recurrence has been described as vascularized solid nodules on color Doppler imaging. The spectra of recurrent tumors have low resistance, high systolic peaks compared with benign lesions. The infiltrated nodes are round and display loss of hilum and a hypoechoic structure. Changes in the appearance of infiltrated nodes may occur due to necrosis and calcification. Partial infiltration of a node produces a heterogeneous echo structure. When nodes show extracapsular invasion, the margins are poorly defined and irregular, and infiltrative growth is observed.

The nodal disease detection rates using ultrasound and CT are low; their main limitation is differentiation between fibrotic and tumor tissue. The use of these imaging methods is based upon the patient symptoms and the physical examination findings and should be individualized.

To evaluate local disease, MRI serves as an optimal method for analyzing disease recurrence. In a site that has been altered by surgery and radiation therapy, MRI is used to differentiate tumor recurrence from fibrosis (Fig. 9.13).

18F-FDG PET-CT has a sensitivity, specificity, and accuracy of 92%, 92.6% and 92.3%, respectively, for the detection of local recurrence as well as lung metastasis, peritoneal spread, paraaortic lymph node spread, and pelvic lymph node metastasis. A complete metabolic response is associated with 3-year disease-free survival. Therefore, women with lesions smaller than 2 cm or with negative lymph nodes do not require follow-up imaging unless they are symptomatic; patients with tumors greater than 2 cm in size with positive lymph nodes are indicated for follow-up via PET-CT13-15.

Approximately 30% of women treated for invasive cervical carcinoma have residual or recurrent disease. Pelvic recurrence is often central, extending from the uterus or cervix after radiotherapy or from the uterine or vaginal bed after surgery. Recurrence can be asymptomatic and can be detected on clinical examination or imaging. Tumor extension may involve the pelvic wall or rectum and can become further complicated by the appearance of a fistula. Recurrence in the pelvic wall can occur via direct extension or metastatic nodal disease, which can manifest as hydronephrosis, edema or pain in the extremities. Patients who received pelvic radiotherapy can have recurrence in extrapelvic sites such as the liver and lungs, despite adequate local control.

CT and MRI play an important role in the detection of recurrence. The accuracy of these modalities in showing recurrence after surgery and/or radiotherapy is 85%. The main limitation of CT and MRI is the differentiation of post-radiation fibrosis from disease recurrence after surgery; the presence of fistulae or rectovesical pouches also limits their usefulness.

MRI has been shown to be more useful than CT after radiotherapy. On MRI, tumor recurrence is detected as a high signal intensity mass within a low signal intensity cervix in the uterine bed or on the wall of the pelvis. Fibrosis usually has low signal intensity on T2 sequences, but high signal intensity areas can also represent inflammation. Thus, inflammation may produce false positives, especially during the first 6 months after radiation therapy. The use of contrast media has not improved the ability of MRI to detect tumor recurrence after radiotherapy, but dynamic imaging sequences have produced better results. Generally, MRI is also preferred for the evaluation of fistulae (Fig. 9.13) [3, 9, 10].

In patients with clinically suspected recurrence, PET-CT has been reported to have a sensitivity of 90.3–92.7% and a specificity of 81–100% for confirming the presence of disease recurrence. The performance of PET-CT on asymptomatic patients has not been shown to improve survival [12, 13].

9.5 The Future of Imaging Methods in the Evaluation of Cervical Cancer

Currently, imaging methods, including tomography, MRI and PET-CT, play a leading role in restaging, response to therapy and treatment failure prognosis in CC.

MRI is especially useful in delineating the extent of the primary tumor to support the planning of radiotherapy. Compared with hybrid PET-CT studies, MRI improves the search for lymphadenopathies with infiltration, enabling a requisite increase in the therapeutic dose [22].

Diffusion sequences have been shown to be useful in assessing the extent of these injuries, responses to therapy and prognosis. Currently, it is considered that the lesion size is ideally evaluated with T2-weighted contrast-enhanced MRI; however, this sequence may be suboptimal in cases of invasive adenocarcinoma, isointense lesions or early stage cancer in which fertility could be preserved. In these cases, considering that the lesions restrict diffusion, these sequences may be useful for disease characterization.

Diffusion MRI sequences can improve the initial staging, facilitating assessment of tumor size, and extrauterine spread of disease. In addition, they can be useful in histologic analysis of CC: the ADC has been suggested to be useful in determining the pathological grade of carcinoma because the ADC represents tumor cell density. The ADC has been reported to be significantly smaller in squamous cell carcinoma than in adenocarcinoma [23].

Considering the recent progress in oncologic PET-CT imaging, it is natural that the search for new applications that combine anatomical and functional imaging, such as PET/MRI fusion, which merges metabolic activity assessment with the spatial resolution of MRI, is promising. Moreover, the efficiency of MRI in local CC staging and the effectiveness of PET in the detection of suspicious lymph nodes and distant disease support the application of PET/MRI fusion. Currently, this hybrid method is limited by its scarce availability and its inherently high cost [24].

Only few studies have demonstrated the effectiveness of PET/MRI in the assessment of gynecological tumors. However, small studies have shown similar effectiveness between PET/MRI and PET-CT in detecting recurrence [24].

References

1. Odicino F, Pecorelli S, Zigliani L, et al. History of the FIGO cancer staging system. Int J Gynaecol Obstet. 2008;101(2):205–10.
2. Okamoto Y, Tanaka YO, Nishida M, et al. MR imaging of the uterine cervix: imaging-pathologic correlation. RadioGraphics. 2003;23(2):425–45.
3. Rauch GM, Kaur H, Choi H, Ernst RD, et al. Optimization of MR imaging for pretreatment evaluation of patients with endometrial and cervical cancer. RadioGraphics. 2014;34:1082–98.
4. Freeman S, Kataoka M, Addley H, et al. The revised FIGO staging system for uterine malignancies: implications for MR imaging. RadioGraphics. 2012;32:1805–27.
5. Fischerova D, Cibula D, Stenhova H, et al. Transrectal ultrasound and magnetic resonance imaging in staging of early cervical cáncer. Int J Gynecol Cancer. 2008;18:766–72.
6. Testa AC, Ludovisi M, Manfredi R, et al. Transvaginal ultrasonography and magnetic resonance imaging for assesment of presence, size and extent of invasive cervical cáncer. Ultrasound Obstet Gynecol. 2009;34:335–44.

7. Alcázar JL, Arribas S, Mínguez JA, Jurado M, et al. The role of ultrasound in the assesment of uterine cervical cáncer. J Obstet Gynaecol India. 2014;64(5):311–6.
8. Fischerova D. Ultrasound scanning of the pelvis and abdomen for staging of gynecologic tumors: a review. Ultrasound Obstet Gynecol. 2011;38(3):246–66.
9. Testa A, Di Legge A, et al. Imaging techniches for the evaluation of cervical cáncer. Best Pract Res Clin Obstet Gynaecol. 2014;28:741–68.
10. Pannu HK, Corl FM, Fishman EK. CT evaluation of cervical cáncer: spectrum of disease. Radiographics. 2001;21(5):1155–68.
11. Yitta S, Hecht EM, Mausner EV, Bennett GL. Normal or abnormal? Demystifying uterine and cervical contrast enhancement at multidetector CT. RadioGraphics. 2011;31(3):647–61.
12. Hildebrandt G, Kodhal R, et al. (18F) fluordeoxyglucose PET/computed tomography in breast cancer and gynecologic cancers, a literature review. PET Clin. 2015;10:89–104.
13. Grant P, Sakellis C. Gynecologic imaging with PET/CT. Semin Nucl Med. 2014;44(6):461–78.
14. Son H, Kositwattanarerk A, Hayes MP, et al. PET/CT evaluation of cervical cancer: spectrum of disease. RadioGraphics. 2010;30(5):1251–68.
15. Tachibana I, Nishimura Y, Shibata T, et al. A prospective clinical trial of tumor hypoxia imaging with 18F-fluoromisonidazole positron emission tomography and computed tomography (F-MISO PET/CT) before and during radiation therapy. J Radiat Res. 2013;54(6):1078–84.
16. Toma-Dasu I, Uhrdin J, Antonovic L, et al. Dose prescription and treatment planning based on FMISO-PET hypoxia. Acta Oncol. 2012;51(2):222–30.
17. Sree H, Alampady S, Srinivasa P. Current concepts in the diagnosis and management of endometrial and cervical carcinomas. Radiol Clin N Am. 2013;51:1087–110.
18. Shaaban. Blodgett. Diagnóstico por Imagen Oncología. Marbán. 2012;Sección 6:726–51.
19. Balleyguier C et al. Staging of uterine cervical cáncer with MRI: guidelines of the European Society of Urogenital Radiology. Eur Radiol. 2011;21:1102–10.
20. Harpreet K, Frank M, Elliot K. CT evaluation of cervical cancer: spectrum of disease. RadioGraphics. 2001;21:1155–68.
21. Welliver M-X, Yuh William TC, et al. Imaging across life span: innovations in imaging and therapy for gynecologic cáncer. Radiographics. 2014;34(4):1062–81.
22. Sunita D, Meenkski T, et al. Diffusion weighted imaging in gynecologic tumors: diagnostic imaging and potential pitfalls. Radiographics. 2014;34(5):1393–416.
23. Sasan P, Andres K, et al. clinical oncologic aplications of PET/MRI: a new horizon. Am J Med Mol Imaging. 2014;4(2):202–12.
24. Bashir U, Mallia A, et al. PET/MRI in oncologic imaging: state of the art. Diagnostics. 2015; doi:10.3390/diagnostics5030333.

Chapter 10
Primary Surgical Treatment of Cervical Cancer

Aarón González-Enciso, Salim Abraham Barquet-Muñoz, and Milagros Pérez-Quintanilla

Abstract Surgery is still the standard treatment for early stage cervix cancer. This form of cancer generally implies the need for a radical hysterectomy with a bilateral pelvic lymphadenectomy (BPL). Patients who benefit from this procedure include those bearing tumors smaller than 4 cm that are confined to the cervix. The goal of these procedures is to resect the entire tumor and to establish, based on pathological analysis, whether the patient possesses pathological risk factors that support adjuvant radiotherapy and chemotherapy. However, surgical treatment is not exempt from complications, which have been reported during the intraoperative period in approximately 2% of cases and during the late postsurgical phase in up to 20%of cases. Over the decades, new minimally invasive methods have been implemented to decrease the appearance of these complications while yielding the same oncological results. Additionally, the sentinel lymph node biopsy in cervical cancer is beginning to be incorporated as an alternative to BPL. Moreover, new techniques that preserve fertility are now used in strictly selected young women who would like to have more children.

Keywords Radical hysterectomy • Laparoscopy • Fertility preservation • Sentinel ganglion • Cervix cancer

A. González-Enciso, MD (✉) • S.A. Barquet-Muñoz, MD • M. Pérez-Quintanilla, MD
Gynecologic Tumors Deparment, Instituto Nacional de Cancerología-México,
Av. San Fernando No 22, Col. Sección XVI, Mexico City, Mexico, 14080
e-mail: agencisonco@hotmail.com

J.G. de la Garza-Salazar et al. (eds.), *Cervical Cancer*,
DOI 10.1007/978-3-319-45231-9_10

10.1 Introduction

Cancer of the cervix is one of the most common malignancies among women, especially in developing countries. Among the therapeutic modalities for cervix cancer, surgery is still the standard treatment, especially in early stage cancer, which displays recovery rates of approximately 90%. However, one must bear in mind that surgery is not exempt from complications or morbidities in both the short term and the long term. Currently, thanks to technological and medical advances, it is possible to perform surgical procedures with reduced morbidity. The current chapter presents the indications, techniques, and complications of cervix surgery, as well as techniques that are currently performed to decrease patient morbidity.

10.2 Indications for a Surgical Procedure

The appropriateness of a surgical procedure to resolve cervical cancer depends on the clinical stage (CS) of the disease, the desire to preserve fertility, the clinical condition of the patient, and resource availability. It is thus necessary to individualize the radicality of the surgical treatment to maximize effectiveness and to minimize the morbidity and, consequently, the patient's quality of life [1].

In 2009, the International Federation of Gynecology and Obstetrics (FIGO) established a clinical staging system for cancer of the cervix, classifying cervical cancer into early and advanced disease [2]. According to the consensus from the international literature, the term early clinical stage (ECS) denotes invasive carcinoma strictly confined to the cervix with a diameter of less than 4 cm without parametrial affection. The stages IA1, IA2, IB1, and IIA1 (smaller than 4 cm in diameter) are considered ECS.

The treatment of choice for ECS cervical cancer is radical hysterectomy, although the clinical indications are not uniform: this procedure is suitable for up to stage IB1 disease, beyond which radical hysterectomy has not been associated with excellent oncological results.

Currently, optimal surgical management of early stage cervical cancer patients consists of decreasing morbidity without compromising the oncological result.

Between 25% and 40% of the patients diagnosed with early stage cervix cancer are of reproductive age or have future pregnancy plans; hence, alternative, less radical treatment options must be considered for these patients [3].

The treatment should be addressed in a systematic manner according to the size of the tumor and the desire to preserve fertility.

10.2.1 Fertility-Sparing Surgery

Fertility-sparing surgery must only be considered for a highly restricted group of patients who satisfy not only oncological criteria but also a set of prenatal and perinatal criteria (Table 10.1).

Table 10.1 Ideal requirements for fertility-sparing surgery in cervical cancer

Confirmed cervical cancer: squamous, adenocarcinoma, or adenosquamous
FIGO stage IA1 with PLV, IA2, or IB1
Desire to preserve fertility
Tumor size < 2 cm
No history of infertility
Limited endocervical affection
Possibility for resection with margins > 5 mm
Cervical length > 1 cm
Negative pelvic ganglia

Microinvasive disease, or stage IA1 disease without lymphovascular permeation (LVP), has an incidence of lymphatic metastasis below 1%; thus, cervical conization is the standard treatment in stage IA1 cervical cancer patients with reproductive wishes. Management of stage IA1 disease with LVP is controversial; the recommendation in most publications is cervical conization with BPL and assessment of sentinel lymph node biopsy.

Patients with stage IA2 or IB1 cervical cancer with a tumor size of less than 2 cm and a favorable histological lineage (epidermoid, adenocarcinoma, or adenosquamous) can be candidates to conservative surgery. Radical trachelectomy with BPL by laparoscopy or by laparotomy with or without sentinel lymph node biopsy in cervical cancer is a treatment option [4]. Wethington et al. reported in a systematic review that the pregnancy rate of patients treated with radical trachelectomy was 52%.

10.2.2 Non-fertility-Preserving Surgery

In women without surgical, technical or medical contraindications and without a desire to preserve fertility, extrafascial, or type A, hysterectomy is the standard treatment for stage IA1 cervical cancer without LVP. In patients with stage IA1 with LPV or stage IA2 disease, radical hysterectomy with BPL, or type B hysterectomy, is the standard treatment option; para-aortic lymphadenectomy (PAL) should also be considered in patients who are suspected to have lymphatic disease in the para-aortic lymph nodes [4].

In patients with stage IB1 disease or with stage IIA1 disease without contraindications, radical hysterectomy with BPL with or without PAL, or type C hysterectomy, is the first treatment option [4].

In young women, it is convenient to preserve the ovaries whenever possible. Radiotherapy shows similar outcome rates to surgery; however, surgical treatment is preferred for young women, given its associated benefits for quality of life, such as the preservation of ovary function, vaginal integrity, and increased lubrication and vaginal elasticity compared to radiotherapy [5].

10.3 Principles of the Surgical Technique

In 1912, Wertheim was the first to popularize the radical hysterectomy technique; after the description of more than 500 cases, associated with a 10% mortality rate, this technique has evolved.

Subsequently, at Harvard Medical School, Meigs modified the radical hysterectomy technique by including complete parametrial excision with BPL. Then, in 1974, Piver, Rutledge and Smith produced the first hysterectomy classification system (Table 10.2) [6]. In 2008, Querleu and Morrow proposed a new classification system that includes a description of the specific anatomic limits and margins of surgical resection (Table 10.3). The resection limits are factors that influence the patient's quality of life [7].

The first and most important surgical principle to be considered before radical pelvic surgery is an exhaustive understanding of pelvic anatomy (Fig. 10.1). This understanding will decrease the incidence of lesions during the procedure, for example perioperative lesions of the hypogastric nerves during the resection of the dorsal portion of the paracervix, or damage to vessels important for the anatomical variants.

Radical hysterectomy includes removal of the uterus as a block together with the parametrium (cardinal and uterosacral ligaments) and one third or one half of the vagina (Fig. 10.2).

Since 1974, according to the Piver-Rutledge-Smith description (Table 10.2), through 2007, according to the new criteria presented by Hidekazu Okabayashi, up to the 2008 Querleu-Morrow classification (Table 10.3), strict anatomical definitions concerning the preservation of autonomous nerves, fertility preservation, and lateral

Table 10.2 Piver-Rutledge-Smith classification of radical hysterectomy [6]

Subtotal/Supracervical The uterus is removed. The superior portion of the cervix is amputated, and the remnant of the cervix is conserved. The uterosacral ligaments are conserved.
Class I Extrafascial hysterectomy. The fascia of the cervix and the inferior segment of the uterus are removed.
Class II Modified radical hysterectomy. The uterine artery is ligated where it bridges over the ureter, and the cardinal and uterosacral ligaments are cut in half at their insertion to the pelvic wall and the sacrum, respectively. One third of the vagina is cut.
Class III Radical hysterectomy. The uterine artery is ligated at its origin to the superior vesical artery or to the iliac artery. The cardinal and uterosacral ligaments are cut at the pelvic and sacral walls. The superior third of the vagina is resected.
Class IV Radical hysterectomy. The ureter is completely dissected from the vesicouterine ligament, the superior vesical artery is sacrificed, and three fourths of the vagina is resected.
Class V Radical hysterectomy. In addition to the above, a portion of the bladder or the distal ureter is resected, followed by the reimplantation of the ureter to the bladder.

Table 10.3 Radical hysterectomy classification system of Querleu and Morrow (2008) [7]

Type A: Extrafascial hysterectomy or minimal paracervix resection The extent of paracervix resection is medial to the ureter but lateral to the cervix, and the uterosacral and vesicouterine ligaments are not resected. The vaginal resection is minimal, and trachelectomy is not performed. This technique includes palpation and observation, but not mobilization, of the uterus.
Type B: Radical modified hysterectomy or paracervix resection at the level of the ureter **B1**: The paracervix is resected at the level of the ureteral tunnel, the uterosacral and vesicouterine ligaments are partially resected, and the neurological component of the paracervix (caudal to the deep uterine vein) is not resected. At least 10 mm of vagina from the cervix to the tumor is removed. A dissection is performed, and the ureter is lateralized without being mobilized. **B2**: The lateral paracervical ganglia are dissected in addition to the procedures described for B1. The edge between the paracervical and parietal ganglia (iliac and obturator lymph nodes) is defined by the obturator nerve. Using this technique, the uterine artery is preserved.
Type C: Radical hysterectomy or paracervical resection at the junction with the vascular iliac system. The cardinal ligaments are resected from the pelvic wall and the uterosacral ligament is resected at the level of the rectum, including a section of the vesicouterine ligament; a 15–20 mm segment of the vagina or the cervix tumor is removed. The ureter is completely mobilized. **C1**: With preservation of the autonomous nerves. **C2**: Without preservation of the autonomous nerves.
Type D: Laterally extending resection **D1**: The parametrium is resected from the pelvic wall with mobilization of the iliac vessels and with exposition of the sciatic nerve roots. **D2**: The parametrium is resected from the pelvic wall together with hypogastric vessels, muscular structures, and adjacent fascia. The ureter is completely mobilized.

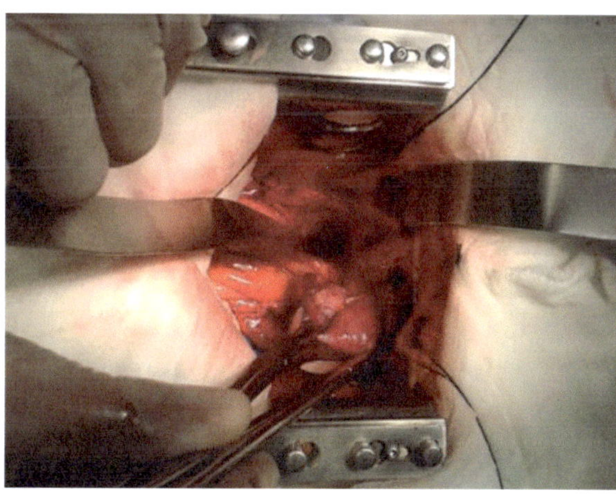

Fig. 10.1 Pararectal and paravesical spaces during a radical hysterectomy. Between both spaces is the parametrium, containing the uterine artery, which is crossed by the ureter

extension are applied to the performance of open, laparoscopic and robotic techniques [8, 9]. The new classification approaches aim to unify traditional concepts and maintain a three-dimentional view of the uterus, the anatomical retroperitoneum, sympathetic innervation and the parasympathetic female pelvis.

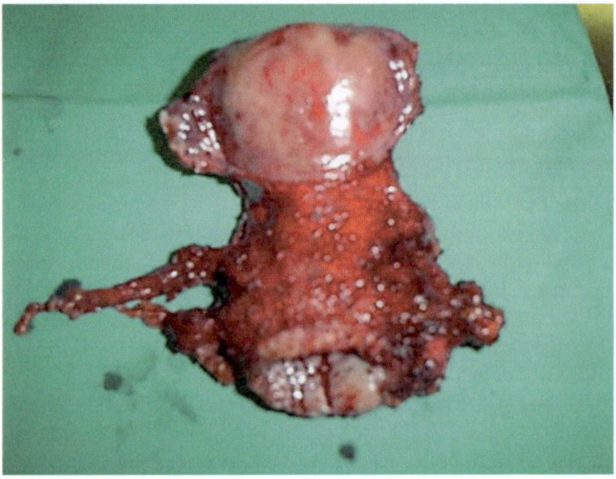

Fig. 10.2 Products of a modified radical hysterectomy. The resected parametrial tissue, uterine artery, and 2 cm of the edge of the vagina are presented

The second surgical principle is radical resection of the parametrium: a decisive parameter for the evaluation of the type of radical hysterectomy. The extent of resection must be defined according to three areas of the parametrium (ventral, dorsal, and lateral) and in three axes (sagittal, frontal, and transverse). These points are described in the Querleu and Morrow classification system, which specifies four types of hysterectomy according to specific anatomical locations. In contrast, the system described by Piver does not distinguish between type II and type III hysterectomy. The main difference lies in the reduction in resection of the vesicouterine ligament, below the ureter, and the dissection in the lateral area of the parametrium. Another difference between these forms of hysterectomy is the performance of uterine artery ligation and pelvic lymphadenectomy [7].

Each step of the procedure must be carefully specified and must have a preoperative and trans-surgical plan for the surgery to succeed. The following must be described.

- The anatomical limits of pelvic ganglionar dissection and the number of lymphatic nodes dissected. Any suspicious lymphatic nodes must be sent for trans-surgical pathological analysis.
- Additional procedures to be performed (bilateral salpingo-oophorectomy or ovarian transposition)
- Type of parametrectomy (B, C1, C2)
- Length of vaginal resection

10.3.1 Bilateral Pelvic Lymphadenectomy

All types of radical hysterectomy include lymph node dissection, which can be classified as level 1, defined as the external and internal iliac lymph nodes (Fig. 10.3); level 2, defined as the common parasacral and iliac lymph nodes; level 3, which corresponds to level 2 and the infra-mesenteric aortic lymph nodes; and level 4, defined as the infra-renal aortic lymph nodes in addition to level 3.

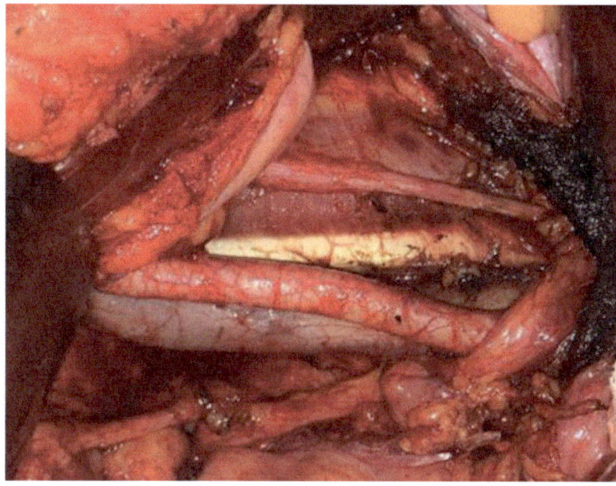

Fig. 10.3 Dissection of the right pelvic lymph nodes. The genitofemoral nerve as well as the iliac external vein and artery crossed by the left ureter are observed

The benefit of pelvic lymphadenectomy has been demonstrated in several retrospective studies showing increased survival and prognostic information after excision of the pelvic lymph nodes with macroscopic or microscopic affection.

In 1996, Benedetti Panici et al. proposed to standardize the radicality of lymphadenectomy for cervical cancer with the purpose of specifying the anatomic limits: cephalic over the common iliac artery bifurcation, caudal to the deep circumflex iliac vein, medial to the superior vesical artery, and lateral to the genitofemoral nerve and the psoas muscle [10].

In a systemic pelvic dissection, between 25 and 35 pelvic lymph nodes are dissected. According to Sakugari, the number of pelvic lymph nodes removed varies from study to study, with the mean between 13 and 56. The European Organization for the Research and Treatment of Cancer (EORTC)-Gynecological Cancer Group (GCG) defined the excision of more than 11 pelvic lymph nodes as an indicator of the quality of pelvic lymphadenectomy [11].

10.3.2 Trachelectomy

In recent decades, there has been an increase in the use of the vaginal trachelectomy with laparoscopic pelvic lymphadenectomy as described in 1994 by Dargent. After that report, several authors have described favorable obstetric and oncologic results in their trachelectomy experience in select patients at early clinical stages, not only using the vaginal approach, but also using the abdominal approach or laparoscopic techniques.

The main goal of trachelectomy is to resect the cervix, 1 or 2 cm of the vagina, the parametrium, and paracervical lymph nodes. This resection is similar to that performed in radical type III or C hysterectomy, exception that in a trachelectomy, the uterine body is conserved. The surgical principles are identical between laparoscopic, open and vaginal abdominal trachelectomy.

During the surgical procedure, the first step before beginning the trachelectomy is to mobilize the ureter; care must be taken in handling the uterine-ovarian pedicle and the uterine horn. The identification of a low-risk group of patients in whom parametrectomy and pelvic lymph nodes dissection can be avoided has been a matter of debate for years; such patients could benefit from a less radical surgery. The concept of the sentinel lymph node biopsy, which is discussed below, emerged from this consideration [1].

10.4 Surgical Complications

Given the anatomic location, the main complications presenting after radical surgery for cervix cancer are those related to nearby structures, such as the bladder, rectum, ureter, and important pelvic vessels.

The main and most documented morbidity involves the urinary tract. Urodynamic changes have been reported after radical hysterectomy; these changes include detrusor muscle hypoactivity, decreased bladder sensation and reduced filling capacity. This morbidity has been reported in 75–85% of patients receiving a type III or C2 hysterectomy. Spontaneous recovery of bladder function is expected within 6–12 months after the surgery. Discomfort, frequently including urgency, urinary incontinence, and bladder emptying difficulties, is reported 6–12 months after the procedure in 30% of patients. Severe bladder dysfunction has been reported in more than 16% of patients [12]. Urinary incontinence is one major complication after radical surgery for cervix cancer. This complication has been observed in 48–53% of women at 6 weeks after the surgical intervention, gradually declining to 30% of patients at 3 months after the surgery [12]. Chuang et al. described detrusor hypoactivity in 85.7% of patients, detrusor hyperactivity in 10.2% and normal function in 4.1% based on follow-up over a period of 6 months to 30 years after the initial treatment [13].

The presence of a vesicovaginal or ureterovaginal fistula after a radical hysterectomy has been reported in 0.9–2.7% of patients [12]. In these cases, the fistula is primarily located in the anterior wall of the vagina. Risk factors of vesical damage, such as hemorrhage, obesity, diabetes, and post-surgical infection, must be considered.

A series of 361 women surgically treated with radical surgery (285 radical hysterectomy, 42 vaginal radical hysterectomy, 30 laparoscopy-assisted radical vaginal hysterectomy, and 4 abdominal radical trachelectomy) revealed intra-operative complications in 6% of the women, transfusion-related complications in 9%, and post-surgical infections in 4% [14].

The extent of anatomic nerve lesions during a radical hysterectomy or trachelectomy plays a crucial role in long-term anorectal dysfunction, such as diarrhea, constipation, fecal incontinence, and flatulence; these complications occur after an extensive dorsal parametrial resection or an extensive colpectomy and are less common, although they can impact a patient's quality of life. Cibula et al. reported significant differences between autonomous nerve-preserving and non-preserving procedures with respect to defecation changes at 6 months after the procedure [15].

Sexual dysfunction often has psychological and functional causes, and anatomic changes play a role in this complication. The current literature is controversial; in women with greater sexual activity, receptivity owing to good vaginal lubrication is achieved when the autonomous nerves are preserved. In addition to bleeding, potential peri- and post-surgical morbidities include the formation of lymph node dissection-related lymphoceles and lymphedema. Lymphoceles are typically incidentally found; they only rarely cause ureteral hydronephrosis or pelvic pain. The incidence of lymphedema has not been specifically studied because of its low incidence after pelvic lymphanedectomy [16].

10.5 Minimally Invasive Approaches

Minimally invasive approaches, such as laparoscopy and robot-assisted surgery, have become more popular over recent decades. These approaches are considered to provide benefits to patients receiving BPL and PAL to treat neoplasias of the cervix without affecting oncological results (Fig. 10.4). No differences in pathological results have been reported between minimally invasive and open surgical approaches. When comparing laparoscopy with open surgery, no difference was found in the size of parametrial resection (1.9 cm versus 1.7 cm, $p = 0.55$), the percentage of patients with negative borders (96% versus 91%, $p = 0.33$), the percentage of patients with lymph node metastasis (26% versus 14%, $p = 0.191$) [17], the 5-year survival rate (92.4% versus 93.6%, $p = 0.29$), or the recurrence rate [18].

The main differences observed for laparoscopy compared to open surgery are a smaller amount of bleeding (55 ml versus 145 ml; $p < 0.01$) [18] and reduced hospitalization time (4 days versus 7 days, $p < 0.01$), although at the expense of longer surgeries (196 min versus 152 min, $p < 0.01$) [18]. Furthermore, the complication rates of these two procedure types are similar.

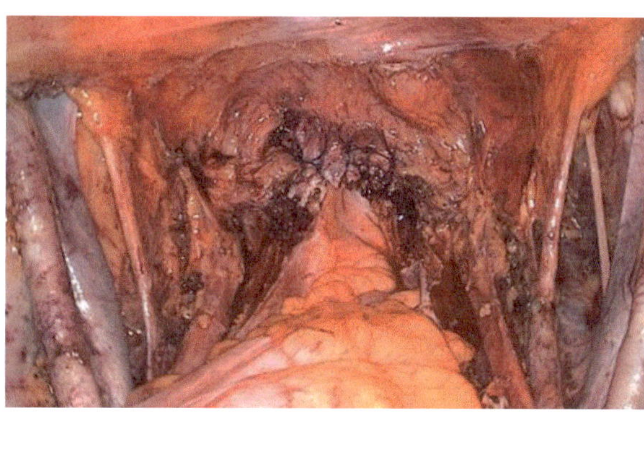

Fig. 10.4 View of the surgical site after a radical hysterectomy with bilateral pelvic lymphadenectomy via laparoscopy in a patient with stage IB1 cervix cancer.

Notably, certain patient groups exhibit better results when treated with a minimally invasive approach. According to Park, the laparoscopic approach has a lower complication rate in obese, elderly women, without sacrificing the oncologic results [19, 20]. Finally, the laparoscopic approach requires formal training and a learning curve of at least 40 procedures to attain a reduction in surgical time (from 307.7 to 266.3 min, $p = 0.022$) or in the complication rate (from 25.7% to 2.9%, $p = 0.013$) [21].

10.6 Oncologic and Obstetric Results of Fertility-Sparing Surgery

The main goal of fertility-sparing surgery is to obtain similar oncologic results to those obtained via radical management of early stage cervix cancer while preserving fertility.

The ideal candidates to undergo a fertility-sparing procedure are cervix cancer patients presenting with histologic types with favorable prognosis at early disease stages, preferably with tumors smaller than 2 cm and without lymph node affection (Table 10.1) [22].

In 1994, Dargent was the first to propose trachelectomy as a fertility-sparing procedure. To date, vaginal, abdominal and laparoscopic approaches of trachelectomy have been described. It is important to always complement this procedure with BPL to rule out lymph node affection. The advantages of the abdominal approach are a larger parametrial resection and a lower recurrence rate, at the expense of a higher rate of early pregnancy loss [16].

The oncological results of fertility-sparing surgery are similar to those reported for radical hysterectomy, with recurrence rates ranging from 1.2% up to 6.8% and neoplasia-related death rates varying between 2.1% and 2.4% [22]. Regarding the obstetric results, fertility preservation (that did not require radiotherapy) rates of 85.1–91.1% were obtained, with pregnancy rates of 16–24% and live birth rates of 11.3–28.3% [23]. Other complications frequently reported in relation to this procedure are amenorrhea, cervical stenosis, abnormal uterine bleeding, endometrial obliteration, postoperative infection, ovarian tube abscess, hematometra, lymphocele and tromboembolism [23].

In tumors larger than more 2 cm, is possible the neoadjuvant chemotherapy before the procedure, in the case reports the results obstetricians and oncological are similarly, but is necessary more evaluation and is recommendable only under protocol and specialized institution in cancer [24].

10.7 Sentinel Lymph Node Biopsy in Cervix Cancer

The sentinel lymph node biopsy has gained acceptance in gynecological cancer in recent years. It is a standard observation in the early stages of other neoplasias, such as breast cancer and melanoma. Presently, the sentinel lymph node is defined as the first lymph node to which the tumor lymphatic supply arrives, and identifying this lymph node can potentially help to determine the risk of lymph node metastasis.

The sentinel node identification technique is recommended in early stage disease, preferably in tumors smaller than 2 cm. Furthermore, a two-step technique must be used, consisting of injecting a radio-colloid such as Tc-99 and a dye such as indocyanine green or patent blue before the procedure. The injection may be peritumoral or within 2–4 quadrants of the cervix and 1 cm deep. Then, using a gamma probe and under direct visualization, the location of the node is determined. The sensitivity of this two-step technique is approximately 92% (95% CI of 84–98%), with a detection rate of 97% (95% CI of 95–98%) [4]. Because the cervix has a bilateral lymphatic system, the pelvic lymph nodes from both sides of the body must be evaluated, even when the sentinel lymph node is detected in a unilateral manner. If a suspicious sentinel lymph node is found and such node must be resected or if the node is metastasis-positive, the surgery is aborted and radiotherapy with concomitant chemotherapy is initiated.

Sentinel lymph node biopsy assessment is associated with short-term and long-term decreases morbidity, mainly in the appearance of pelvic inferior member lymphocysts and lymphedema [1]. Currently, sentinel lymph node analysis is not a standard for cervix cancer; therefore, determination of the status of the sentinel lymph node is exclusively recommended in research protocols.

10.8 Conclusions

Over time, cervix cancer treatment has evolved. Surgical treatment is still the curative choice for early stage disease. The oncological results of surgical treatment are similar to those of other treatments. Updates to the classification of surgical techniques have facilitated the incorporation of novel techniques that have decreased surgery-related morbidities. At present, the implementation of less invasive surgical procedures that decrease the extent of bleeding and the length of hospital stay is widely accepted. Similarly, the incorporation of fertility-sparing techniques has increased the range of treatment options for women of all ages. Finally, although these techniques have not yet been standardized, the use of less invasive techniques, such as sentinel ganglion analysis, have supported the establishment of new treatment options that decrease procedure-related short- and long-term complications with equivalent oncological results.

References

1. Salicrú SR, de la Torre JF, Gil-Moreno A. The surgical management of early-stage cervical cancer. Curr Opin Obstet Gynecol. 2013;25:312–9. doi:10.1097/GCO.0b013e3283630d6a.
2. Pecorelli S. International Journal of Gynecology and Obstetrics Revised FIGO staging for carcinoma of the vulva, cervix, and endometrium. Int J Gynecol Obstet. 2009;105:103–4. doi:10.1016/j.ijgo.2009.02.012.
3. Arbyn M, Autier P, Ferlay J. Burden of cervical cancer in the 27 member states of the European Union: Estimates for 2004. Ann Oncol. 2007;18:1423–5. doi:10.1093/annonc/mdm377.
4. Reade CJ, Eiriksson LR, Covens A. Surgery for early stage cervical cancer: how radical should it be. Gynecol Oncol. 2013;131:222–30. doi:10.1016/j.ygyno.2013.07.078.

5. Landoni F, Maneo A, Colombo A, et al. Randomised study of radical surgery versus radiotherapy for stage Ib-IIa cervical cancer. Lancet. 1997;350:535–40. doi:10.1016/S0140-6736(97)02250-2.
6. Piver MS, Rutledge F, Smith JP. Five classes of extended hysterectomy for women with cervical cancer. Obstet Gynecol. 1974;44:265–72. doi:10.1097/00006254-197503000-00027.
7. Querleu D, Morrow CP. Classification of radical hysterectomy. Lancet Oncol. 2008;9:297–303. doi:10.1016/S1470-2045(08)70074-3.
8. Long Y, Yao D-S, Pan X-W, Ou T-Y. Clinical efficacy and safety of nerve-sparing radical hysterectomy for cervical cancer: a systematic review and meta-analysis. PLoS One. 2014;9:e94116. doi:10.1371/journal.pone.0094116.
9. Wang WW, Bin L, Jing Z, et al. Evaluation of pelvic visceral functions after modified nerve-sparing radical hysterectomy. Chin Med J. 2014;127:696–701. doi:10.3760/cma.j.issn.0366-6999.20132485.
10. Benedetti Panici P, Basile S, Angioli R. Pelvic and aortic lymphadenectomy in cervical cancer: The standardization of surgical procedure and its clinical impact. Gynecol Oncol. 2009;113:284–90. doi:10.1016/j.ygyno.2008.12.014.
11. Verleye L, Vergote I, Reed NOP. Quality assurance for radical hysterectomy for cervical cancer: the view of the AEuropean Organization for Research and Treatment of Cancer–Gynecological Cancer Group (EORTC-GCG). Ann Oncol. 2009;20:1631–8.
12. Wit EMK, Horenblas S. Urological complications after treatment of cervical cancer. Nat Rev Urol. 2014;11:110–7. doi:10.1038/nrurol.2013.323.
13. Chuang F, Kuo H. Management of lower urinary tract dysfunction after radical hysterectomy with or without radiotherapy for. J Formos Med Assoc. 2009;108:619–26. doi:10.1016/S0929-6646(09)60382-X.
14. Covens RB, Murphy J, et al. Changes in the demographics and perioperative care of stage IA(2)/IB(1) cervical cancer over the past 16 years. Gynecol Oncol. 2001;81:133–7. doi:10.1006/gyno.2001.6158.
15. Cibula D, Velechovska PJ, et al. Late morbidity following nerve-sparing radical hysterectomy. Gynecol Oncol. 2010;116:506–11. doi:10.1016/j.ygyno.2009.10.061.
16. Shepherd JH. Cervical cancer. Best Pr Res Clin Obs Gynaecol. 2012;26:293–309.
17. Yin XH, Wang ZQ, Yang SZ, et al. Clinical observation of laparoscopic radical hysterectomy for cervical cancer. Int J Clin Exp Med. 2014;7:1373–7.
18. Malzoni M, Tinelli R, Cosentino F, et al. Total laparoscopic radical hysterectomy versus abdominal radical hysterectomy with lymphadenectomy in patients with early cervical cancer: our experience. Ann Surg Oncol. 2009;16:1316–23. doi:10.1245/s10434-009-0342-7.
19. Park JY, Kim DY, Kim JH, et al. Laparoscopic compared with open radical hysterectomy in obese women with early-stage cervical cancer. Obstet Gynecol. 2012;119:1201–9. doi:10.1097/AOG.0b013e318256ccc5.
20. Park JY, Kim DY, Kim JH, et al. Laparoscopic versus open radical hysterectomy for elderly patients with early-stage cervical cancer. Am J Obstet Gynecol. 2012;207:195.e1–8. doi:10.1016/j.ajog.2012.06.081.
21. Hwang JH, Yoo HJ, Joo J, et al. Learning curve analysis of laparoscopic radical hysterectomy and lymph node dissection in early cervical cancer. Eur J Obstet Gynecol Reprod Biol. 2012;163:219–23. doi:10.1016/j.ejogrb.2012.05.005.
22. Schneider A, Erdemoglu E, Chiantera V, et al. Clinical recommendation radical trachelectomy for fertility preservation in patients with early-stage cervical cancer. Int J Gynecol Cancer. 2012;22:659–66. doi:10.1097/IGC.0b013e3182466a0e.
23. Pareja R, Rendón GJ, Sanz-Lomana CM, et al. Surgical, oncological, and obstetrical outcomes after abdominal radical trachelectomy – a systematic literature review. Gynecol Oncol. 2013;131:77–82. doi:10.1016/j.ygyno.2013.06.010.
24. Osman M. The role of neoadjuvant chemotherapy in the management of locally advanced cervix cancer: a systematic review. Oncol Rev. 2014;8:250. doi:10.4081/oncol.2014.250.

Chapter 11
Surgical Treatment for Advanced or Recurrent Disease in Cervical Cancer

Gonzalo Montalvo-Esquivel, Milagros C. Pérez-Quintanilla, Angel Herrera-Gómez, Francisco Javier Alcalá-Prieto, Flavia Morales-Vásquez, and Horacio Noé López Basave

Abstract In patients with locally recurrent cervical cancer, pelvic exenteration is a viable option with long-term survival in over one third of patients. Depending on the survival disease-free, the site and size of recurrence can be set 5-year survivals of 48–60%. Since it was first reported in 1948, pelvic exenteration has been used in the treatment of advanced pelvic cancers. The original procedure has been modified in an attempt to preserve urinary or fecal continence. The subclassification of the exenteration groups into type I (supralevator), type II (infralevator), and type III (with vulvectomy) is helpful to facilitate understanding of the extent of resection of the pelvic structures and the anatomical changes associated with each operation. Pelvic exenteration should only be undertaken by experienced surgeons at specialized centers. Restorative techniques for both urinary and gastrointestinal tracts can diminish the need for stomas and, along with vaginal reconstruction, can significantly improve quality of life for many patients afterexenteration. These advances in surgery and radiotherapy help make the procedure a viable option for patients with otherwise incurable elvic malignancy.

Keywords Exenteration • Recurrent cervical cancer • Type I (supralevator) • Type II (infralevator) • and Type III

G. Montalvo-Esquivel, MD (✉) • A. Herrera-Gómez, MD
F.J. Alcalá-Prieto, MD • H.N.L. Basave, MD
Department Surgical Oncology, Instituto Nacional de Cancerología-México,
Av. San Fernando No 22, Col. Sección XVI, Mexico City, zip code 14080, Mexico
e-mail: drgmonty@yahoo.com.mx

M.C. Pérez-Quintanilla, MD
Gynecologic Tumors Deparment, Instituto Nacional de Cancerología-México,
Mexico City, Mexico

F. Morales-Vásquez, MD
Department Medical Oncology, Instituto Nacional de Cancerología-México,
Mexico City, Mexico

J.G. de la Garza-Salazar et al. (eds.), *Cervical Cancer*,
DOI 10.1007/978-3-319-45231-9_11

11.1 Introduction

The term Pelvic Exenteration (PE) refers to an ultraradical procedure of en bloc resection of multiple endopelvic organs, followed by surgical reconstruction, in order to re-establish the abolished visceral and parietal functions. It has a curative, and local control goal in patients with gynecological cancer; its main indication is in recurrent cervix cancer (CC) patients that cannot be treated with less invasive procedures [1].

Between 1985 and 2015, at the National Cancer Institute of Mexico, 115 recurrent CC-related PE procedures were performed, with a disease-free period of 18 months. Of these women, 85 (73.9%) undertook total PE, and 19% suffered from complications. This is less than the international literature mean, which is between 22 and 32%, with a global survival of 18 months in a 2-year follow up. Currently, the procedure is designed for recurrent disease and is used in this way mainly in America. Nonetheless, it is used for both primary and recurrent disease in Europe.

11.2 Historical Perspective

The PE was first described in 1948 by Dr. Alexander Brunschwig, director of the Gynecology service of the New York Memorial Hospital, USA, as a palliative procedure for the abdominalperineal resection of recurrent or persistent gynecological tumors. In its beginnings, the procedure consisted of three steps: first the colostomy, second, the transcutaneous nephrostomies, and third, the pelvic viscera scission. However, after the disappointing results obtained, this procedure was replaced by a one-step resection included the rectosigmoids, the genital tract, and bladder, including the suspensory structures, regional lymph nodes of these organs, the ureter, anus, and vulva, with the implantation of the ureters to the Colon, and terminal colostomy; temporarily packing the empty pelvis with gauze, and closing the wound with adaptation of the tissues. Dr. Brunsshwig performed the procedure in 22 patients, reporting 5 perioperative deaths (23% of the series), four late deaths, and 14 patients who survived up to 8 months [2].

Complications on the long run mainly consisted of infections of the urinary tract, hyperchloraemic acidosis, and difficulty in the management of stomas and feces-collection devices [1].

Later, Ernest M. Bricker importantly improved the technique, with the development of an ileal conduit that separated the urinary and fecal stomas, thus avoiding hyperchloraemic acidosis and reducing the risk of pyelonephritis and renal failure [3]. This way, the procedure purpose changed from palliative to potentially curative, in adequately selected patients [4].

The experience in this procedure, such as the advances in radiotherapy and chemotherapy, allowed its adjustment to each particular case, making it possible to preserve some pelvic organs that had no evidence of tumoral affection and, in some cases, to extend the surgery to include the pelvic wall. As a result, different types of partial PE were developed (supraelevator, anterior, posterior), as well as extensions towards the sacrum and coccyx in some cases, such as colorectal tumors [5, 6].

From 1950 to 1965, the surgical mortality rate reduced from 13.4 to 1.8% with a mortality rate of 7.8% in patients with CC after radiotherapy. Total mortality of the series was 10%. A literature review of that times that included 932 patients reported a surgical mortality rate of 17% and 5 year survival rates of 21% [7].

During the 1970s and the 1980s, with the purpose of solving morbidities, such as abscess formation and fistulae in the empty pelvis (mainly associated to radiotherapy and intestinal obstruction) the use of non-radiated tissue flaps was implemented as major omentum, made of muscular-cutaneous flaps from the hips or the abdominal wall. These were transposed into the interior pelvis or perineum, thus reducing the procedure morbidity [7, 8].

During the 1990s, the main PE advances were in the area of reconstruction, mainly of the deep colorectal anastomoses, the formation of new continent urinary reservoirs, and the formation of neo-vaginas, with the use of muscular-cutaneous flaps [1].

11.3 PE Classification

The original classification divided the PE in three main groups: total, anterior, and posterior (Fig. 11.1); it depended on the position and type of resected pelvic organs. Thus, the anterior included the bladder, uretra, and genital tract; the posterior included the genital tract, and rectum sigmoids; and the total included the genital tract, bladder, uretra, and rectum sigmoids. Among the PE, there is another subtype: the PE with lateral endopelvic extended resection (LEER) which refers to a total PE that includes resection of the internal obturator muscle, pubococcygeus and iliococcygeus muscles [1].

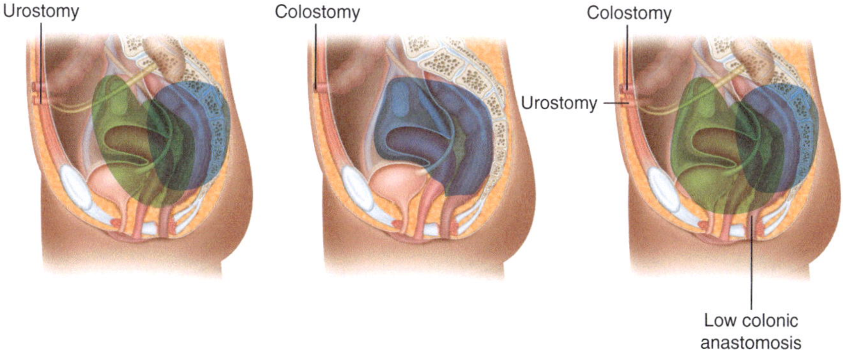

Fig. 11.1. Types of pelvic exenteration ((**a**) Anterior. (**b**) Posterior. (**c**) Total)

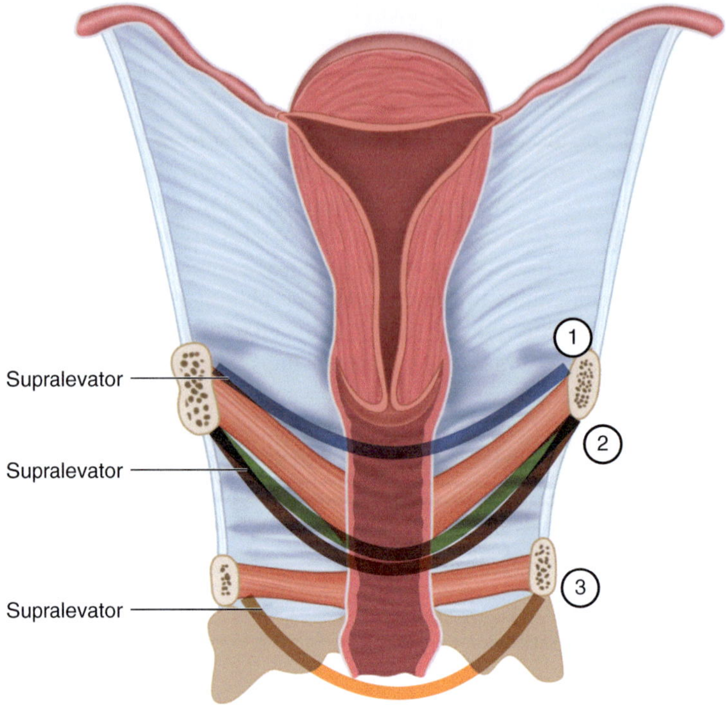

Fig. 11.2. Types of pelvic exenteration. (*I*. Supralevator, *II*: Infralevator, *III*, with vulvectomy)

Notwithstanding, this classification was considered very restricted, since it is based on the nature of the resected organs, without providing an estimated level of resection, the preservation or scission of the elevator muscles of the anus, the size of the resection of the urogenital diaphragm and of the vulvoperineal tissues, or the removal of other pelvic or extrapelvic structures [9].

As a result, in the year 1990, a classification dividing the PE in three different types was published: I (supraelevator), II (infralevator), and III (including vulvectomy) in relation to the resected tissue extension and the anatomic changes in each PE group (Fig. 11.2); likewise, the group "extended PE" was added, which refers to the PE that include additional procedures (bone resection, small intestine, groin, paraortic nodes, soft tissues) [6]. The anatomical differences between the types of exenterative procedures are described by structures involved in the Table 11.1.

11.4 Indications and Contraindications in Pelvic Exenteration

EP is an ultra-radical procedure which shall must only be used as "the last chance", other options implying less morbidity must always be considered before choosing this procedure, since it has the highest morbidity and mortality, while its reported

Table 11.1 Types of pelvic exenteration

Type 1	Type 2	Type 3
• ABOVE THE LEVATOR MUSCLE	• UNDER THE LEVATOR MUSCLE	• UNDER THE LEVATOR MUSCLE
• Levator muscles:	• Levator muscles:	• Levator muscles:
• NONE	• LIMITED	• COMPLETE
• Urogenital diaphragm:	• Urogenital diaphragm:	• Urogenital diaphragm:
• NONE	• LIMITED	• COMPLETE
• Vulvoperineal structures:	• Vulvoperineal structures:	• Vulvoperineal structures:
• NONE	• LIMITED	• COMPLETE

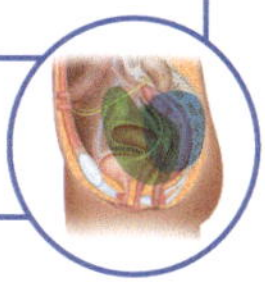
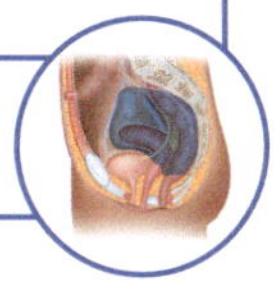
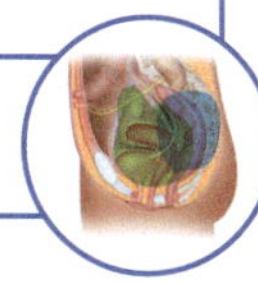

curation rates do not exceed 45% [10]. The most common indication (70%) for PE is in recurrent or persistent CC, followed by advanced colorectal cancer (20%), and 10% in other gynecologic cancers [1].

Accordingly, indications for PE [11–13] are as follows:

- Recurrent or persistent CC, after central level radiotherapy (with previous hysterectomy)
- Primary metastatic CC

The indications of this procedure as a palliative treatment are controversial due to its per se high morbidity.

The following must be considered:

- Resectability of the tumor and ability to obtain negative margins
- Tumor localization
- Previous treatments, such as pelvic radiotherapy

The contraindications of this procedure are:

Absolute
- Pelvic wall involvement
- Sacral plexum or sciatic nerve involvement
- Large vessel affection
- Extrapelvic metastases (40–50% detected during the approach)
- Poor functional study

Relative
- Obstructive unilateral or bilateral uropathy
- Advanced age
- Major systemic disease
- Psychologic distress
- Impossibility to take care of stomas
- Morbid obesity and malnutrition

The clinical unresectability triad must be considered [8]:

- Unilateral obstructive uropathy
- Inferior ipsilateral member edema
- Edema and pain in the ipsilateral inferior member

Brunschiwg and Barber define certain unresectability criteria based upon clinical and imaging studies [5]:

- Pelvic wall lesion
- Recurrence in previously radiated nodes
- Paraortic positive lymph nodes
- Evidence of intra-abdominal tumor

In 2006, Michael Hökel, made a systematic review of 21 previous studies on gynecologic cancer, and found that 40–63% of the patients who undertook PE were suspended because of unresectability. As for theoretical results, only 50 out of 200 recurrent patients will be candidate to a radical procedure with curative purposes [1].

11.5 Recurrent Cervical Cancer

The main PE indication in gynecological cancer in is recurrent CC, which is the most common site of recurrence at the local level. At the level of the vaginal vault, it represents 30–45% in patients who previously undertook radical hysterectomy, or to pelvis, without lateral pelvic wall affection. In patients who received radiation therapy, with uterus conversion, the recurrence sites are, ordered by frequency: 43% parametria and pelvic wall, 27% cervix, uterus and superior third of the vagina, and 16% distant sites.

Candidates to surgical resection must be carefully selected, taking into consideration that disease-free minimum acceptable time is 12 months, and the size of the tumor less than 3 cm, to achieve 5 year success rates of 50–60% [13].

11.6 Palliative Pelvic Exenteration

Its use is still controversial. In the series of published cases, 2-year survival rate is 10.5–47%. The objective is not only to obtain margins, or increase its overall survival, but to improve patients' quality of life. The use of neoadjuvant chemotherapy, with the goal of reducing tumor size, but very few series of patients have been published on this subject [14].

The main indications of palliative PE are:

- Intestinal or uretral obstruction
- Recto-vaginal or vesico-vaginal fistulae
- Post-radiotherapy cistitis or proctitis

11.7 Diagnosis and Selection of the Patient

In the preoperative evaluation, the adequate selection of the patient consists of three crucial principles:

- Medical evaluation
- Psychological apects
- Imaging studies

Medical Evaluation
Adequate medical condition for a long surgical procedure, with the changes that can occur during the transoperative, as well as the right liquid management, possibility to need blood transfusions, and nutritional help are vital considerations to take in account; thus, the presence of chronic diseases must also be considered.

Studies published by the MD. Anderson suggest that chronologic age and obesity must not be considered as a contraindication to a curative surgical procedure, since such factors do not affect the duration of the surgery, blood loss, hospital stay or complcations [15, 16].

The objective of the medical evaluation (full history and a physical examination, laboratory and imaging studies) is to find evidence of unresectable or metastatic disease. The presence of one or two of the clinical previously mentioned unresectability triad signs suggests pelvic lateral wall metastatic disease, which makes it unresectable, as well as the presence of palpable lymph nodes.

Histologic confirmation is vital before decision making, since clinical findings may be done, that can be considered as tumoral activity data, such as post-radiation therapy fibrosis, cellulites, and endometriosis.

Clinical studies to be performed in addition to general examination, electrolytes test, and uroanalysis, are a viral detection panel that includes hepatitis virus and HPV, as well as renal and hepatic function assessment.

Cytoscopy and rectosigmoidoscopy are exclusive for patients who will undertake less radical resections (anterior or posterior exenteration).

Psychological Aspects
Nowadays, the role of psychologic support in a patient undertaking PE has been underscored. Candidate patients must be capable of accepting important changes in her body's shape that occur despite the strongest surgeon's efforts in anatomical reconstruction. Moreover, the patient must have intact mentales faculties, and have access to continuous medical and psychological assistance, stoma care. Furthermore, she must be aware of alterations that will take place in her sexual function, possible complications of the disease, and long hospital stays [17].

Moreover, the patient must also be familiar with the notion that the PE operative mortality rate is of 3–5%. On the other hand, the surgeon must be aware of the psychological syndromes that may arise in this kind of patients. Psychological support is crucial, not only during the preoperative, but also in the immediate and long-term postoperative.

Reported psychiatric syndromes, according to a study by Danielle Turns in 2001 are [17]:

Postoperative syndromes Delirium, depression, and brief reactive psychosis.

Long-term syndromes Post-traumatic stress, somatoform disorders, and sexual dysfunction.

Imaging Studies
Imaging studies have the purposes of evaluating local recurrence and distant metastasis.

Abdominal and pelvic Computerized Axial Tomography (ACT) has the goal of valuaing lesion resectability and extension.

Pelvic Magnetic Resonance Imaging (MRI) is the study of choice to determine tumor size and anatomic extension to adjacent organs. This imaging technique has an invasion-evaluation sensitivity of 88–92% in the bladder, 81–96% to the rectum, and 87–97% to the pelvic wall, and a specificity of 66.7–77.6% [18].

Positron Emission Tomography with FDG (PET-CT-FDG) has currently gained a significative value in the detection of distant metastasis, with a sensitivity of 100%, and specificity of 73% [19].

Apart from conventional studies, medical evaluation and physical examination under anesthesia, laparoscopic exploration has an additional value to identify the disease, to determine its exact location and extension, and to exclude peritoneal carcinoma.

11.8 Surgical Procedure

Generally, the surgical procedure can be divided in three steps: exploration, ablation, and reconstruction [1].

Exploration Step
The exploration step is traditionally performed through an incision in the middle line. If the presence of peritoneal carcinomatosis or liver metastasis is ruled out, the retroperitoneum must be reviewed in a creanial-caudal direction, starting by a systematic dissection of the paraortic lymph nodes to rule out the presence of disease at such level, since their involvement constitutes a contraindication to the procedure: it is considered to decrease survival [20, 21].

Lateral resectability is also valuated during the exploration step: if the disease is extended to the pelvic wall, the procedure must be aborpted [22]. Nonetheless, Hockel described in 1994 the lateral extended endopelvic resection, which implies the en bloc resection of muscular structures and lateral endopelvic fascia; this allows for the resection of tumors fixed to the pelvic wall, giving enough free-margin (R0) in up to 96% of the cases, with over 61% survival rates [23].

Laparoscopic exploration has also been used to substitute laparotomy: Kohler showed, in 41 candidates of PE, a 95.2% sensitivity, 100% specificity, 95.2%

negative predictive value, thus avoiding unnecessary laparatomies, diminishing morbidity and decreasing patient recovery. However, the exploration provides limited access to evaluate the caudal portion of the parametrium, which is exclusively accessible during the procedure [24].

But still, lateral resectability pre-surgical evaluation can be achieved by means of exploration under anesthesia, or by imaging methods, such as MRI.

Ablative Step

In 2006, Höckel stated that the ablative step must be performed with two main goals: enhance the control over the pelvic tumor, which increases survival; and decrease treatment-associated morbidities as much as possible [1].

PE is the combination of three different monovisceral radical diseases (abdomino-perineal resection, hysteron-colpectomy, and cystectomy). With the use of conventional techniques, only central tumors are resectable with free margins. In spite of the exclusion of patients with pelvic wall extension, positive margins are present in the pathological definitive report in 10–20% of the cases [1]. It is widely recognized that accomplishing negative margins correlates with survival. In an attempt to determine the correct margin amplitude to achieve local control, Westin et al. confirmed the importance of the negative margin. However, they were unable to define such amplitude; most studies, on the other hand, define positive margins as those between >1 and 10 mm, and negative margins as those > 10 mm [25, 26].

As previously mentioned, lateral extended endopelvic resection has allowed for the resection of tumors fixed to the pelvic wall. This procedure is characterized by the en bloc scission of the pelvic visceral compartment with some of the following parietal structures: para-visceral fat, internal iliac vessels, internal obturator muscle, pubococcygen, iliococcygen, or coccygen. Nonetheless, it is associated to an elevated morbidity of up to 70%, most commonly implying wound dehiscence, and anastomosis leak [27].

Complications resulting from the ablative step are reported in 51–82% of the cases. The most common of them are bleeding, infection, and dehiscence (the most frequent in up to 39% of the cases), urinary or intestinal fistulae formation, obstruction, pulmonary embolism, among others. Surgical re-intervention is reported in up to 31% of the cases. The patients that most commonly present such complications are those that have undergone radiation therapy (61% vs 33.5%) [28].

In 2014, Chinatera et al. described and classified by frequency the complications presented by the patients: in the case of infectious complications (18.7%) the most common are originated in the abdomen, followed by pulmonary infections. As for the complications related to the surgical procedure on itself, the colorectal anastomosis leakage is present in 20% of the cases, followed by wound dehiscence in 17% of them [28].

Thanks to the careful selection of patients, improvement in surgical technique and postsurgical care, and the use of antibiotics, the procedure-associated mortality has decreased by 37%, presenting rates of 2–3% in the first series of the last decade [27].

Currently, the use of laparoscopy combined with perineal or vaginal access, followed by mini-laparotomy to reconstruct the pelvic functions has reported perioperative morbidity reductions, including a lower amount of blood loss, early roaming and early hospital exit, less scars, and better cosmesis, without compromising pelvic control or surival [29, 30].

Reconstruction Step

There are multiple techniques to re-establish the pelvic functions lost during the exenteration. One of the main issues concerning the reconstruction are, the unpredictable cicatrization capacity of the radiated tissues, and the determination of the balance between increasing the complication risk versus the potential benefit of the use of complex reconstruction techniques.

As for the rectal function, if the anal sphincter cannot be preserved, a terminal colonostomy is required. In case of anal sphincter preservation with the use of supraelevator exenteration, the intestinal continuity can be preserved in some occasions, and may be restored with the use of colorectal or co-anal anastomosis, when technically possible. Nevertheless, anastomosis failure is as high as 30–40% despite good technical maneuvers, mainly due to radiation therapy-related side effects. The use of stoma has not reduced the risk of fistula formation, but rather allows a more benign course: in some studies a decrease in the number of interventions and a higher rate of recoveries from fistulae have been reported. Thus, the use of colorectal anastomosis is not recommended in radiated tissue [31, 32].

As for the vesico-uretral function restitution, one of the options is the use of an orthotopic neo-bladder, supra-vesical urinary diversion, through a continent bag, or an incontinent conduct. Among such options, the conducts present less technical complexity but require the patient to permanently use a urinary bag, resulting in a negative impact on her image and quality of life.

Diverse surgical techniques have been described and validated for the formation of a urinary reservoir, with the use of a segment of ileum or colon. The poor methodology of the studies comparing both techniques up to date make it difficult to make any conclusions on the superiority of any specific technique in terms of complications, functional results, or quality of life.

The ilial conduct was the standard method for years, in which a piece of the distal ileum on which the ureters were anastomosed and later, a stoma was created towards the abdominal wall was firt described by Bricker in 1950 [3]. In a 131 patient analysis with ileum conduct, a complication rate of 66% was discovered, among which the most common was stenosis, para-estomal hernia, and bladder infection (24%, 24%, and 23%, respectively), reporting a renal function undermining of 27% [33].

There are multiple continent urinary derivation techniques described, like the Kock, Miami, Florida, Camey II, among others. These have a valve mechanism and thus, are useful when the uretra preservation is not possible [34].

One such technique was described in Miami University, and it uses the segment 12 cm–14 cm of the terminal ileum, ascendant colon, and proximal transverse colon. With this technique, ureteral stenosis has been reported in up to 22% of the cases, pyelonephritis in 16.9%, and gastrointestinal complications in 26% [35]. In one of the largest series published about the Miami-type reservoir experiences, 90 patients were analyzed, 90% of which had radiation therapy records. The most common early complication was urinary duct infection (40%), followed by anastomosis (14%). Among the late complications, (>60 days) the most common was again urinary duct infection, followed by uretral stenosis (42 and 11%, respectively). The conclusion was that 80% of the complications can be solved in a conservative way, in addition of being a simple technique, effective even in patients with radiation therapy records, with which continence preservation can be achieved in 93% of the cases [36].

Pelvic and vulvovaginal structures reconstruction can be achieved using straight abdominal muscle flaps, major gluteus, or gracilis, with which the dead pelvic space is obliterated. As a result, small intestine hernias, and adherence or abscess formation are prevented. Additionally, the cicatrization process is improved thanks to the presence of healthy, vascularized tissue inside the radiated area. Otherwise, omentoplasty can be performed, which on its own, improves the cicatrization process. Among these, the vertical straight abdominal muscle is preferrable, since it has a larger volume, and is more vascularized, with a big pedicle. Furthermore, it does not interfere with the use of urinary or intestinal stomas, and can be obtained from the laparatomy's same vertical scission [8].

11.9 Prognostic Factors

In a retrospective study by Westin et al. it was shown that factors that impact the most on disease-free, and overall survival are the margin size, lympho-vascular invasion, peri-neural invasion, and the presence of positive lymph nodes [25]. Baiocchi et al. al reported a higher recurrence risk in patients with nodal affection and peri-neural invasion; higher risk of death in patients with grade three tumors, nodal affection, and the resection of more than three organs during the procedure. The lapse between primary treatment and exenteration had a significative impact on survival, if it was longer than 24 months; Moreover, it was also found that patients with endometrial pathology have a better 5-year global survival, when compared to cancer of the cervix (64.2% vs 23.1%) [12]. In 2007, Park discovered that tumor size, taking 4 cm as a cut-off value, significatively influences on recurrence, without having any significative impact on survival [37].

11.10 Global and Disease-free Survival

With the correct patient selection that takes in account the previously mentioned unfavorable prognostic factors, PE use as a primary or secondary procedure has been reported in 41–70% range, with 5-year survival rates of 20–73%. As a palliative treatment, 5-year global survival has been reported at 10–27% [8].

As for disease-free survival and recurrence, it has been steady, at 48–55% in spite of the years, and application of new surgical techniques and patient selection criteria [1].

Reference	Year	No. patients	Survival (%)
Rutledge et al	1977	296	42
Averette et al	1984	92	58
Lawhead e al	1987	65	23
Cuevas et al	1988	252	44
Morley et al	1989	100	66
Soper y et al	1989	69	40
Goldberg et al	1998	154	24
Total/Mean		**1028**	**43**

11.11 Quality of Life

Most of the studies that evaluate quality of life in patients with PE are retrospective, and report a decrease in quality of life, unless when it is used as a palliative procedure, where patients' quality of life actually improves. Recent prospective information on the evaluation of physical and psychological welfare report that after an initial decrease, there is a return to the basal state, in the 9–12 months. This suggests an adaptation process undertaken by the patient, to her new health state [38].

References

1. Höckel M, Dornhöfer N. Pelvic exenteration for gynaecological tumours: achievements and unanswered questions. Lancet Oncol. 2006;7(10):837–47.
2. Brunschwig A. Complete excision of pelvic viscera for abdominal carcinoma. Cancer. 1948;1:177–88.
3. Bricker EM. Bladder substitution after pelvic evisceration. Surg Clin North Am. 1950;30:1511–21.
4. Brunschwig A. What are the indications and results of pelvic exenteration? JAMA. 1965;194(3):274.
5. Brunschwig A, Barber HRK. Pelvic exenteration combined with resection of segments of bony pelvis. Surgery. 1969;65:417–20.
6. Magrina JF. Types of pelvic exenterations: a reappraisal. Gynecol Oncol. 1990;37:363–6.
7. Sevin B-U. Pelvic exenteration. Surg Clin North Am. 2001;81(4):771–80.
8. Kaur M, Joniau S, D'Hoore A, Vergote I. Indications, techniques and outcomes for pelvic exenteration in gynecological malignancy. Curr Opin Oncol. 2014;26(5):514–20.
9. Buchsbaum HJ, White AJ. Omental sling for management of the pelvic floor following exenteration. Am J Obstet Gynecol. 1973;117:407–12.
10. Soper JT, Berchuck A, Creasman WT, Clarke-Pearson DL. Pelvic exenteration: factors associated with major surgical morbidity. Gynecol Oncol. 1989;35:93–8.

11. Magrina JF et al. Pelvic Exenterations: supralevator, infralevator, and with vulvectomy. Gynecol Oncol. 1997;64:130–5.
12. Baiocchi G, Guimaraes GC, Oliveira RA, Kumagai LY, Faloppa CC, Aguiar S, Begnami MD, Soares FA, Lopes A. Prognostic factors in pelvic exenteration for gynecological malignancies. Eur J Surg Oncol. 2012;38(10):948–54.
13. Peiretti M et al. Management of recurrent cervical cancer: a review of the literature. Surg Oncol. 2012;21(2):59–66.
14. Landoni F et al. Neoadjuvant chemotherapy prior to pelvic exenteration in patients with recurrent cervical cancer: single institution experience. Gynecol Oncol. 2013;130(1):69–74.
15. Iglesias DA et al. The effect of body mass index on surgical outcomes and survival following pelvic exenteration. Gynecol Oncol. 2012;125:336–42.
16. Huang M, Iglesias DA, Westin SN, et al. Pelvic exenteration: impact of age on surgical and oncologic outcomes. Gynecol Oncol. 2014;132:114–8.
17. Turns D. Psychosocial issues: pelvic exenterative surgery. J Surg Oncol. 2001;76:224–36.
18. Kaur M, Joniau S, et al. Pelvic exenteration for gynecological malignancies: a study of 36 cases. Int J Gynecol Cancer. 2012;22:889–96.
19. Vargas H. Magnetic resonance imagin/ positron emission tomography provides a roadmap for surgical planning and serves as predictive biomarker in patients with recurrent gynecological cancer undergoing pelvic exenteration. Int J Gynecol Cancer. 2013;23(8):1512–9.
20. Rutledge FN, McGuffee VB. Pelvic exenteration: prognostic significance of regional lymph node metastasis. Gynecol Oncol. 1987;26(3):374–80.
21. Schmidt AM, Imesch P, Fink D, Egger H. Indications and long-term clinical outcomes in 282 patients with pelvic exenteration for advanced or recurrent cervical cancer. Gynecol Oncol. 2012;25(3):604–9.
22. Berek JS, Howe C, Lagasse LD, Hacker NF. Pelvic exenteration for recurrent gynecologic malignancy: survival and morbidity analysis of the 45-year experience at UCLA. Gynecol Oncol. 2005;99:153–9.
23. Höckel M, Horn LC, Einenkel J. (Laterally) extended endopelvic resection: surgical treatment of locally advanced and recurrent cancer of the uterine cervix and vagina based on ontogenetic anatomy. Gynecol Oncol. 2012;127(2):297–302.
24. Köhler C, Tozzi R, Possover M, Schneider A. Explorative laparoscopy prior to exenterative surgery. Gynecol Oncol. 2002;86(3):311–5.
25. Westin SN, Rallapalli V, Fellman B. Overall survival after pelvic exenteration for gynecologic malignancy. Gynecol Oncol. 2014;134(3):546–51.
26. Jurado M, Alcázar JL, Martinez-Monge R. Resectability rates of previously irradiated recurrent cervical cancer (PIRCC) treated with pelvic exenteration: is still the clinical involvement of the pelvis wall a real contraindication? a twenty-year experience. Gynecol Oncol. 2010;116(1):38–43.
27. Höckel M. Laterally extended endopelvic resection (LEER)--principles and practice. Gynecol Oncol. 2008;111(2 Suppl):S13–7.
28. Chiantera V, Rossi M, De Laco P. Morbidity after pelvic exenteration for gynecological malignancies: a retrospective multicentric study of 230 patients. Int J Gynecol Cancer. 2014;24(1):156–64.
29. Martínez A, Filleron T, Vitse L, Querleu D. Laparoscopic pelvic exenteration for gynaecological malignancy: is there any advantage? Gynecol Oncol. 2011;120(3):374–9.
30. Puntambekar S, Rajamanickam S. Laparoscopic posterior exenteration in advanced gynecologic malignant disease. J Minim Invasive Gynecol. 2011;18(1):59–63.
31. Hatch KD, Gelder MS, Soong SJ, et al. Pelvic exenteration with low rectal anastomosis: survival, complications, and prognostic factors. Gynecol Oncol. 1990;38:462–7.
32. Moutardier V, Houvenaeghel G, Lelong B. Colorectal function preservation in posterior and total supralevator exenteration for gynecologic malignancies: an 89-patient series. Gynecol Oncol. 2003;89(1):155–9.

33. Madersbacher S, Schmidt J, Eberle JM. Long-term outcome of ileal conduit diversion. J Urol. 2003;169(3):985–90.
34. Bloch WE, Bejany DE, Penalver MA, Politano VA. Complications of the Miami pouch. J Urol. 1992;147(4):1017–9.
35. Mirhashemi R, Im S, Yazdani T. Urinary diversion following radical pelvic surgery. Curr Opin Obstet Gynecol. 2004;16(5):419–22.
36. Salom EM, Mendez LE, Schey D, Lambrou N, Kassira N, Gómez-Marn O, Averette H, Peñalver M. Continent ileocolonic urinary reservoir (Miami pouch): the University of Miami experience over 15 years. Am J Obstet Gynecol. 2004;190(4):994–1003.
37. Park JY, Choi HJ, Jeong SY, Chung J, Park JK, Park SY. The role of pelvic exenteration and reconstruction for treatment of advanced or recurrent gynecologic malignancies: analysis of risk factors predicting recurrence and survival. J Surg Oncol. 2007;96(7):560–8.
38. Rezk YA, Hurley KE, Carter J, Dao F, Bochner BH, Aubey JJ, Caceres A, Einstein MH, Abu-Rustum NR, Barakat RR, Makker V, Chi DS. A prospective study of quality of life in patients undergoing pelvic exenteration: interim results. Gynecol Oncol. 2013;128(2):191–7.

Chapter 12
Radiotherapy in Cervical Cancer

Aida Mota-García, Monika Blake-Cerda, Bonifacio Ramón-Ortega, Roque Alberto Guadarrama-Fleites, and Guadalupe Elizabeth Trejo-Durán

Abstract Cervical Cancer is one of the most common types of cancer in the female Mexican population, and unfortunately, in almost half of all cases, the patient presents with locally advanced clinical stage, therefore being familiar with all radiotherapy techniques is crucial in order to give our patients the best possible outcome. Stage by stage the possibilities with radiotherapy treatment are so many: from conformal radiotherapy to the most modern techniques such as stereotaxic radiotherapy and IMRT are tools that we can use depending on the clinical scenario, and all those type of treatments are described and discussed in this chapter. What is the most important thing to remember is that every patient is a different case and we always have to individualize treatment to get best results.

Keywords Cervical cancer • Radiotherapy • Brachytherapy • Adjuvant radiotherapy • Point A • Intensity modulated radiotherapy

12.1 Early-Stage Cervical Cancer

Treatments for early-stage cervical cancer are mainly surgical because the control rate is high and the expected toxicity in surgery is low. When surgery is compared to radical radiotherapy, the data show that toxicity is lower after surgery than what is expected following radiation therapy. The main advantage of surgery over radiotherapy lies in the fact that it preserves the ovaries and sexual functions of young patients, which improves patient quality of life and avoids early menopause. We

A. Mota-García, MD (✉) • B. Ramón-Ortega, MD • R.A. Guadarrama-Fleites, MD
G.E. Trejo-Durán, MD
Department of Radiation Oncology, Instituto Nacional de Cancerología-México,
Av. San Fernando No 22, Col. Sección XVI, Mexico City 14080, Mexico
e-mail: aidamota_2000@yahoo.com.mx

M. Blake-Cerda, MD
Department of Radiation Oncology, Instituto Nacional de Cancerología-México,
Av. San Fernando No 22, Col. Sección XVI, Mexico City 14080, Mexico

Department of Radiation Oncology, Centro Médico ABC, Mexico City, Mexico

J.G. de la Garza-Salazar et al. (eds.), *Cervical Cancer*,
DOI 10.1007/978-3-319-45231-9_12

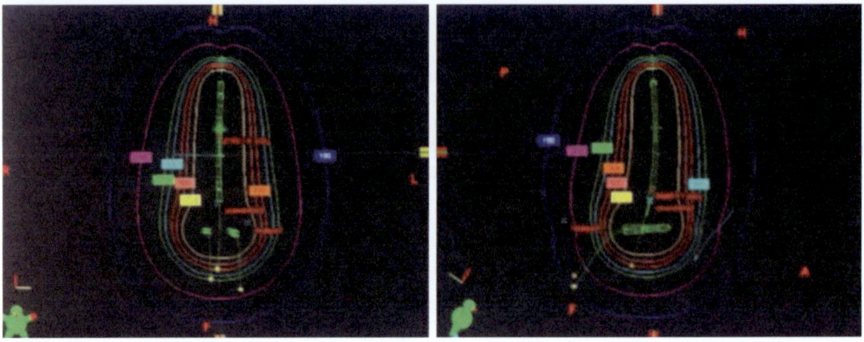

Fig. 12.1 Point A location. A pre-defined point that was located 2 cm above and 2 cm lateral to the external cervical orifice

cannot ignore the fact that morbidity is also lower and, finally, that the surgical procedure provides the surgeon with the possibility of obtaining a complete evaluation of the pelvis to identify implants or suspicious lesions outside of the cervix.

Studies have compared the results of surgery vs. radical radiotherapy in early stage cervical cancer. These studies have been mainly retrospective, and they have provided results that are comparable for local control and overall survival (OS) (80–90%) in a 5-year follow up [1].

However, this study showed that there were higher rates of toxicity in patients who were treated with radiation therapy. In 1997, the first randomized clinical study was published that compared radical radiotherapy to surgery. This study included patients with cervical cancer in stages IB-IIA. The patients were randomized to treatment with surgery or radiotherapy. In the surgical group, adjuvant radiotherapy was indicated for patients with a clinical stage above IIA, positive margins, positive lymph nodes or less than 3 mm of non-compromised cervical stromal tissue. External radiotherapy consisted of administering 47 Gy to the pelvic area followed by low-dose brachytherapy for a total dose of 76 Gy (point A). Point A was defined as a point located 2 cm above and 2 cm lateral to an external cervical orifice. This point represents where the ureter crosses the uterine artery (Fig. 12.1). There was no significant difference in OS (83 vs. 83%), progression-free survival (PFS) (74 vs. 74%) or local recurrence. The only difference was in the morbidity associated with the treatments: 28% of the patients in the surgical group received adjuvant radiotherapy, suggesting that the treatment choice should be based on the clinical stage, menopausal state, age, and, more importantly, cervical diameter to reduce complications secondary to treatment [2].

The treatment of choice for patients with early-stage cervical cancer is surgery, especially when the possibility of needing adjuvant radiation is low. In the opposite scenario, when adjuvant radiotherapy is thought to be required after surgery (e.g., because of large tumors, the risk of leaving residual tumors after surgery, of lymph node involvement) radical radiotherapy should instead be consider as a first option.

12.2 Adjuvant Radiotherapy for Cervical Cancer

As we discussed in a previous section, the treatment of choice for patients with early-stage cervical cancer in early stages is surgery. However, approximately one-third of the patients who going into surgery have one or more high risk factors for recurrence in their pathology report. The GOG-49 study [3] showed that having a tumor size larger than 4 cm, lympho-vascular invasion or invasion into more than one-third of the cervical stroma and exhibiting positive pelvic lymph nodes, positive surgical margins and parametrial involvement are predictive markers. In 1990, the GOG classified patients into the following three risk subgroups: low, intermediate and high-risk, with the latter having a 41% risk of recurrence.

To reduce this risk, postoperative radiotherapy treatments are recommended in the following two clinical situations: first, when there is an intermediate risk of recurrence, in which case, radiation therapy treatment alone is recommended (i.e., when lympho-vascular invasion is observed or the tumor size larger than 4 cm and involves more than one-third of stromal invasion); and second, when there is a high risk of recurrence, in which case, adjuvant treatment with chemo-radiotherapy is suggested (i.e. in the presence of positive pelvic lymph nodes, positive margins and positive parametrial invasion). In absence of macroscopic disease, a 45–50 Gy dose applied to the pelvis is typically prescribed as an adjuvant treatment. After external radiotherapy, the brachytherapy boost must be individualized. Once these factors were determined, several randomized trials that used adjuvant radiation to reduce local recurrence after surgery were performed.

In the first such trial, GOG-92 [4], the researchers analyzed results in patients with an intermediate risk of recurrence who received postoperative radiotherapy. The experimental group received 50.4 Gy of external radiotherapy to the pelvis. The control group was observed only after surgery. The results favored the treatment group, in which local recurrence was 14%, whereas it was 21% in the control group. As expected, higher toxicity was observed in the group that received radiotherapy (6% vs. 2.1%). An update after a 10 year follow-up confirmed that the patients who underwent external radiotherapy had a higher PFS (HR 0.58; p:0.009). However, no differences were found in OS [5].

The second randomized study, the GOG-109 study [6], included high risk patients. These patients were defined by the presence of positive parametrial invasion, positive margins or lymph node involvement. Patients were randomly assigned to receive either pelvic external radiotherapy at a total dose of 49.3 Gy (with 45 Gy to the para-aortic region whenever the iliac common nodes were positive) or chemo- and radiotherapy. The chemotherapy scheme was cisplatin- and 5-fluorouracyl-based. In this study, OS was higher in the group that received the combined treatment (71% vs 81%) after a 4-year follow-up, and the combined group also had a higher PFS (63% vs 80%). This information was confirmed in several trials after that publication [7].

The last randomized study to explore adjuvant therapy in cervical cancer was published in 2012 by the NOGGO-AGO Intergroup. Their study evaluated the use of neo-adjuvant therapy in patients with a high risk of recurrence. A total of 271 of such CxCa patients were treated with either carboplatin and paclitaxel followed by radiotherapy or with standard chemo-radiotherapy. The study found that there was no significant difference in OS (86% vs 79%). They did demonstrate that the toxicity profile was different in every scheme, with nausea, vomit and hematologic toxicity displayed in the chemo-radiotherapy group and balding and neurotoxicity displayed in the group in which carboplatin and paclitaxel were sequentially administered [8].

It is reasonable to consider the use of brachytherapy in margin-positive patients [9]. In patients with broad residual disease, treatment with interstitial brachytherapy is the right choice. Furthermore, brachytherapy can be considered in cases where the parametrial tissue or the vagina has been compromised.

12.3 Irradiation Techniques

If a patient has early-stage cervical cancer (i.e. pre-invasive stages and up to 1A2) and refuses or cannot be taken into surgery because of a comorbidity, treatment with radiation therapy is feasible. However, in these cases, brachytherapy as a sole modality is preferred because the risk of lymph node involvement is low. The installation of brachytherapy devices is performed in the operation room, often while the patient is under sedation. The choice of device depends on the anatomy of the vagina (i.e., its size, length and compliance) and especially the target volume that needs to be covered.

There are several treatment schemes for brachytherapy. The choice should be based upon whether the treatment is going involve low dose rate (LDR) or high dose rate (HDR) brachytherapy. For LDR, the prescribed dose is approximately 65–75 Gy to the vaginal vault, and with HDR, the dose is 35–45 Gy and is given in fractions of 6–7 Gy. Using Manchester and GEC-ESTRO Systems, the treatment is administered at a 5 mm depth from the vaginal mucosa.

For patients with stages IB to IIA, the treatment consists of pelvic external radiotherapy and intracavitary brachytherapy with a prescription to point A. Two-dimensional treatment (2D) is based on predefined bone limits, which are localized using fluoroscopy. The tumor, uterus and pelvic lymph node tissue should be covered. The field's arrangement more commonly uses an anterior, posterior and two lateral (pelvic box) approaches. The superior border, which is determined based on bone anatomy, is delimited by L4-L5. This is the level at which the bifurcation of the aorta most commonly takes place. The lower border is marked by the inferior limit of the Obturator Foramen. The lateral border of the posterior and anterior fields is indicated by a line that is marked as an imaginary line 2 cm beyond the true pelvic ring. For the lateral fields, the anterior border is 1 cm beyond the pubic symphysis, and the posterior border is along an imaginary vertical line that is traced at the level of S2. The superior and lower borders of the lateral fields are the same as the ones for the anterior and posterior fields.

Three-dimensional radiotherapy treatment is based on anatomical limits according to the lymph node region and the extension of the tumor, which are observed on tomography. The region should cover the common, internal and external iliac lymph nodes and the pre-sacral lymph nodes, and the dose should be localized in the Obturator foramen. It also should cover the whole cervix, the uterus, the parametrial tissue that lies on the way from the cervix to the pelvic wall, the uterus-sacral ligaments and the upper half of the vagina. The peri-rectal lymph nodes should be covered if the pelvic lymph nodes are affected. Prophylactic radiation to the para-aortic lymph nodes is not routinely indicated unless these nodes appear to be affected. If that is the case, these nodes should be covered above the renal vessels, at approximately the T12-L1 level [10].

Brachytherapy should be administered during or after treatment with external radiotherapy. The protocol will depend on the preferences of the oncologic center, the patient's vaginal capacity, the grade of tumor regression and the concomitant use of chemotherapy. If the patient was not previously treated with surgery, treatment with brachytherapy should be performed using a uterine probe and ovoids (Tandem) to cover the entire cervix. If the patient no longer has a uterus, the treatment should be performed using a cylinder or ovoids, depending on anatomy and the volume that needs to be treated.

According to the Manchester System, which is evaluated by the ICRU 38, the dose should be administered to the A point. When using the GEC-ESTRO System, the dose should be targeted to the affected region regardless of pre-determined points of administration. This indicates that the residual tumor and the area presenting a high risk of recurrence should be covered. The final dose of radiotherapy to the A point or PTV (according to the type of brachytherapy) will depend on the clinical stage, which can vary from 65 to 75 Gy in stage IA1 and up to 85 Gy in stage IB and IIA [11].

12.4 Locally Advanced Cervical Cancer

Cervical Cancer is one of the most common types of cancer in the female Mexican population, and unfortunately, in almost half of all cases, the patient presents in a locally advanced clinical stage [12]. The reason for this is probably related to a lack of coverage by Pap-smear tests and, in many other cases, the fact that women tend to seek medical attention long after the appearance of the first symptoms. This results in the fact that surgical treatment can only be offered to a small percentage of presenting patients. The reason for this is that beginning with clinical stage IB2, treatment should preferably involve concomitant chemo-radiotherapy followed by brachytherapy. This protocol has already been described in several works, which have shown that there is an inverse relationship between size of the tumor and the probability of controlling the cancer. That is, the larger the tumor size, the less likely the treatment will be successful. This is because the effect of radiation depends on the amount of oxygen in the tissue. A large tumor generally has extended areas of necrosis and decreased blood flow. This results in a compromised oxygen supply, which means that less oxidation damage is applied to malignant tissues. At the end of the 1990s, a series of publications changed the standard treatment for locally advanced cervical cancer patients, making concomitant chemo-radiotherapy the primary treatment option because it proved that it provided better results than when radiotherapy was used as the sole modality [14–17]. The fundamental idea behind the use of combined treatment is based on the synergistic effect between both modalities: chemotherapy acts as a radio-sensitizing agent that increases the tumor's susceptibility to the effects of radiation. This complicity between both treatments has several mechanisms of action, but it mainly inhibits the repair of sub-lethal damage and synchronizes cells in a particular radio-sensitive phase [18]. Also, the combined use of these treatments makes the effects of radiation less oxygen-dependent. The first concomitance studies were performed using hydroxy-urea [14]. However, hematological toxicity was considerably high, and a randomized study was therefore carried out that compared the results of treatment with pelvic radiotherapy (at a mean dose of 50 Gy in conventional fractioning, i.e. 2 Gy) combined with the following three chemotherapy agents: cisplatin, fluorouracil and hydroxyurea or with hydroxyurea alone [13]. In all, 526 patients with stages IIB-IVA were included, and the results demonstrated that in both of the groups in which Cisplatin was administered, there was an improvement in OS and PFS, whereas more toxicity was observed in the group that received all three drugs than in the group that received cisplatin as the only drug. This is the reason why the standard treatment for locally advanced cervical cancer is currently radiotherapy plus cisplatin, with both treatments used concomitantly [13]. In a different study that was aimed at patients with a voluminous IB clinical stage, two groups were compared: patients that underwent hysterectomy after radiotherapy and those who were treated with chemo-radiotherapy. In this study, OS and PFS were better in the patients who were treated with the combined treatment (CT and RT) [16]. Finally, another study supported the superiority of treatment results gained using pelvic radiotherapy (50 Gy medium dose) combined with chemotherapy compared with pelvic and para-aortic region radiotherapy treatment without chemotherapy [15]. These results were confirmed in an updated publication on 2004 [19]. These studies are the basis for what is currently considered the standard treatment for locally advanced Cervical Cancer (Fig. 12.2).

Regarding the choice of treatment technique, several factors can be outlined. In patients with disease confined to the pelvic region (e.g., the cervix, pre-sacral region and high-risk lymph regions such as the iliac lymph nodes and obturator foramen), the four field technique can be used (e.g., AP-PA and opposing laterals) until 45–50 Gy is administered in conventional fractionations (e.g., 1.8 to 2 Gy per fraction), and in case of an enlarged lymph node (determined using imaging), these could be treated with a booster dose of 60–70 Gy. To achieve this high dose, we can use intensity-modulated radiotherapy (IMRT) because we need high dose gradients. In the absence of the availability of this technique, 3D conformal RT with medial-line

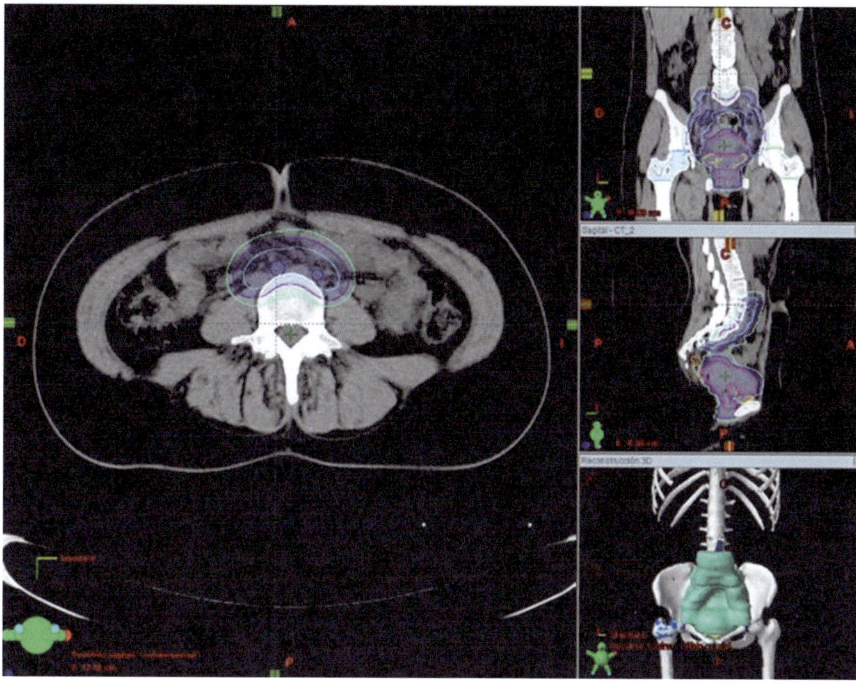

Fig. 12.2 Treatment volume in a patient with locally advanced cervical cancer. A contour has been drawn around the uterus, the cervix, the proximal one-third of the vagina, and the lymph node regions at risk (i.e., the iliac, presacrum and Obturator Foramen). In a head to tail orientation, the field extends traditionally from the bifurcation of the aorta (common iliac chain) to the point at which the tumor mass finishes with a 2 cm margin or down to Obturator Foramen. Lateral fields covered the region from the pubic symphysis to an imaginary line that was drawn at the level of S2. It is worth mentioning that these limits are the same that were used when planning with fluoroscopy (2D). Tomography is currently widely used to define treatment volumes

structure blockade (e.g., of the rectum, vagina and intestine) can also be performed [15]. It is worth mentioning that even though the availability of IMRT is increasing around the world, its use is not considered standard for this type of tumor because of the ongoing debate concerning factors that negatively affect local-regional control, such as how the target tissue is outlined, inter and intra-fraction movement, and tumoral regression during treatment [20–22]. Another alternative treatment that is increasingly accessible is stereotaxic radiotherapy (SBRT). This treatment consists of delivering high doses of radiation to a small target over a few sessions (generally no more than five). There are already reports of this technique being used on patients who are not candidates for brachytherapy after external radiotherapy. One of the largest series that has been performed reported highly motivating results in which no 3 or 4 toxicities were reported and satisfactory local control rates were achieved Fig. 12.3 [23].

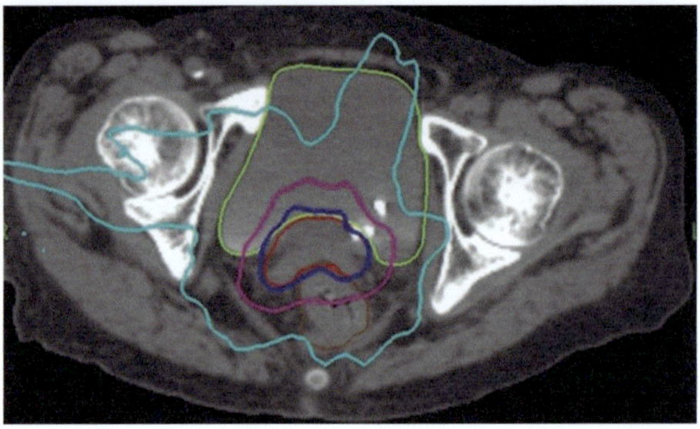

Fig. 12.3. Stereotactic radiation therapy after receiving conventional pelvic radiotherapy [23]

Table 12.1 The three risk stratification groups into which patients with cervical cancer were assigned

Low risk	Intermediate risk	High risk
Clinical stage IA and 1B1 patients with additional risk factors	Deep stromal invasion Lymphovascular invasion Tumor size >4 cm	Positive lymph nodes Positive margins Parametrial invasion
↓	↓	↓
No further treatment	Adjuvant radiotherapy	Adjuvant chemo-radiotherapy

Each group underwent surgical treatment. It was recommended that patients in the lower risk group did not need to receive any adjuvant treatment, whereas intermediate risk patients should receive adjuvant radiotherapy (tele-therapy and brachytherapy), and high-risk patients must be treated with adjuvant chemo- and radiotherapy (tele-therapy and brachytherapy)

12.5 Adjuvant Treatment in Locally Advanced Cervical Cancer

Approximately 80% of the cervical cancer cases in clinical stage I are cured by surgery and require no further treatment [24]. However, some well-known factors increase the risk of recurrence, thereby negatively impacting OS in these patients. The presence of positive lymph nodes is associated with a reduced 5-year survival rate [25]. A tumor size higher than >4 cm, deep invasion into the cervical stromal tissue and lympho-vascular invasion are all prognostic factors that increase the risk of recurrence and therefore affect LC and OS [26–29]. To achieve a more straight forward decision regarding whether a patient needs adjuvant therapy or not and whether this adjuvant treatment will be radiotherapy alone or radiotherapy concurrent with chemotherapy. A stratification risk has been develop to help the oncologist taking the decision. As shown in Table 12.1, low, intermediate and high risk of recurrence has been established.

In conclusion, approximately 20–25% of the patients that undergo surgery will possess an unfavorable prognostic factor that will dictate their need for adjuvant treatment. The adequate selection of such patients, both before and after surgery, is extremely important so that we can always offer the best treatment options according to the clinical and pathological characteristics of each patient. This allows us to guarantee the best possible oncological.

12.6 Brachytherapy

Radiotherapy has been successfully used in cervical cancer for approximately a century. Cervical tissues are particular sensitive to radiation. A combination consisting of external radiotherapy and brachytherapy has been shown to be an effective treatment option [30, 31]. Several studies have reported that brachytherapy as a boost after tele-therapy decreases the risk of recurrence and increases the survival rate. In selected cases, it may be used as the only component of a treatment scheme during the early stages of cervical cancer, and it is characterized by a close disposition between the radiation source and the tumor or vaginal vault [2]. The ICRU 38 defines the brachytherapy dose rates as follows: low dose rate (LDR) 0.4–2 Gy/hr., medium dose rate 2–12 Gy/hr. and high dose rate over 12 Gy/hr [32].

Low dose rate brachytherapy
This scheme has a long history as a treatment for cervical cancer. Initially, Radium 226 was used, but it was then replaced by Cesium 137, a radioisotope with similar physical characteristics, except that it has a lower half-life (30 years) than radium 226 (>1000 years) and results in health care providers being exposed to less radiation. According to ICRU 38, the permitted dose rate range for low dose brachytherapy is from 0.4 to 2 Gy/hr [33].

Pulsed dose brachytherapy
This is the most recent modality, and it was first used in San Francisco in 1992. It combines the physical advantages of a high dose rate and the radiobiological advantages of a low dose rate. It delivered radiation pulses in pre-established time intervals using Iridium 192 and the dose ranges described by the ICRU 28 are from 2 to 12 Gy/hr [34, 35].

High dose rate brachytherapy
This technique was first used on 1950, and the used of this treatment modality has increased considerably during recent decades. Currently, iridium 192 is used, and the ICRU 38 approves a dose from 12 Gy/hr. Among the advantages acquired with this kind of treatment in comparison with the low dose rate is that it avoids exposing the personnel in charge of patient care, allows dose optimization and higher reproducibility and is an ambulatory treatment. Several studies and meta-analyses found no difference in oncologic results or toxicity between the low dose and high dose rates [35]. Hence, independent of the absolute dose, the equivalent biological dose is the same for both modalities.

Applicators

Different applicator systems have been used to position the source of radiation inside the uterus and the vagina. These have included ovoids, a ring and a probe, a cylinder and a probe, and ovoids and a probe, but the most widely used ones are the Fletcher-Suit-Delclos.

The position of the applicators is a critical determinant. Conditions required for an adequate intracavitary insertion include:

1. The geometry of the insertion should avoid sub-dosification around the cervix.
2. The parametrial tissue most receive an adequate dose.
3. Doses to the vaginal mucosa, bladder and rectum should be monitored and maintained as the lowest possible level to decrease the risk of toxicity.

During the patient's initial evaluation, a determination is made regarding which applicators will be uses for the brachytherapy treatment, but the final evaluation will take place once external radiotherapy has concluded, and the ideal applicators will be selected based on the obtained response [34].

Planning of the treatment

Diverse methods have been used to determine the prescription points to be dosed during the evolution of brachytherapy. However, because of the limited availability of 3D images, most of the international instruction manuals continue to use orthogonal radiographies based on the definition of Point A and dose restrictions for the bladder (absolute <75 Gy, relative <90%) and rectum (absolute of 70% Gy and relative <80%). This was the nomenclature that was approved by ICRU 38 [36]. Fig. 12.4 shows treatment performed in tandem in patients with a uterus.

Dose

The American Brachytherapy Society (ABS) recognizes that the dose of external radiotherapy to the whole pelvis varies from one institution to another and that size of the dose and the number of fractions of a high dose rate of brachytherapy will depend on the doses given before in radiotherapy to the wholes pelvis. Some institutions limit the dose of external pelvic radiotherapy in early-stage patients to 20 Gy before performing the programmed brachytherapy. These institutions then complete the dose to the whole pelvis in a second round while using central protection. Nonetheless, most institutions prefer to first administer a 40–50 Gy dose of pelvic external radiotherapy and then lower the brachytherapy dose [37].

The optimal high dose rate brachytherapy scheme remains undefined, and the dose per fraction may vary by +/– 0.25 Gy. However, it goes higher than 7 Gy per fraction, then special care should be taken with the organs that are at risk (especially the rectum and bladder), given the long-term complications that exposure could present. It is also recommend that the length of treatment should not exceed 8 weeks to obtain the best results [34, 36]. The decision to use a higher dose in the external radiotherapy than in the brachytherapy will depend on the initial volume of the disease, the ability to separate the bladder and the rectum, the degree of tumor regression observed during external radiotherapy and the preference of the institution [37]. The most widely used dose schemes, each of which is recommended by the ABS, are listed below (Tables 12.2 and 12.3).

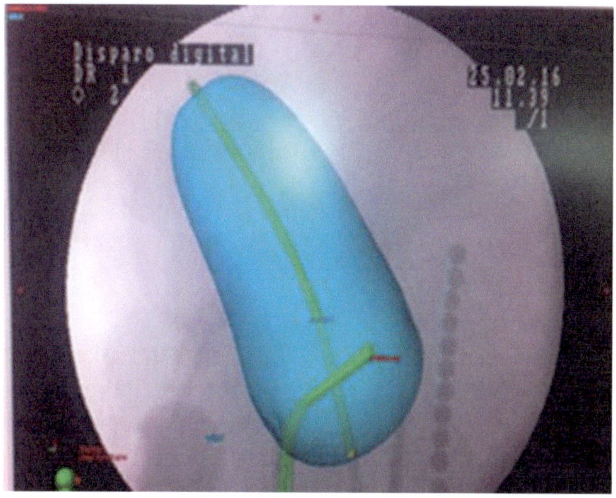

Fig. 12.4 Planning of a high dose rate brachytherapy treatment using a probe and ovoids. Note the position of the bladder (*left of the blue dose curve*) and rectal (*right to the blue dose curve*) probes. These two structures assist in defining the dose to give to the bladder and the rectal wall while determining dose tolerance limits

Table 12.2 Radiotherapy schemes recommended by the ABS to treat early-stage cervical cancer

External radiotherapy dose (Gy)	Number of fractions (brachytherapy)	Dose per fraction (brachytherapy)
20	6	7.5
20	7	6.5
20	8	6
45	5	6
45	6	5.3

Table 12.3 Radiotherapy schemes recommended by the ABS to treat locally advanced cervical cancer

External radiotherapy dose (Gy)	Number of fractions (brachytherapy)	Dose per fraction (brachytherapy)
45	5	6.5
45	6	5.8
50.4	4	7
50.4	5	6
50.4	6	5.3

Another gynecological brachytherapy planning technique is one that is guided by an image (3D). This is possible in both HDR and PDR. The localization of target structures is carried out using tomography, simulation and sometimes magnetic resonance imaging. The full GTV and CTV coverage is crucial and one of the most important prognosis factors that is directly related with the final results. Instead of choosing a prescription point, as in fluoroscopy panning methods, a prescription is made to treat the volume involved, and dose restrictions for organs are made in association with the maximum prescribed dose (D2cc) [11].

The final dose of radiotherapy to point A or to the CTV (depending on the type of brachytherapy) will depend on the clinical stage and can vary from 65 to 75 Gy in stages IA1 and up to 85 Gy in locally advanced stages [11, 36].

12.7 Re-irradiation

It is estimated that approximately 35% of all patients with a cervical cancer diagnosis who are treated with radiotherapy will recur during the first 5 years after they finish treatment. In young patients with good status performance and small central recurrence, exenteration is the standard treatment. Complete resection (R0) significantly impacts the outcome of treatment. R1 resection, especially in tumors that are close to pelvic wall, can be treated with intra-operative radiotherapy [38]. However, the majority of patients with local recurrences after radiotherapy have an advanced age and severe comorbidities. For this reason, re-irradiation is often the preferred option in these patients. In fact, there are time when this is the only curative option. Whether external radiotherapy or brachytherapy is preferred generally depends on the conformal dose distribution offered by each technique, with the optimal strategy being the one with the possibility of delivering very high doses to the affected zone and smaller doses to surrounding tissues. There is currently not enough information available in the literature regarding the restriction of doses to at-risk organs 9, 10. In a previously published small retrospective series, a dose that included a total of +/− 48 Gy in conventional fractionation was found to be safe. This study reported disease-free survival and 5-year local control rates of 46 and 45%, respectively. Severe complications were reduced by the implementation of 3D planning for brachytherapy and IMRT. Nonetheless, there are adverse prognosis factors, such as a short period before recurrence (< 6 months) and a tumor size larger than 3 cm. It is very important to analyze the technique that was used previous to a recurrence (e.g., energy, volume, external radiotherapy dose and brachytherapy dose) and the time that has elapsed between treatments to determine the feasibility of re-irradiation [39]·

High dose rate brachytherapy, rate can be applied either in intracavitary or interstitial form for re-irradiation but must be considered with extreme caution to reduce the potential complications.

Conclusions

Intra-cavitary brachytherapy is a very important part of treatments for cervical cancer, whether it is used as a sole modality or in combination with external beam radiotherapy. In multiple studies, a decrease in recurrence and an increase in survival have been reported when brachytherapy has been applied, given its capacity to deliver very high, localized doses while reducing the amount of radiation delivered to the surrounding tissues. This technique and dose fractionation schemes frequently vary between different institutions [38].

12.8 Toxicity and Complications Post-radiotherapy in Cervical Cancer

In 1999, the National Cancer Institute (NCI) announced that the concurrent use of chemotherapy and radiotherapy improved OS in locally advanced cervical cancer, and this treatment method was subsequently considered the standard treatment option. Pelvic radiotherapy plays a definitive roll in patients, but we cannot ignore the toxicity that is often associated with it. Because complications normally arise between 3–5 years after treatment, there is still much to investigate regarding long-term morbidity in this patients [40]. As radiation oncologists, we must be aware that even though our main concern and efforts are focused on controlling malignant cells, we must understand that the complications associated with these treatments can impact our patients' quality of life in a negative way.

The definitions of acute and late toxicity vary in the literature. In some cases, acute toxicity is defined as the presence of adverse effects that take place during treatment and up to 42, 60 and 90 days after radiotherapy is complete. Late toxicity refers to effects that present after 90 days or even years later. The incidence of late sequelae in patients with early-stage cervical cancer who were treated with radiotherapy is approximately 3.5%, whereas in patients with locally advanced disease, the rate of complications is reported to be slightly higher (10–15%). The reason for this difference is simple: the total dose to central structures tends to increase as the clinical stage of the patient increases (e.g., 85–90 Gy are administered to the cervix in clinical stage III and IV patients). We can conclude that the probability of complications arising is directly related to the clinical stage, the volume of tissue being treated, the patient's anatomy and the total dose administered to individual tissues [43].

Genitourinary toxicity
In cervical cancer, pelvic radiotherapy can result in complications in the lower urinary tract. Acute toxicity (G1–2) is relatively common following external beam radiotherapy (17–40%), depending on the report being described [41]. The risk of developing adverse urinary effects (e.g., grade 3 or 4) is higher in the first 3 years but has an actuarial risk of 0.25% per year for the next 25 years 44, and the annual incidence increases between 18 and 28% after 3 and 5 years post-radiotherapy, respectively [42].

It is estimated that 44% of these patients will develop adverse acute urinary effects (<9 days post-radiotherapy), while only 7–9.5% will develop adverse late effects44. However, the time required for these adverse effects to manifest can be substantial. For instance, the presence of urethral stenosis and spontaneous bladder rupture have been observed up to 30 years after radiotherapy is complete. From a physio-pathological point of view, this technique results in damage to the basal membranes of blood vessels, which can lead to occlusion, thrombosis, neovascularization and an increase in the proliferation of fibroblasts [44]. These events can subsequently lead to lesions in the urinary tract, with the bladder and the point at which the ureter inserts into bladder being the most susceptible to damage, given their anatomical positions. Neo-vascularization is an important factor that contributes to radiation cystitis and the later development of hemorrhagic cystitis. The most common urinary adverse effects (grade three or higher) are urethral stenosis, vesicle-vaginal fistula, ureter-arterial fistula and hemorrhagic cystitis [43]. The risk of severe toxicity after radiotherapy is significantly associated with higher radiotherapy doses and the number of administered treatments [43, 44]. Urethral stenosis has been reported in 5% of pre-operative radiotherapy patients and in 25% of patients treated with definitive radiotherapy alone.

Gastrointestinal toxicity

Acute gastrointestinal toxicity can appear up to 90 days after radiotherapy treatment and is characterized mainly by diarrhea, tenesmus, and pain or hemorrhoids with rectal bleeding that can be controlled with symptomatic medication. Late toxicity could appear during the first 2 years or more after radiotherapy and is characterized mainly by proctitis, stenosis and rectal fistula.

Several risk factors can increase the chances of a patient experiencing toxicity due to radiation. Prior abdominal or pelvic surgery can increase the risk of intestinal obstruction or adherence formation in patients treated with radiation therapy (> 50 Gy). Additionally, patients with coexisting comorbidities, including previous pelvic inflammatory disease, atherosclerosis, diabetes, vascular disease, collagen disease, tobacco consumption history or intestinal inflammatory disease, might have an increased risk of developing acute or long-term secondary effects following radiation therapy [45].

Eifel et al. [43] reported increase in toxicity and a higher risk of chronic adverse effects in patients with cervical cancer who were treated with radiotherapy. The risk was higher during the first 3 years of treatment, with 7.7% of patients presenting with G3 complications within 3 years. The incidence of rectal complications was 1% during the first 2 years and lowered to 0.68% from 2 to 25 years. The incidence of fistula was approximately twice as high in patients who were subjected to extrafascial hysterectomy and adjuvant treatment. These patients presented with this complication at rates of 5.3% and 2.3%, respectively, at 20 years post-radiation, and 5.2% and 2.9%, respectively, in patients who were previously subjected to laparotomy. The risk of intestinal obstruction is also increased in patients subjected to laparotomy (14.5% and 3.7%, respectively, after 10 years), and patients who weighted <120 lb. (8.2% and 3.6%, respectively). The cumulative risk of complications was higher in young patients because they had a stronger probability of survival and were therefore exposed for a longer period of time.

Mitchel et al. [46] evaluated 398 patients with clinical stage I-III cervical cancer who were treated with definitive radiotherapy. The patients were divided into two groups, as follows: those who were 35–69 years old and those who were >70 years old. The frequency and severity of acute and late adverse effects were equivalent in both groups. Age was therefore not associated with higher rates of acute or chronic toxicity.

There is a direct correlation between the incidence of complications and the dose administered. Pérez et al. [47] reported that with doses <75–80 Gy the risk of G2–3 complications in the urinary tract and rectum is approximately 5%. However, this percentage increased >10% when higher doses of radiation were applied. In the small intestine, the incidence of morbidity was lower (2%) in patients treated with less than 50 Gy than in those treated with >50–60 Gy (5%). It has been demonstrated that patients who experienced treatment sequelae had slightly better survival rates than patients without complications. This result was associated with better tumor control when administering high doses of radiotherapy.

The effects of the total dose of radiotherapy on the bladder, rectum and point A are also correlated with the severity of the complications. Eiffel et al. evaluated 1456 patients who were treated with external radiotherapy and LDR brachytherapy consisting of a total dose of 70–90 Gy. The frequency of G2 morbidity in these patients was 10–12%, and the frequency of G3 morbidity was 10%. The most important adverse effects ere cystitis and proctitis (G2) (0.7–3%), vesicle-vaginal fistula (G3) (0.6–2%), rectal-vaginal fistula (0.8–3%) and intestinal obstruction (0.8–4%). In the bladder, doses <80 Gy were correlated with a <3% incidence of morbidity, and this incidence increased to 5% with higher doses. In the rectal wall, the incidence of morbidity was <4% when <75 Gy was applied. In the small intestine, the incidence of morbidity was <1% when 50 Gy or less was administered, 2% for 50–60 Gy and 5% for higher doses [48].

There are a variety of dosimetry parameters that are tightly correlated with the incidence of morbidity in patients who were treated with definitive radiotherapy. Hence, we should pay special care and attention to these related factors, which will help us reduce morbidity to a minimum without compromising tumor control.

The correlation between tobacco and late complications following radiotherapy is of particularly interest. A significant difference has been observed in the incidence of intestinal complications between smokers and non-smokers, and this difference was associated with the intensity of tobacco consumption. These data provide evidence regarding a synergistic effect between tobacco use and the effects of normal tissue radiation [13].

Sexual function after pelvic radiotherapy

The most common gynecological complications following radiotherapy are ovarian insufficiency in pre-menopause patients and vaginal stenosis in patients that receive vaginal radiation. Vaginal stenosis is defined as a tightening or reduction of the vaginal canal that can interfere with a physical exam or sexual function. Its incidence varies between 20 and 88%. In patients who are initially subjected to surgery and then later receive vaginal HDR brachytherapy, the incidence is lower 2.5% [16]. It is most common for this complication to occur during the first year post-radiotherapy, but it has been observed at intervals ranging from 26 days up to 5.5 years. The risk factors associated with vaginal stenosis include high doses of radiation, patients who are >50 years old, insufficient use of the dilator, and concomitant chemoradiotherapy. Doses >80 Gy have been associated with a 10–15% increase in the risk of G2 vaginal toxicity, including vaginal stenosis [49]. Radiation-induced menopause generally occurs within 6 months after treatment.

Hematologic toxicity
High doses of radiation can induce chronic myelo-suppressive effects and lower tolerance to chemotherapy by damaging the bone marrow micro-environment. The results of prospective studies have reported a 25% incidence of hematological toxicity >G3 when using cisplatinum-based chemo-radiotherapy. Irradiating an extended field that includes the covering over the para-aortic lymph nodes results in more irradiation of total bone marrow and therefore a higher rate of hematological toxicity. It is important to consider this complication and to monitor hematological toxicity because it predisposes patients to infections, frequent hospitalizations, multiple transfusions and delays in receiving chemotherapy [50, 51].

Brachytherapy toxicity
In a meta-analysis published by Cochrane in 2010, LDR and HDR intracavitary brachytherapy were compared in locally advanced cervical cancer. All of the included studies, which involved 1265 patients, provided detailed information regarding the complications that presented. The tissues found to be at risk of late complications were the bladder, sigmoid rectum and small intestine. The relative risk for late complications was 1.33 in the bladder, 1.0 in the sigmoid rectum and 3.37 in the small intestine. These results indicate that except for a slight increase in the complications that presented in the small intestine, there were no significant difference in complication in patients treated with a high dose [31].

Complications of concomitant radiotherapy/chemotherapy
Concerning the recent application of chemo-radiotherapy, it has been clearly demonstrated that this combination results in higher rates of acute toxicity, particularly hematologic and gastrointestinal complications, than radiotherapy alone.

Kiran et al. [52] carried out a review of acute and late toxicology following chemo-radiotherapy in 1766 patients. They found that G1 and G2 hematologic toxicity effects occurred more often in the chemo-radiotherapy group. A significant difference was observed in G3 and G4 hematological and gastrointestinal toxicity. Late toxicity has been described in eight assays, seven of which reported a significant difference. However, the survival benefit obtained from applying chemo-radiotherapy makes up for the toxicity observed in these patients, and this makes this strategy an acceptable option.

In spite of the fact that there is not sufficient data on late toxicity to support its results, the data obtained from meta-analyses performed in the RTOG 900198 study [53, 54] suggests that there may not be any significant difference in the type or severity of the late effects produced by chemo-radiotherapy or radiotherapy alone. Only a small percentage of women (1–3%) presented with severe late toxicity, and these complication primarily affected the rectum, bladder, intestines and vagina.

New radiation techniques aim to improve toxicity
As new radiation techniques have been developed, it has now become possible to minimize or substantially prevent G1 toxicity. The use of multiple fields avoids a lack of homogeneity in drug dose delivery. Additionally, the physical displacement

of the intestines can be optimized by using a "belly board" while the patient lies in a prone position, and the procedure is now generally performed while the patient has a full bladder. Improved moderate radiotherapy treatment (IMRT) may contribute even further to reducing the rate of G1 toxicity. Moderate radiotherapy treatment is highly conformal and uses many angles to better adjust the treatment to the tumor's geometry and minimize the dose applied to the normal surrounding tissues. The most recent technique, image-guided radiotherapy (IGRT), permits some adjustments during treatment and enables the practitioner to reduce the dose delivered to normal tissues by a higher percentage [55].

Ghandi et al. [56] published the results of a randomized study that evaluated toxicity and clinical results in 44 patients with locally advanced cervical cancer who received 3D pelvic radiotherapy vs IMRT with a dose of 50.4 Gy, which was delivered in 28 fractions that were administered concomitant with 40 mg/m2 cisplatin and followed by HDR intracavitary brachytherapy. IMRT was associated with a lower rate of acute G1, >G2 (63.3% vs 31.8%) and >G3 (27.3% vs 4.5%) toxicity in addition to a lower rate of late G1 toxicity (50 vs. 13.6%). In a dosimetric comparison between both groups, IMRT applied a significantly lower dose to the small intestine and rectum.

New techniques that involve 3D imaging, either with TAC or with IMR, help us to better delimit the form of the surrounding tissues in patients that receive a high dose of brachytherapy, which allows us to achieve reductions in toxicity.

References

1. Kielbinska S, Ludwika T, Fraczek O. Studies of mortality and health status in women cured of cancer of the cervix uteri: comparison of long-term results of radiotherapy and combined surgery and radiotherapy. Cancer. 1973;32:245–52. doi:10.1002/1097-0142(197307)32:1<245.
2. Landoni F, Maneo A, Colombo A, Placa F, Milani R, Perego P, Favini G, Ferri L, Mangioni C. Randomised study of radical surgery versus radiotherapy for stage Ib-IIa cervical cancer. Lancet. 1997;350:535–40. doi:10.1016/S0140-6736(97)02250-2.
3. Delgado G, Bundy B, Zaino R, Sevin BU, Creasman WT, Major F. Prospective surgi- cal–pathological study of disease-free interval in patients with stage IB squamous cell carcinoma of the cervix: a Gynecologic Oncology Group study. Gynecol Oncol. 1990;38(3):352–7. PMID: 2227547
4. Sedlis A, Bundy BN, Rotman MZ, Lentz SS, Muderspach LI, Zaino RJ. A Randomized trial of pelvic radiation therapy versus no further therapy in selected patients with stage IB carcinoma of the cervix after radical hysterectomy and pelvic lymphadenect- omy: a Gynecologic Oncology Group Study. Gynecol Oncol. 1999;73(2):177–83. doi:10.1006/gyno.1999.5387.
5. Rotman M, Sedlis A, Piedmonte MR, Bundy B, Lentz SS, Muderspach LI, Zaino RJ. A phase III randomized trial of postop- erative pelvic irradiation in Stage IB cervical carcinoma with poor prognostic fea- tures: follow-up of a Gynecologic Oncology Group study. Int J Radiat Oncol Biol Phys. 2006;65(1):169–76. doi:10.1016/j.ijrobp.2005.10.019.
6. Peters 3rd WA, Liu PY, Barrett 2nd RJ, Stock RJ, Monk BJ, Berek JS, Souhami L, Grigsby P, Gordon Jr W, Alberts DS. Concurrent chemotherapy and pelvic radiation therapy compared with pelvic radiation therapy alone as adjuvant therapy after radical surgery in high-risk early-stage cancer of the cervix. J Clin Oncol. 2000;18(8):1606–13. PMID: 10764420

7. Carballo N, González-Cortijo L, González-Martín A, Rojo A, Chiva L. Indications for adjuvant radiotherapy treatment after surgery and novel modalities for treatment. Gynecol Oncol. 2008;110(3 Suppl 2):S41–4. doi:10.1016/j.ygyno.2008.07.009.
8. Sehouli J, Runnebaum IB, Fotopoulou C, Blohmer U, Belau A, Leber H, Hanker LC, Hartmann W, Richter R, Keyver-Paik MD, Oberhoff C, Heinrich G, du Bois A, Olbrich C, Simon E, Friese K, Kimmig R, Boehmer D, Lichtenegger W, Kuemmel S. A randomized phase III adjuvant study in high-risk cervical cancer: simultaneous radiochemotherapy with cisplatin (S-RC) versus systemic paclitaxel and carboplatin followed by percutaneous radiation (PC-R): a NOGGO-AGO Intergroup Study. Ann Oncol. 2012;23:2259–64. doi:10.1093/annonc/mdr628.
9. Version 1. National Comprehensive Cancer Network (NCCN) clinical practice guidelines in oncology, cervical cancer. 2015.
10. Small W, Mell LK, Anderson P, Cruetzberg C, De Los Santos J, De Los Santos J, Gaffney D, Jhingran A, Portelance L, Schefter T, Iyer R, Varia M, Winter K, Mundt AJ. Consensus guidelines for delineation of CTV for intensity-modulated pelvic radiotherapy in postoperative treatment of endometrial and cervical cancer. Int J Radiat Oncol Biol. 2008;71(2):428–34. doi:10.1016/j.ijrobp.2007.09.042.
11. Haie-Meder C, Potter R, Van Limbergen E, Briot E, De Brabandere M, Dimopoulos J, Dumas I, Hellebust TP, Kirisits C, Lang S, Muschitz S, Nevinson J, Nulens A, Petrow P, Wachter-Gerstner N, Gynaecological (GYN) GEC-ESTRO Working Group. Recommendations from Gynaecological (GYN) GEC-ESTRO Working Group (I): Concepts and terms in 3D image based 3D treatment planning in cervix cancer brachytherapy with emphasis on MRI assessment of GTV and CTV. Radiother Oncol. 2005;74(3):235–45. doi:10.1016/j.radonc.2004.12.015.
12. Primer consenso nacional de prevención, diagnóstico y tratamiento del cáncer cervicouterino . Gaceta Mexicana de Oncología. 2014;13(Suppl 4):1–3.
13. Rose PG, Bundy BN, Watkins EB, Tate Thigpen J, Deppe G, Maiman MA, Clarke-Pearson DL, Insalaco S. Concurrent cisplatin-based radiotherapy and chemotherapy for locally advanced cervical cancer. New Engl J Med. 1999;340:1144–53. doi:10.1056/NEJM199904153401502.
14. Whitney CW, Sause W, Bundy BN, Malfetano JH, Hannigan EV, Fowler Jr WC, Clarke-Pearson DL, Liao SY. Randomized comparison of fluorouracil plus cisplatin versus hydroxyurea as an adjunct to radiation therapy in stage IIb-IVa carcinoma of the cervix with negative para-aortic lymph nodes: a gynecologic oncology group and southwest oncology group study. J Clin Oncol. 1999;17:1339–48. PMID: 10334517
15. Morris M, Eifel P, Lu J, Grigsby PW, Levenbac C, Stevens RE, Marvin Rotman MD, Gershenson DM, Mutch DG. Pelvic radiation with concurrent chemotherapy compared with pelvic and para-aortic radiation for high-risk cervical cancer. N Engl J Med. 1999;340:1137–4. doi:10.1056/NEJM199904153401501.
16. Keys HM, Bundy BN, Stehman FB, Muderspach LI, Chafe WE, Suggs CL, Walker JL, Gersell D. Cisplatin, radiation, and adjuvant hysterectomy compared with radiation and adjuvant hysterectomy for bulky stage IB cervical carcinoma. N Engl J Med. 1999;340:1154–61. doi:10.1056/NEJM199904153401503.
17. Peters 3rd WA, Liu PY, Barrett 2nd RJ, Stock RJ, Monk BJ, Berek JS, Souhami L, Grigsby P, Gordon Jr W, Alberts DS. Concurrent chemotherapy and pelvic radiation therapy compared with pelvic radiation therapy alone as adjuvant therapy after radical surgery in high-risk early-stage cancer of the cervix. J Clin Oncol. 18:1606–13. PMID: 10764420
18. Fu KK. Biological basis for the interaction of chemotherapeutic agents and radiation therapy. Cancer. 1985;55(9 Suppl):2123–30. PMID: 3884135
19. Eifel PJ, Winter K, Morris M, Levenback C, Grigsby PW, Cooper J, Rotman M, Gershenson D, Mutch DG. Pelvic Irradiation With Concurrent Chemotherapy Versus Pelvic and Para-Aortic Irradiation for High-Risk Cervical Cancer: An Update of Radiation Therapy Oncology Group Trial (RTOG) 90-01. J Clin Oncol. 2004;22:872–80. doi:10.1200/JCO.2004.07.197.
20. Van de Bunt L, van der Heide UA, Ketelaars M, de Kort GA, Jürgenliemk-Schulz IM. Conventional, conformal, and intensity-modulated radiation therapy treatment planning of

external beam radiotherapy for cervical cancer: The impact of tumor regression. Int J Radiat Oncol Biol Phys. 2006;64(1):189–96. doi:10.1016/j.ijrobp.2005.04.025.
21. Van de Bunt L, Jurgenliemk-Schulz IM, de Kort GA, Roesink JM, Tersteeg RJ, van der Heide UA. Motion and deformation of the target volumes during IMRT for cervical cancer: What margins do we need? Radiother Oncol. 2008;88(2):233–40. doi:10.1016/j.radonc.2007.12.017.
22. Taylor A, Powell ME. An assessment of interfractional uterine and cervical motion: implications for radiotherapy target volume definition in gynecological cancer. Radiother Oncol. 2008;88(2):250–7. doi:10.1016/j.radonc.2008.04.016.
23. Haas JA, Witten MR, Clancey O, Episcopia K, Accordino D, Chalas E. CyberKnife Boost for Patients with Cervical Cancer Unable to Undergo Brachytherapy. Front Oncol. 2012;2:25. doi:10.3389/fonc.2012.00025.
24. Petterson F. Annual report of the results of treatment in gynecologic cancer (FIGO). Int J Gynecol Obstet. 2006;95(sup 1):23. doi:http://dx.doi.org/10.1016/S0020-7292(06)60043-X
25. Delgado G. Stage IB squamous cancer of the cervix: the choice of treatment. Obstet Gynecol Surv. 1978;33:174–83. PMID: 343017
26. Chung CK, Nahhas WA, Stryker JA, Curry SL, Abt AS, Mortel R. Analysis of factors contributing to treatment failure in stage IB and IIA carcinoma of the cervix. Am J Obstet Gynecol. 1980;138(5):550–6. doi:10.1016/0002-9378(80)90285-9.
27. Boyce J, Fruchter RG, Nicastri A, Ambiavagar P, Reinis MS, Nelson J. Prognostic factors in stage I carcinoma of the cervix. Gynecol Oncol. 1981;12:154–65. PMID: 7297927
28. Van Nagell JR, Donaldson ES, Parker J. The significance of vascular invasion and lymphocytic infiltration in invasive cervical cancer. Cancer. 1978;41(1):228–34. PMID: 626931
29. Abdulhayoglu S, Rich WM, Reynold J, DiSaia PJ. Selective radiation therapy in Stage IB uterine cervical carcinoma following radical pelvic surgery. Gynecol Oncol. 1980;10(1):84–92. doi:10.1016/0090-8258(80)90068-2.
30. Boyce J, Fruchter R, Nicastri AD, De Regt R, Ambiavagar P, Reinis M, Macassaet M, Rotman M. Vascular invasion in stage I carcinoma of the cervix. Cancer. 1984;53:1175–80. doi:10.1002/1097-0142(19840301)53:5<1175::AID-CNCR2820530524>3.0.CO;2-Y.
31. Wang X, Liu R, Ma B, Yang K, Tian J, Jiang L, Bai ZG, Hao XY, Wang J, Li J, Sun SL, Yin H. High dose rate versus low dose rate intracavity brachytherapy for locally advanced uterine cervix cancer. Cochrane Database Syst Rev. 2010;7(7):CD007563. doi:10.1002/14651858.CD007563.pub2.
32. Halperin Edward C, Pérez C, et al. Endometrial cáncer. In: Pérez and Brady's principles and practice of radiation oncology. 6th ed. Copyright 2013. p. 1426–48.
33. Lertsanguansinchai P, Lertbutsayanukul C, Shotelersuk K, Khorprasert C, Rojpornpradit P,Chottetanaprasith T, Srisuthep A, Suriyapee S, Jumpangern C, Tresukosol D, Charoonsantikul C (2004) Phase III Randomized trial comparing LDR and HDR brachytherapy in treatment of cervical carcinoma. Int J Radiat Oncol Biol Phys 59 (5)1424–1431. doi: 10.1016/j.ijrobp.2004.01.034
34. Viswanathan AN, Thomadsen B, American Brachytherapy Society Cervical Cancer Recommendations Committee; American Brachytherapy Society. American Brachytherapy Society consensus guidelines for locally advanced carcinoma of the cervix. Part I: General principles. Brachytherapy. 2012;11(1):33–46. doi:10.1016/j.brachy.2011.07.003.
35. Viswanathan AN, Beriwal S, De Los Santos JF, Demanes DJ, Gaffney D, Hansen J, Jones E, Kirisits C, Thomadsen B, Erickson B, American Brachytherapy Society. American Brachytherapy Society consensus guidelines for locally advanced carcinoma of the cervix. Part II: High-dose-rate brachytherapy. Brachytherapy. 2012;11(1):47–52. doi:10.1016/j.brachy.2011.07.002.
36. International Commission of Radiation Units and Mea- surements. Dose and volume specifications for reporting intracavitary therapy in gynecology. ICRU Report 38. Bethesda: International Commission on Radiation Units; 1985.
37. Nag S, Erickson B, Thomadsen B, Orton C, Demanes JD, Petereit D. The American Brachytherapy society recommendations for high-Dose-Right brachytherapy for carcinoma of the cervix. Int J Radiat Oncol Biol Phys. 2000;48(1):201–11. PMID: 10924990

38. Viswanathan A, Erickson B. Seeing is saving: the benefit of 3D imaging in gynecologic brachytherapy. Gynecol Oncol. 2015;138:207–15. doi:10.1016/j.ygyno.2015.02.025.
39. Xiang- E, Shu-mo C, Ya-qin D, Ke W. Treatment of late recurrent vaginal malignancy after initial radiotherapy for carcinoma of the cervix: an analysis of 73 cases. Gynecol Oncol. 1998;69:125–9. doi:10.1006/gyno.1998.4975.
40. National Institute of Health. NCI issues clinical announcement on cervical cancer: chemotherapy plus radiation improves survival. 22 Feb 1999. Article 01826.
41. Georg P, Potter R, Georg D, Lang S, Dimopoulos JC, Sturdza AE, Berger D, Kirisits C, Dörr W. Dose effect relationship for late side effects of the rectum and urinary bladder in magnetic resonance image-guided adaptive cervix cancer brachytherapy. Int J Radiat Oncol Biol Phys. 2012;82(2):653–7. doi:10.1016/j.ijrobp.2010.12.029.
42. Georg P, Boni A, Ghabuous A, Goldner G, Schmid MP, Georg D, Pötter R, Dörr W. Time course of late rectal- and urinary bladder side effects after MRI-guided adaptive brachytherapy for cervical cancer. Strahlenther Onkol. 2013;189:535–40. doi:10.1007/s00066-013-0365-7.
43. Eifel PJ, Levenback C, Wharton JT, Oswald MJ. Time course and incidence of late complications in patients treated with radiation therapy for FIGO stage IB carcinoma of the uterine cervix. Int J Radiat Oncol Biol Phys. 1995;32(5):1289–300. doi:10.1016/0360-3016(95)00118-I.
44. Lorvidhaya V, Tonusin A, Changwiwit W, Chitapanarux I, Srisomboon J, Wanwilairat S, Chawapun N, Sukthomya V. High-dose-rate afterloading brachytherapy in carcinoma of the cervix: an experience of 1992 patients. Int J Radiat Oncol Biol Phys. 2000;46:1185–91. PMID: 10725630
45. Charra-Brunaud C, Harter V, Delannes M, Haie-Meder C, Quetin P, Kerr C, Castelain B, Thomas L, Peiffert D. Impact of 3D image-based PDR brachytherapy on outcome of patients treated for cervix carcinoma in France: results of the French STIC prospective study. Radiother Oncol. 2012;103(3):305–13. doi:10.1016/j.radonc.2012.04.007.
46. Mitchell PA, Waggoner S, Rotmensch J, Mundt AJ. Cervical cancer in the elderly treated with radiation therapy. Gynecol Oncol. 1998;71(2):291–8. doi:10.1006/gyno.1998.5180.
47. Perez CA, Grigsby PW, Lockett MA, Chao KS, Williamson J. Radiation therapy morbidity in carcinoma of the uterine cervix: dosimetric and clinical correlation. Int J Radiat Oncol Biol Phys. 1999;44(4):855–66. PMID: 10386643
48. Eifel PJ, Jhingran A, Bodurka DC, Levenback C, Thames H. Correlation of smoking history and other patient characteristics with major complications of pelvic radiation therapy for cervical cancer. J Clin Oncol. 2002;20(17):3651–7. PMID: 12202666
49. Perez CA, Breaux S, Bedwinek JM, Madoc-Jones H, Camel HM, Purdy JA, Walz BJ. Radiation therapy alone in the treatment of carcinoma of the uterine cervix II. Analysis of complications. Cancer. 1984;54(2):235–46. PMID: 6722748
50. Mauch P, Constine L, Greenberger J, Knospe W, Sullivan J, Liesveld JL, Deeg HJ. Hematopoietic stem cell compartment: acute and late effects of radiation therapy and chemotherapy. Int J Radiat Oncol Biol Phys. 1995;31(5):1319–39. doi:10.1016/0360-3016(94)00430-S.
51. Small Jr W, Winter K, Levenback C, Iyer R, Hymes SR, Jhingran A, Gaffney D, Erickson B, Greven K. Extended-field irradiation and intracavitary brachytherapy combined with cisplatin chemotherapy for cervical cancer with positive para-aortic or high common iliac lymph nodes: results of ARM 1 of RTOG 0116. Int J Radiat Oncol Biol Phys. 2007;68(4):1081–7. doi:10.1016/j.ijrobp.2007.01.026.
52. Kirwan JM, Symonds P, Green JA, Tierney J, Collingwood M, William CJ. A systematic review of acute and late toxicity of concomitant chemoradiation for cervical cancer. Radiother Oncol. 2003;68(3):217–26. PMID: 13129628
53. Chemoradiation for Cervical Cancer Meta-Analysis Collaboration. Reducing uncertainties about the effects of chemoradiotherapy for cervical cancer: a systematic review and meta-analysis of individual patient data from 18 randomized trials. J Clin Oncol. 2008;26:5802–12.
54. Chemoradiation for Cervical Cancer Meta-Analysis Collaboration (CCCMAC). Reducing uncertainties about the effects of chemoradiotherapy for cervical cancer: individual patient

data meta-analysis [serial online]. Cochrane Database Syst Rev. 2010;20(1):CD008285. doi:10.1002/14651858.CD008285.

55. Viswanathan AN, Lee LJ, Eswara JR, Horowitz NS, Konstantinopoulos PA, Mirabeau-Beale KL, Rose BS, von Keudell AG, Wo JY. Complications of pelvic radiation in patients treated for gynecologic malignancies. Cancer. 2014;120(24):3870–83. doi:10.1002/cncr.28849.
56. Gandhi AK, Sharma DN, Rath GK, Julka PK, Subramani V, Sharma S, Manigandan D, Laviraj MA, Kumar S, Thulkar S. Early clinical outcomes and toxicity of intensity modulated versus conventional pelvic radiation therapy for locally advanced cervix carcinoma: a prospective randomized study. Int J Radiat Oncol Biol Phys. 2013;87(3):542–8. doi:10.1016/j.ijrobp.2013.06.2059.

Chapter 13
Systemic Treatment of Cervical Cancer

Flavia Morales-Vásquez, Claudia Cano-Blanco, Jaime Alberto Coronel-Martínez, Lucely Cetina-Pérez, Jorge Martínez-Tlahuel, Julio César Velasco-Rodríguez, Horacio N. López-Basave, and Jaime G. de la Garza-Salazar

Abstract In this section, we review the systemic management of patients with cervical cancer (CC) at different stages of disease: locally advanced, metastatic, or recurrent. The roles of chemoradiotherapy, neoadjuvant chemotherapy, and palliative chemotherapy, as well as of biological therapy, in this pathology are also discussed.

Since the end of the 1990s, different meta-analyses have supported the use of combination chemoradiotherapy based on evidence of an increase in overall survival.

Certain studies have reported that neoadjuvant chemotherapy offers a benefit similar to that obtained with chemoradiotherapy in patients with advanced tumors (larger than 4 cm) or complications such as hydronephrosis but with fewer side effects; however, these inferiority data do not support a change in the standard treatment.

Angiogenesis inhibitors are an efficacious, promising therapy in CC. Recent clinical studies in metastatic and/or recurrent cancer suggest that new signaling pathways in CC can be explored to identify novel molecular targeted therapies in order to obtain better outcomes for patients with this disease.

Some of the therapies for infrequent histologic types are also briefly reviewed.

F. Morales-Vásquez, MD, MSc (✉) • C. Cano-Blanco, MD • J. Martínez-Tlahuel, MD
Department of Medical Oncology, Instituto Nacional de Cancerología-México,
Av. San Fernando No 22, Col. Toriello Guerra, Tlalpan, Mexico City, Mexico, 14070

J.A. Coronel-Martínez, MSc • L. Cetina-Pérez, MSc
Clinical Research Department, Instituto Nacional de Cancerología-México,
Mexico City, Mexico

J.C. Velasco-Rodríguez, MD
Department of Medical Oncology, Hospital Español de México, Mexico City, Mexico

H.N. López-Basave, MD, MSc
Department Surgical Oncology, Instituto Nacional de Cancerología-México, Mexico City, Mexico

J.G. de la Garza-Salazar, MD
Department of Clinical Investigation, Instituto Nacional de Cancerología-México,
Mexico City, Mexico

J.G. de la Garza-Salazar et al. (eds.), *Cervical Cancer*,
DOI 10.1007/978-3-319-45231-9_13

Keywords Cervical Cancer (CC) • Chemotherapy • Chemoradiotherapy • and Targeted therapy

13.1 Introduction

For centuries, surgery has rarely been the only therapeutic option for cervical cancer (CC). For several decades beginning in 1903, radiotherapy alone was considered the superior option for the management of CC. Margaret Claves started treating patients with radiotherapy in 1903 in New York. In 1913, Abbe reported a case of patient with disease-free 8 years after treatment. Radium was the first element utilized in radiotherapy [1].

With the advent of chemotherapy, small exploratory studies were performed to test the efficacy of chemotherapeutic agents. However, epidermoid cancer is one of the least chemosensitive types of cancer, but the few CC-active agents (Table 13.1) were tested in patients receiving palliative care due to recurrent disease in previously radiated areas; such tumors are surrounded by avascular and fibrous zones that impede drug penetration.

Some clinical trials were performed in patients with locally advanced disease to reduce tumor size and ease surgical management. Although these trials revealed an 18% response rate for cisplatin-based monotherapy and a 29% response rate for combination schemes, the responses only lasted for 4 months in the best scenarios, and the impact on patient survival did not seem relevant; furthermore, there were no significant differences in postoperative complications. Because there was no real improvement compared to radiotherapy alone, these treatment regimens were not pursued.

In the 1990s, the use of chemotherapy-associated radiotherapy was expanded. Prospective randomized clinical trials provided solid evidence for the benefits of adding concurrent cisplatin to radiotherapy. Finally, in 1999, based on some of these studies, the National Cancer Institute of the United States of America published a statement on the benefits of concurrent chemoradiotherapy (QT/RT) compared to radiotherapy alone [2–6], thereby permanently changing the way CC was treated.

Systemic treatment, integrating radiotherapy and concurrent chemotherapy, is administered to all patients with locally advanced (stages IB2 to IVA) CC.

13.2 Standard Treatment: Chemoradiotherapy

Because of the previously mentioned series of studies published in the 1990s showing the absolute benefit of combination QT/RT, we no longer consider radiotherapy- or chemotherapy-free management of CC: combining these strategies is the new standard [7]. Previous clinical trials evaluated platinum vs non-platinum schemes, as well as the application periodicity (weekly vs more than once per week) and the dose intensity (<25 vs >25 mg/m^2/week cisplatin). These studies aimed to evaluate

Table 13.1 Active agents in cervical cancer. Epidermoid lineage, single agent

Drug	Patients	Response (%)
Alkylating agents		
Cyclophosphamide	251	15
Chlorambucil	44	25
Dibromodulcitol	102	23
Galactitol	36	19
Ifosfamide	157	22
Melphalan	20	20
Heavy metal complexes		
Carboplatin	175	15
Cisplatin	815	23
Antibiotics		
Doxorubicin	266	17
Porfiromycin	78	22
Antimetabolites		
Baker's antifol	32	16
5-fluoracil	142	20
Methotrexate	96	18
Plat alkaloids		
Vincristine	55	18
Vindesine	21	24
Other agents		
CPT-11	55	24
Hexamethylmelamine	64	19
Paclitaxel	52	17
Topotecan	45	22
Gemcitabine	18	8

overall survival, the recurrence-free interval, and toxicity. The >25 mg/m^2/week cisplatin dosage was found to be the best radiosensitizer because it reduced the risk of death by 20%.

The best radiotherapy scheme was also ascertained by comparing >45 Gy with brachytherapy, >45 Gy without brachytherapy, and <45 Gy with brachytherapy. The optimal duration of radiotherapy (≤8 weeks vs >8 weeks) was also assessed. The best results were obtained with a dose greater than 45 Gy for fewer than 8 weeks; hence, the established radiotherapy dose is 50.4 Gy in 28 sessions, with a 4 field "box" technique and an isocentric technique. Brachytherapy has two modalities: low dose (with cesium 137; 35 Gy dose) and high dose (with iridium 192) at four applications of 6 Gy twice a week.

In total, 4818 patients participated in the trials showing that simultaneous chemoradiotherapy provided a clear benefit in overall survival and the recurrence-free interval with tolerable toxicity. Specifically, there was a 6% increase in overall survival and an 8% increase in 5-year recurrence-free survival [8].

The conclusions of these studies are as follows:

1. The standard treatment for locally advanced CC is 40 mg/m^2 cisplatin starting on day 1 and given every 7 days and radiotherapy at a maximum dose of 50 Gy in combination with brachytherapy (8500–9000 cGy).
2. Combination treatment increases overall survival and the recurrence-free interval. The risk of recurrence in patients with early-stage disease is 16–30%, with the risk increasing to 70% in patients with advanced disease, for an overall risk of recurrence of 50% [9].
3. Toxicity is manageable, and cases of grade 3–4 toxicity are infrequent.

Given the complexity of this pathology, there were various questions regarding the therapeutic options and some controversies concerning the entire treatment regimen; the primary question was whether additional therapeutic agents could achieve greater radiosensitization to produce a higher response rate. The use of doublets has been explored in concurrent chemoradiotherapy, and such doublets have yielded higher complete pathological response rates (77.5% vs 55%), albeit with higher rates of toxicity [10].

Are there alternatives to brachytherapy? Certain studies have compared brachytherapy to hysterectomy after chemoradiotherapy, and the results are similar in terms of overall survival and recurrence-free survival. In 2013, a clinical trial was published in which brachytherapy was compared to hysterectomy after chemoradiotherapy. In this study, 211 patients with stage IB2-IIB disease who were treated with cisplatin/gemcitabine concurrent with external radiotherapy were randomized to receive brachytherapy or hysterectomy. Although the study failed to demonstrate that hysterectomy is superior to brachytherapy, proper interpretation of the data indicates that hysterectomy is an alternative in health centers where brachytherapy systems are unavailable [11].

13.3 Neoadjuvant or Adjuvant Therapy

In spite of the impact of recently implemented therapeutics on overall and recurrence-free survival, considerable challenges remain because we are far from curing all patients. Thus, questions arise as to whether neoadjuvant chemotherapy before definitive chemoradiotherapy has utility and whether adjuvant chemotherapy after definitive chemoradiotherapy offers an increase in overall survival or progression-free survival.

A series of studies attempted to answer these questions and demonstrated the benefit of adjuvant chemotherapy after chemoradiotherapy: they reported an increase of up to 19% in overall survival, although there was an increase in toxicity.

Given the response rates to combination chemotherapy schemes, it was assumed that these new studies would show more responses that would impact recurrence-free survival and overall survival.

Five of the seven studies failed to demonstrate a benefit of neoadjuvant therapy, and only two studies reported a significant benefit in survival compared to radiotherapy alone [9].

In a review of 323 patients with locally advanced disease who participated in controlled clinical trials of carboplatin plus paclitaxel-based neoadjuvant chemotherapy, the response to neoadjuvant chemotherapy was approximately 67.8–70%, without a significant impact on survival compared to the concurrent chemoradiotherapy strategy [12].

As previously mentioned, small phase II studies have shown that adjuvant chemotherapy after chemoradiotherapy has a modest impact on progression-free survival but is associated with increased toxicity.

13.4 Chemotherapy in Recurrent or Persistent Disease

Most cases of recurrent disease occur in the first 2 years after diagnosis, and 50–60% of recurrences are located outside the pelvis; in these situations, palliative chemotherapy plays a fundamental role. Distant CC metastases are diagnosed in 8–17% of cases. Historically, women with recurrent or persistent metastatic CC have had few therapeutic options.

Recurrent disease is defined as local or distant tumor growth after a complete response; if the disease is detected within the first 6 months of treatment or a response, it is defined as persistent disease. The percentages of recurrent disease are as follows for each clinical stage: IB: 10%; IIA: 17%; IIB: 23%; III: 42%; and IVA: 74%. The median survival is 24 weeks for patients with nodal recurrence and 12 weeks for those with visceral disease.

Treatment options depend on the affected anatomical site and previous treatment. Four different disease patterns can be distinguished: central lesion, pelvic wall recurrence up to the pelvic bones, loco-regional nodal recurrence, and distant metastasis, primarily to the supraclavicular lymph nodes (21%), bone (16%), liver (8%), and lungs (7%). In all cases, a confirmation biopsy is recommended, especially if the lesions are small or isolated [13–15].

In patients who have not previously received radiotherapy or in whom the recurrence is outside the radiated field, the recommended treatments are radiotherapy, cisplatin-based chemotherapy, and, in some cases, brachytherapy [15].

In patients with a central recurrence, pelvic exenteration must be considered after radiotherapy; in properly selected cases, this treatment is associated with a 5-year survival rate of up to 50% [16]. Pre-exenteration chemotherapy has been employed in an attempt to improve tumor resectability or prognosis in women who are not initially candidates for exenteration. A study reported the outcomes of 17 patients treated with platinum-based chemotherapy: the clinical response rate was 53%, and 50% of the patients achieved a complete pathological response. Another retrospective study reported the outcomes of 61 patients: 30 were treated with surgery alone, and 31 received chemotherapy prior to surgery; no differences were observed in terms of survival or complications. This is not the standard option, and it must be considered in the context of clinical trials. However, clinical reports describe experience with a limited number of patients; hence, their conclusions must not be considered universal. For patients with a non-central, local recurrence, the preferred treatment options include resection with intraoperative radiotherapy and chemotherapy or medical support, depending on tumor location and patient condition [16, 17].

13.5 Chemotherapy in Metastatic Disease

In women with metastatic disease, chemotherapy has been shown to improve progression-free survival and quality of life; it can even improve overall survival when combined with targeted therapy.

The patient's condition must be clearly established before treatment planning, and the objectives of highest chance of survival and best quality of life must always be considered. The clinicians must become acquainted with the patient and consider her environment, resources, and treatment background. There are more treatment possibilities for a patient with de novo metastatic disease than for a previously treated patient with recurrent metastatic disease because poorer response and higher toxicity rates are observed in the latter group.

Various chemotherapeutic agents have demonstrated activity as single drugs or in combination. In the last 30 years, cisplatin has been the most utilized chemotherapeutic, with associated response rates of 18–38%. The response rate to cisplatin is lower in the recurrent disease setting; thus, other drugs have been tested, including carboplatin, capecitabine, docetaxel, 5-fluorouracil, gemcitabine, ifosfamide, irinotecan, oxaliplatin, mitomycin C, paclitaxel, liposomal doxorubicin, pemetrexed, topotecan, and vinorelbine [18].

Given the poor responses obtained with single-agent cisplatin, diverse strategies and combinations have been tested. The first strategy consisted of increasing the cisplatin dose; a phase III trial by the Gynecologic Oncology Group (GOG; Randomized Trial of Three Cisplatin Dose Schedules in Squamous-Cell Carcinoma of the Cervix) established 50 mg/m^2 every 3 weeks as the standard treatment regimen because higher doses were associated with increased toxicity without improved overall survival [19].

Two randomized GOG studies supported important changes in treatment strategies. The patients in GOG 169 and GOG 264 were randomized to receive 50 mg/m^2 cisplatin or 50 mg/m^2 cisplatin + 135 mg/m^2 paclitaxel. A clinical response was observed in 19% and 36% of the cases, respectively ($p = 0.002$). The median progression-free survival was 2.8 vs 4.8 months, respectively ($p < 0.001$). There were no significant differences in overall survival (8.8 months vs 9.4 months) or quality of life [20]. In GOG 179, patients were randomized to receive 50 mg/m^2 cisplatin every 3 weeks; 50 mg/m^2 cisplatin + 0.75 mg topotecan on days 1–3 every 3 weeks; or 30 mg/m^2 methotrexate on days 1, 15 and 22, 3 mg/m^2 vinblastine on days 2, 15 and 22, 30 mg/m^2 doxorubicin on day 2 and 70 mg/m^2 cisplatin on day 2 every 4 weeks (M-VAC). The outcome objectives were survival, response rate, and progression-free survival, and quality of life was also assessed. The M-VAC arm was prematurely closed because of patient deaths. Patients who received cisplatin + topotecan had a significantly better outcome than those who received cisplatin alone: overall survival: 9.4 vs 6.5 months ($p = 0.017$); median overall survival: 4.6 vs 2.9 months ($p = 0.14$) and response rates: 27% and 13%. The FDA approved the cisplatin + topotecan scheme as a treatment option for patients with advanced cancer in 2006 [21]. Later, GOG 204 [22] was designed to evaluate the most efficient

Table 13.2 Noninferiority trial of carboplatin plus paclitaxel

Arm	N	Events	Median (m) [95% CI]	1-yr. OS	2-yr. OS	3-yr. OS
TP	123	106	18.3 m [16.1–22.9]	72.4%	38.8%	18.3%
TC	121	98	17.5 m [14.2–20.3]	67.6%	31.5%	21.3%

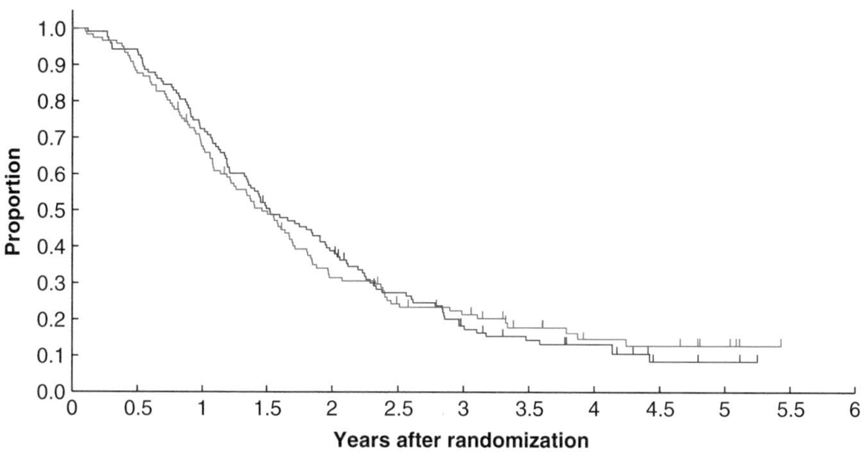

Fig. 13.1 Progress in survival in advanced and recurrent cervical cancer

doublet. Three cisplatin-based schemes were compared (combinations with vinorelbine, gemcitabine or topotecan) to the standard treatment of 50 mg/m^2 cisplatin + 135 mg/m^2 paclitaxel. In total, 513 patients were included in this study; no scheme was superior to cisplatin + paclitaxel in terms of overall survival. There was a positive trend in response rate, progression-free survival and overall survival for cisplatin and paclitaxel (Table 13.2) [22]. However, the median survival remained at 12 months. Based on these studies, clinicians began to add targeted therapies to chemotherapy, which will be discussed in another section.

A Japanese group performed the next study (JCOG0505) comparing 135 mg/m^2 paclitaxel + 5 AUC carboplatin to 135 mg/m^2 paclitaxel + 50 mg/m^2 cisplatin.

Two hundred fifty-three patients were included in this study. The median overall survival was 18.3 months for paclitaxel + cisplatin and 17.5 months for carboplatin + paclitaxel. Therefore, the carboplatin/paclitaxel combination was not inferior to the cisplatin/paclitaxel combination in terms of overall survival and clinical benefit, and thus, it constitutes a viable alternative considering its toxicity profile (Fig. 13.1) [23].

Palliative treatment in second- and third-line regimens is based on phase II studies and case series; before administering palliative treatment, a clinician should evaluate the functional physical state, proper organ function, disease sites, and previous chemotherapeutic schemes, while also considering the patient's desires.

13.6 Targeted Therapy in Cervical Cancer

Patients with CC who are not candidates for surgery/radiotherapy and those with advanced stage, metastatic, recurrent and persistent disease have a very poor prognosis with a limited median survival of between 10 and 12.9 months [21, 22] upon treatment with current chemotherapeutic agents, underscoring the need to design and develop novel drugs.

Since the introduction of molecular targeted therapy in the realm of cancer therapeutics, there have been great expectations. However, with the exception of a few select cases of spectacular results in a small proportion of solid tumors, the results have been underwhelming, most likely because of the "gene addiction phenomenon". Unfortunately, this phenomenon appears to be the rule rather than the exception [24].

The novel biological agents that modulate different signal transduction pathways include those that target the epidermal growth factor receptor (EGFR) and those that inhibit angiogenesis, cell cycle progression, metalloproteases, cyclooxygenase-2 (COX-2), mTOR, the proteasome, and epigenetic mechanisms. In the present chapter, we will discuss the most commonly used biological agents [25].

13.6.1 Targeting the Epidermal Growth Factor Receptor

The 170-kDa glycoprotein EGFR, also known as HER-1, is one of the four members of the HER receptor family; these receptors are activated by ligand binding (e.g., EGF) and subsequent homo- or hetero-dimerization, which enables self-phosphorylation of the receptor and subsequent recruitment of specific intracellular proteins. This receptor protein scaffold transduces the signal downstream through the Ras/Raf/Mek or the phosphatidylinositol 4,5-biphosphate 3-kinase (PI3K) signaling pathway, while phospholipase C-gamma (PLCγ) and signal transducer and activator of transcription (STAT), as well as other transcription factors, bind directly to the receptor. PI3K can also directly bind to any of the erbB (HER-2, HER-3 and HER-4) or EGFR heterodimers. Receptor endocytosis occurs via three different routes: recycling, lysosomal degradation, or nuclear translocation. Once inside the nucleus, EGFR can act as a transcription factor or a co-regulator to transactivate the expression of genes associated with cellular proliferation, apoptosis evasion, and metastasis [25]. Interestingly, at least three of the early HPV oncogenic proteins (E5, E6, and E7) lead to the upregulation of EGFR in CC through transcriptional and post-transcriptional mechanisms [25].

In CC, EGFR positivity ranges between 6% and 90%, depending on methodology [26, 27]. EGFR overexpression has been associated with poor prognosis in some studies, but these data were not reproducible by other authors [26]. Currently, there are two pharmacological types of EGFR inhibitors: tyrosine kinase (TK) inhibitors and anti-EGFR monoclonal antibodies. Goncalves et al. reported the efficacy and tolerability of 500 mg/day gefitinib in the second- or third-line treatment of patients with CC with loco-regional recurrent metastatic disease in a multicenter study. Twenty percent of the patients had stable disease, with a median duration of 111.5 days; the median time to progression was 37 days, and the median overall survival was 107 days. A potential correlation between EGFR expression and antitumor activity was not established [26].

Erlotinib is another EGFR small molecule inhibitor. In a study of 28 patients with squamous cell CC, erlotinib was administered at 150 mg/day until disease progression or any adverse event. No objective responses were observed, although 16% of the women achieved stable disease, and only one patient experienced progression-free survival for 6 months or longer (4%). Erlotinib was well tolerated, and the most commonly reported adverse events were gastrointestinal toxicity, fatigue, and pruritus [27].

Erlotinib was also evaluated in a phase I study as a radiosensitizer in combination with cisplatin in locally advanced CC: erlotinib (50/100/150 mg) combined with cisplatin (40 mg/m^2, weekly, 5 cycles) and conventional radiotherapy. Fifteen patients were included in this study, and overall, the combination was well tolerated. The authors concluded that the maximum tolerated dose of erlotinib is 150 mg. In a subsequent phase II trial of the same treatment scheme, the authors reported complete responses in 23 patients (91.3%) with locally advanced CC (IIB-IIIB). The treatment was again well tolerated, with grade 3 toxicities of diarrhea and pruritus in 12% [3] and 20% [5] of the patients, respectively. The complete response rate was within the range obtained with chemoradiotherapy, with a median follow-up of 9 (3–25) months. None of the patients progressed during the study, but the follow-up period was short.

Lapatinib, a dual TK inhibitor that targets both HER-1 and HER-2, has also been used in CC therapy. Another double-blind, randomized trial compared lapatinib and pazopanib (a multikinase inhibitor of angiogenesis) alone or in combination. However, the combination group was cancelled for toxicity reasons. The response rates for lapatinib and pazopanib were 5% and 9%, respectively, with a median overall survival of 39.1 vs 50.7 weeks, thus demonstrating the superiority of antiangiogenic agents [28].

Monoclonal antibodies against EGFR are also being investigated for use in CC. One of the best studied drugs in this group is cetuximab, which was evaluated by the GOG as a single agent at conventional doses in a phase II trial in recurrent or persistent CC.

As a single agent, cetuximab was well tolerated, and five patients (14.3%) achieved stable disease; however, no objective responses were obtained in 36 evaluable patients. In a phase II multicenter study, cisplatin-based chemotherapy + conventional topotecan was assessed; cetuximab was added at an initial 400 mg/m^2 dose, followed by subsequent 250 mg/m^2 weekly doses, for patients with advanced disease or prior treatment. This study was stopped due to excessive toxicity, mainly myelosuppression. Although no complete clinical responses were reported, six partial responses were observed (32%), as well as six cases of stable disease (32%). The role of cetuximab in combination with chemotherapy requires further exploration.

Nimotuzumab was assessed in a phase II study (nimotuzumab + gemcitabine vs nimotuzumab alone) in patients with recurrent or persistent CC who had received 2 or 3 prior lines of chemotherapy. Nimotuzumab was effective in maintaining stable disease with little toxicity [29]. A randomized, double-blind phase III study is underway to evaluate the efficacy of nimotuzumab in combination with cisplatin and vinorelbine at conventional doses (NCT02083211). The results of this study are eagerly anticipated.

13.6.2 Anti-angiogenic Therapy in Cervical Cancer

Angiogenesis plays a critical role in tumor growth and survival in various types of cancer and is thus considered an attractive therapeutic target. Vascular endothelial growth factor (VEGF) plays an important role in regulating angiogenesis, tumor growth, and metastasis [30].

VEGF production is upregulated in CC by many mechanisms. There is evidence that HPV (human papilloma virus) directly stimulates VEGF production. Overexpression of the oncogenic protein E6 is associated with VEGF production, and E6 apparently promotes VEGF production in a p53-independent manner. Furthermore, HPV 16 E6 and E7 have been shown to decrease the expression of anti-angiogenic factors, such as thrombospondin-1 and mas-pin [30]. Pre-clinical studies of the monoclonal antibody bevacizumab, which is currently used to treat colon, lung, breast, and renal cell cancer, have been reported in CC. In a retrospective study, six women with metastatic disease who received 5-fluorouracil and then bevacizumab had a 67% clinical benefit with a median time to progression of 4.3 months [31].

In a phase II study by the GOG that evaluated bevacizumab efficacy and tolerability, 15 mg/kg bevacizumab was administered intravenously every 3 weeks until disease progression or intolerance due to toxicity. This study reported five partial responses (10.9%) and 11 cases of stable disease (23.9%) in the cohort of 46 patients, for an average progression-free survival and overall survival of 3.4 and 7.9 months, respectively. The treatment was well tolerated [31]. These GOG results prompted a phase III trial in advanced CC with three experimental groups and a standard treatment group: group 1, cisplatin + paclitaxel; group 2, cisplatin + paclitaxel followed by bevacizumab; group 3, paclitaxel + topotecan (without cisplatin); and group 4, paclitaxel + topotecan followed by bevacizumab. This study, GOG 240, showed increases in overall survival (17 vs 13.3 months) and progression-free survival (8.2 vs 5.3 months) favoring the chemotherapy and bevacizumab group (see Fig. 13.1). There was a tolerable increase in toxicity in this group [32].

Bevacizumab has also been studied as a radiosensitizer. The Radiotherapeutic Oncology Group (RTOG) completed a phase II study in which bevacizumab was followed by radiotherapy and cisplatin in patients with locally advanced CC (stages IIB and IIIB). This treatment scheme achieved an overall survival rate of 81.3% and a disease-free survival (DFS) rate of 67.8% in a 3-year period with tolerable toxicity; thrombotic events and fistulae were not mentioned [33].

Pazopanib is a second generation TK inhibitor that targets VEGFR-1, VEGFR-2, VEGFR-3, PDGFR-alpha, PDGFR-beta, and c-kit. In pre-clinical studies, pazopanib showed excellent anti-angiogenic and anti-tumor activity [34]. Pazopanib and lapatinib (a HER-1 and HER-2 TK inhibitor), alone and in combination, were evaluated in 230 patients with recurrent CC as first- or second-line chemotherapy. The combination group was stopped, and the final analysis exclusively compared pazopanib to lapatinib. Pazopanib was well tolerated and showed improvements in the main study objectives, DFS (HR, 0.66; 90% CI, 0.48–0.91; p = 0.013) and overall survival (HR, 0.67; 90% CI, 0.46–0.99; p = 0.045). The response rate was 9% for pazopanib and 5% for lapatinib [35]. Although this study did not have the power to detect a difference in overall survival, an independent publication reported a median patient survival of 44.1 weeks for lapatinib and 49.7 weeks for pazopanib (HR, 0.96; 90% CI, 0.71–1.30; p = 0.407).

13.6.3 Epigenetic Therapy

Targeting epigenetics is a promising approach for cancer therapeutics that predominantly relies on the use of DNA methyltransferase (DNMT) and histone deacetylase (HDAC) inhibitors as single agents or in combination. Currently, two different HDAC inhibitors, vorinostat and depsipeptide, have been approved for use in cutaneous and T cell lymphoma, and two DNMT inhibitors, decitabine and azacitidine, have been approved for use in myelodysplastic syndromes. The presence of epigenetic alterations in CC has been established. We currently know that the HPV E6 and E7 proteins interact with DNMTs and HDACs. In addition to cellular transformation, this could impact the inactivation of certain tumor suppressor genes. Pilot studies on DNMT inhibitors alone or in combination with cisplatin in advanced CC showed modest antineoplastic activity. However, myelosuppression was a limiting factor [33, 34]. Moreover, we currently have limited information on HDAC inhibitors in CC; there is a report of sustained stable disease in a patient treated in a phase I trial of the HDAC inhibitor MS-275 and a prolonged response in a patient with refractory CC who was treated with an HDAC inhibitor and epirubicin [36]. Hydralazine, a hypertensive agent repositioned as a DNA methylation inhibitor, showed a growth inhibitory effect in vivo and in vitro in combination with valproic acid; furthermore, it exhibited chemosensitizing activity, had a synergistic effect on global gene expression, and upregulated class I human leukocyte antigen expression and the antigen-specific cytotoxic T lymphocyte response in CC cells. In a pilot study in locally advanced CC, valproate plus hydralazine in combination with cisplatin showed a 100% complete clinical response rate after radiotherapy, thus confirming the previously mentioned radiosensitization characteristic of epigenetic drugs in experimental models.

A phase III first-line trial of 36 patients with advanced CC evaluated cisplatin + topotecan with or without hydralazine and valproic acid (HV): 17 patients were assigned chemotherapy + HV, and 19 were given chemotherapy + placebo. The treatment was well tolerated, although more haematologic toxicities were observed in the experimental group, independently of toxicity the results in terms of response are better. There were increases in the response rate and the achievement of stable disease in the HV group during a median 7-month follow-up period (range: 1–22 months), with a progression-free survival of 6 months in the chemotherapy + placebo group and 10 months in the chemotherapy + HV group ($p = 0.0384$, two-way analysis) [37]. Although these results are preliminary, this was the first randomized clinical trial to show a significant advantage in terms of progression-free survival for an epigenetic drug plus chemotherapy regimen in advanced CC. These results suggest that epigenetics-targeted treatments could play an important role in CC. Nonetheless, it is necessary to confirm these results in future clinical trials.

13.7 Systemic Treatment in Special Histologies

13.7.1 Small Cell Cervical Carcinoma

The reported annual incidence of small cell CC is 0.6 in 100,000 women, compared to an incidence of 6.6 and 1.2 for the squamous cell and adenocarcinoma types, respectively [38].

Neuroendocrine tumors constitute a rare histology that represents 2% of all cervical neoplasias. They can be characterized as well differentiated (typical and atypical carcinoids) or poorly differentiated (small and large cells), with different biological behaviors. The small cell type is the most frequent variant. This form of CC is usually diagnosed in young women, and its prognosis is worse compared to the corresponding clinical stages of the squamous and adenocarcinoma histologies. Small cell CC has a higher propensity for lymphovascular invasion, nodal and hematogenous dissemination, and early metastasis to liver, lung, bone, and brain. It also has a shorter 5-year overall survival of 36% compared to 61% and 70% for the squamous cell and adenocarcinoma histologies, respectively [39].

Small cell CC may be difficult to diagnose because the expression of classical neuroendocrine markers may be focal or negative. TTF1 has shown positive expression in 71% of nuclei, and the expression of AE1/3, chromogranin, synaptophysin, CD56, and CK7 has also been reported. Similar to the epidermoid histology, small cell CC has been associated with the presence of HPV 16 and 18 [40].

Treatment strategies are based on series and case reports. In the early treatment stages, radical surgery is preferred, but this treatment modality has a reported distant recurrence rate of up to 43% and a mortality rate of up to 85% in a 30-month period. This observation highlights the need for aggressive multimodal treatments [41].

Most published series have included systemic treatment, surgical treatment and radiotherapy, even in early-stage disease. Zivanovic et al. analyzed progression-free survival and overall survival in 17 patients to determine whether cisplatin chemotherapy offered a real benefit. In the early-stage group, the 3-year recurrence-free survival was 83% for those who received chemotherapy and 0% for those who did not receive chemotherapy as part of their initial treatment regimen ($p = 0.025$). Therefore, the benefit of chemotherapy and radiotherapy in small cell lung carcinoma can be extrapolated to small cell CC.

Cohen et al. analyzed 188 patients from different series, including 135 patients with stage I-IIA disease, 45 with stage IIB-IVA disease, and 8 with stage IVB disease. Overall, 55.3% of the patients underwent surgery, 16% received chemotherapy in combination with other treatment, 12.8% had radiation, and 3.2% received chemotherapy alone. The 5-year survival decreased according to clinical stage progression: 36.8%, 9.8%, and 0% for I-IIA, IIB-IVA, and IVB, respectively ($p = 0.001$). Adjuvant chemotherapy or adjuvant chemoradiotherapy was associated with increased survival in patients with stage IIB-IVA disease compared to those who did not receive chemotherapy (17.8% vs 6%; $p = 0.04$). The most frequently utilized chemotherapy regimens were cisplatin + etoposide, VAC, and carboplatin + paclitaxel.

Skull prophylactic radiotherapy is not recommended [42–45].

13.7.2 *Other Histologies*

Clear Cell Carcinoma

This histology represents 4–9% of all cases of cervical adenocarcinoma and, in some cases (mostly in young women), is associated with in utero exposure to diethylstilbestrol. Other etiologic factors include microsatellite instability, HPV infection, Bcl-2 overexpression, and p53 mutation. The literature does not support the fact that this entity has a worse prognosis than its epidermoid equivalent, and thus, specific therapeutic approaches are not being pursued [46].

Glassy Cell Carcinoma

This histology represents 1–5% of all cases of CC. It is a poorly differentiated variant of the adenosquamous histology that is associated with earlier age at onset, Her2/neu overexpression (45% of cases), and recurrence in the first 2 years after treatment. According to the reported cases, multimodal treatment is beneficial; carboplatin and paclitaxel neoadjuvant therapy achieved a 67% response rate when administered to patients with locally advanced disease [47].

13.8 Conclusions

The systemic management of patients with CC poses considerable challenges.

1. For well-functioning patients with locally advanced CC, platinum-based schemes with single-agent radiosensitizers are proposed. The use of doublet therapies, including chemotherapy and molecular targeted therapy, must be further explored.
2. Hysterectomy is an alternative to brachytherapy after chemoradiotherapy in health centers where brachytherapy is unavailable. The two most important factors to

consider are the skills of the oncology surgeon and the time between the end of combination therapy and surgery, which must not exceed 6 weeks.
3. The implementation of concurrent chemoradiotherapy as the standard treatment for locally advanced cancer has decreased the risk of recurrence.
4. Neoadjuvant or adjuvant chemotherapy has not been proven superior to chemotherapy alone.
5. In metastatic or recurrent disease, combinations of chemotherapy and molecular targeted therapy have the most potential; the combination of bevacizumab and an anti-angiogenic agent offers the greatest increase in overall survival to date. However, there are numerous opportunities for drug discovery in CC therapeutics.
6. In general, the rarer histologies are treated in the same way as the predominant lineages (epidermoid and adenocarcinoma) because cases of the other histologies are infrequent. Although some lineages have been proposed to exhibit more aggressive biological behavior, there are not enough clinical studies to support changes in their management recommendations. As a general rule, the rarer histologies require a multimodal approach, and it is acceptable for clinicians to adjust the systemic management of these CC subtypes depending on the patient's situation. Nonetheless, currently, there are no strict guidelines for each variant.

References

1. Abbe R. The use of radium in malignant disease. Lancet. 1913;2:524.
2. Keys HM, Bundy BN, Stehman FB, et al. Cisplatin, radiation and adjuvant hysterectomy compared with radiation and adjuvant hysterectomy for bulky stage IB cervical carcinoma. N Engl J Med. 1999;340(15):1154–61.
3. Morris M, Eifel PJ, Lu J, et al. Pelvic radiation with concurrent chemotherapy compared with pelvic and para-aortic radiation for high-risk cervical cancer. N Engl J Med. 1999;340:1137–43.
4. Peters WA, Liu PY, Barrett RGW. Cisplatin, 5-Fluorouracil plus radiation therapy are superior to radiation therapy as adjunctive therapy in high risk, early stage carcinoma of the cervix after radical hysterectomy and pelvic lymphadenectomy: report of a Phase III inter group study. Presented at Society of Gynecologic Oncologists 30th annual meeting; San Francisco; 5–9 Feb 1999.
5. Rose PG, Bundy BN, Watkins EB, et al. Concurrent cisplatin-based radiotherapy and chemotherapy for locally advanced cervical cancer. N Engl J Med. 1999;340:1144–53.
6. Whitney CW, Sause W, Bundy BN, et al. Randomised comparison of fluorouracil plus cisplatin versus hydroxyurea in stage IIB/IVA in carcinoma of the cervix. J Clin Oncol. 1999;17:1339–48.
7. Tzioras S, Pavlidis N, Paraskevaidis E, et al. Effects of different chemotherapy regimens on survival for advanced cervical cancer: systematic review and meta-analysis. Cancer Treat Rev. 2007;33:24–38.
8. Claire Vale, Meta-Analysis Group. Collaborators 27. Reducing uncertainties about the effects of chemoradiotherapy for cervical cancer: a systematic review and meta-analysis of individual patient data from 18 randomized trials. J Clin Oncol. 2008;26:5802–12.

9. DeVita Jr VT, Lawrence TS, Rosenberg SA. Cancer of the cervix, vagina and vulva. In: Cancer principles and practice of oncology. 9th ed. Philadelphia: Lippincott Williams and Wilkins, a Wolters Kluwer Business; 2011.
10. Dueñas-González A, Cetina-Perez L, Lopez-Graniel C, et al. Pathologic response and toxicity assessment of chemoradiotherapy with cisplatin versus cisplatin plus gemcitabine in cervical cancer: a randomized Phase II study. Int J Radiat Oncol Biol Phys. 2005;61(3):817–23.
11. Cetina L, González-Enciso A, Cantú D, et al. Brachytherapy versus radical hysterectomy after external beam chemoradiation with gemcitabine plus cisplatin: a randomized, phase III study in IB2-IIB cervical cancer patients. Ann Oncol. 2013;24(8):2043–7.
12. De Azevedo CR, Thuler LC, de Mello MJ, Ferreira CG. Neoadjuvant chemotherapy followed by chemoradiation in cervical carcinoma: a review. Int J Gynecol Cancer. 2016;26:729–36.
13. Tewari KS, Monk BJ. Development of a platform for systemic antiangiogenesis therapy for advanced cervical cancer. Clin Adv Hematol Oncol. 2014;12:737–48.
14. Choi JL, Kim SH. Recurrent uterine cervical carcinoma: spectrum of imaging findings. Korean J Radiol. 2000;1:198–207.
15. Peiriti M, Zapardiel I, Zanagnolo V. Management of recurrent cervical cancer: a review of the literatura. Surg Oncol. 2012;21:e59–66.
16. Sardain H, Lavoue V, Redpath M, et al. Curative pelvic exenteration for recurrent cervical carcinoma in the era of concurrent chemotherapy and radiation therapy. A systematic review. Eur J Surg Oncol. 2015;41(8):975–85.
17. López-Graniel C, Dolores R, Cetina L, et al. Pre-exenterative chemotherapy, a novel therapeutic approach for patients with persistent or recurrent cervical cancer. BMC Cancer. 2005;5:118.
18. Long HJ. Management of metastatic cervical cancer: review of the literatura. J Clin Oncol. 2007;25:2966–74.
19. Bononi P, Blessing JA, McQuellon. Randomized trial of three of cisplatin dose schedules in squamous cell carcinoma of the cervix: a Gynecologic Oncology Group study. J Clin Oncol. 1985;3:79–85.
20. Moore DH, Blessing JA, McQuellon RP. Phase III study of cisplatin with or without paclitaxel in stage IVB, recurrent, or persistent squeamous cell carcinoma of the cervix: a Gynecologic Oncology Group study. J Clin Oncol. 2004;22:3113–9.
21. Long HJ, Bundy BN, Grendys EC. Randomized phase III trial of cisplatin with or without topotecan in carcinoma of the uterine cervix: a Gynecologic Oncology Group Study. J Clin Oncol. 2005;23(21):4626–33.
22. Monk BJ, Sill MW, McMeekin S, et al. Phase III trial of four cisplatin-containing doublet combinations in stage IVB recurrent, or persistent cervical carcinoma: a gynecologic Oncology Group Study. J Clin Oncol. 2009;27:4649–55.
23. Kitagawa R, Katsumata N, Shibata T. Paclitaxel plus carboplatin versus paclitaxel plus cisplatin in metastatic or recurrent cervical cancer: the open-label randomize phase III trial: JCOGO 0505. J Clin Oncol. 2015;33:2129–35.
24. Weinstein IB, Begemann M, Zhou P, et al. Disorders in cell circuitry associated with multistage carcinogenesis: exploitable targets for cancer prevention and therapy. Clin Cancer Res. 1997;3:2696–702.
25. Zagouri F, Sergentains T, Chrysikos D, et al. Molecularly targeted therapies in cervical cáncer. A systematic review. Gynecol Oncol. 2012;126:291–303.
26. Goncalves A, Fabbro M, Lhomme C, et al. A phase II trial to evaluate gefitinib as second- or third-line treatment in patients with recurring locoregionally advanced or metastatic cervical cancer. Gynecol Oncol. 2008;108:42–6.
27. Schilder RJ, Sill MW, Lee YC, et al. A phase II trial of erlotinib in recurrent squamous cell carcinoma of the cervix: a Gynecologic Oncology Group study. Int J Gynecol Cancer. 2009;19:929–33.
28. Monk BJ, Mas Lopez L, Zarba JJ, et al. Phase II, open-label study of pazopanib or lapatinib monotherapy compared with pazopanib plus lapatinib combination therapy in patients with advanced and recurrent cervical cancer. J Clin Oncol. 2010;28:3562–9.

29. Cetina L, Crombet T, Jiménez R, et al. A phase II trial to evaluate Nimotuzumab as second- or third-line treatment or more in patients with recurring or persistent locorregionally advanced or metastatic cervical cancer. Cancer Biol Ther. 2015;16(5):684–9.
30. Guidi AJ, Abu-Jawdeh G, Berse B, et al. Vascular permeability factor (vascular endothelial growth factor) expression and angiogenesis in cervical neoplasia. J Natl Cancer Inst. 1995;87:1237–45.
31. Wright JD, Viviano D, Powell MA, et al. Bevacizumab combination therapy in heavily pretreated, recurrent cervical cancer. Gynecol Oncol. 2006;103:489–93.
32. Monk BJ, Sill MW, Burger RA, et al. Phase II trial of bevacizumab in the treatment of persistent or recurrent squamous cell carcinoma of the cervix: a Gynecology Oncology Group study. J Clin Oncol. 2009;27:1069–74.
33. Shefter TE, Winter K, Kwon JS, et al. A phase II study of bevacizumab in combination with definitive radiotherapy and cisplatin chemotherapy in untreated patients with locally advanced cervical carcinoma: preliminary results of RTOG 0417. Int J Radiat Oncol Biol Phys. 2012;83(4):1179–84.
34. Sonpavde G, Hutson TE. Pazopanib: a novel multitargeted tyrosine kinase inhibitor. Curr Oncol Rep. 2007;9:115–9.
35. Monk BJ, Pandite LN. Survival data from a phase II, open-label study of pazopanib or lapatinib monotherapy in patients with advanced and recurrent cervical cancer. J Clin Oncol. 2011;29:4845.
36. Munster P, Marchion D, Bicaku E, et al. Phase I trial of histone deacetylase inhibition by valproic acid followed by the topoisomerase II inhibitor epirubicin in advanced solid tumors: a clinical and translational study. J Clin Oncol. 2007;25:1979–85.
37. Coronel J, Cetina L, Pacheco I, et al. A double-blind, placebo-controlled, randomized phase III trial of chemotherapy plus epigenetic therapy with hydralazine valproate for advanced cervical cancer. Preliminary results. Med Oncol. 2011;28(S1):540–6.
38. Chen J, Macdonald OK, Gaffner DK. Incidence, mortality, and prognostic factors of small cell carcinoma of the cérvix. Obstet Gynecol. 2008;111:1394–402.
39. McCusker ME, Coté TR, Clegg LX, et al. Endocrine tumors of the uterine cérvix: incidence demographics, and survival with comparison to squeamous cell carcinoma. Gynecol Oncol. 2003;88:333–9.
40. Albores-Saavedra J, Gersell D, Gilks CB, et al. Terminology of endocrine tumors of the uterine cervix. results of a workshop sponsored by the College of American Pathologist and the National Cancer Institute. Arch Pathol Lab Med. 1997;121:34–9.
41. Sheets EE, Berman ML, Hrountas CK, et al. Surgical treated, early-stage neuroendocrine small-cell cervical carcarcinoma. Obstet Gynecol. 1988;71:10–6.
42. Viswanathan AN, Deavers MT, Jhingran A, et al. Small cell neuroendocrine carcinoma of the cervix:outcome and patterns of recurrence. Gynecol Oncol. 2004;93:27–33.
43. Zivanovic O, Leitao Jr MM, Park KJ, et al. Small cell neuroendocrine carcinoma of the cervix: analysis of outcome, recurrencia pattern and the impact of platinum-base combination chemotherapy. Gynecol Oncol. 2009;112:590–3.
44. Cohen JP, Kapp DS, Shin JY, et al. Small cell carcinoma of the cervix: treatment and survival outcomes of 188 patients. Am J Obstet Gynecol. 2010;203:347.e1–6.
45. Hoskins PJ, Swenerton KD, Pike JA, et al. Small cell carcinoma of the cervix: fourteen years of experience at a single institution using a combined-modality régimen of involved-field irradiation and platinum-based combination chemotherapy. J Clin Oncol. 2003;21:3495–501.
46. Melnick S, Cole P, Anderson D, et al. Rates and risks of diethylstilbestrol-related clear-cell adenocarcinoma of the vagina and cervix. N Engl J Med. 1987;316:514–6.
47. Nasu K, Takai N, Narahara H. Multimodal treatment for glassy cell carcinoma of the uterine cervix. J Obstet Gynaecol Res. 2009;35(3):584–7.

Chapter 14
Immuno-Oncology in Cervical Cancer

Juan P. Marquez-Manriquez, Erik Ramos, and Dolores Gallardo-Rincón

Abstract Cervical cancer (CC) remains a challenging disease despite the approved preventive vaccines against HPV, which is the cause of this type of tumor. Immune-mediated treatments, or immuno-oncology, currently represent 6% of cancer therapies, and in the next 10 years, this percentage is expected to increase up to 70%. There are ongoing efforts to develop specific immunotherapies, such as immunomodulatory drugs and antibodies, to treat CC in combination with standard-of-care regimens. However, currently, there are no clinically available active antigen-specific immunotherapies that effectively treat CC, despite multiple studies in animal models that have mainly focused on the viral early proteins (E2, E5, E6, and E7). There are data from clinical trials using DNA, proteins, and peptide vaccines targeting these viral early proteins as treatments for CC, but there has been limited clinical success. It is clear that the adaptive immune system plays an important role in CC; multiple studies have shown that immune infiltration is related to prognosis. Non-viral targets are also potential candidates for targeting by next-generation immunotherapies for CC and vaccines to prevent relapse.

Keywords Cervical cancer antigens • Checkpoint inhibitors • Active antigen-specific immunotherapy • Combination immune therapies • HPV antigens for cervical cancer treatment • Non-viral biological oncogenic drivers • Clinically relevant antigens and immune infiltration

J.P. Marquez-Manriquez, MD • E. Ramos, MD
Tumor Vaccine Group, University of Washington, Seattle, WA, USA

D. Gallardo-Rincón, MD (✉)
Department of Medical Oncology, Instituto Nacional de Cancerología-México,
Av. San Fernando No 22, Col Sección XVI, Tlalpan, Mexico City, Mexico, 14080
e-mail: dgallardorincon@gmail.com

J.G. de la Garza-Salazar et al. (eds.), *Cervical Cancer*,
DOI 10.1007/978-3-319-45231-9_14

14.1 Introduction

Cervical cancer (CC) remains an important disease despite the approval of preventive vaccines against human papillomavirus (HPV) in 2006 and 2009 [1]. However, the available prophylactic vaccines against HPV do not protect against established pre-malignant lesions, such as cervical intraepithelial neoplasia (CIN) grades I, II and III, or against CC [1], as they target proteins that are no longer relevant in these clinical conditions. In order to treat CIN and CC, we need a vaccine that can elicit an active antigen-specific response against proteins that are important in established disease.

There are several pre-clinical and clinical efforts underway to develop active antigen-specific immunotherapy (immunotherapy) to treat established pre-malignant lesions and CC [2]. Most of the studies have focused on HPV proteins, such as E2, E5, E6 and E7, which are known to be involved in HPV-induced cancer. However, the clinical results have been mixed, and there is not yet a clinically approved immunotherapy for CC [2] (Fig. 14.1).

Clinical trials for HPV-associated cancer

Vaccine	Antigen(s)	Phase	
ADXS11 -001:	HPV-16	I	Cervical cancer
Lm seceting fusion to LLO-HPV-16 E7 protein (Lm-LLO-E7)	E7	I	HPV-oropharyngeal cancer
		II	Recurrent cervical carcinoma
TA-HPV: Recombinant vaccinia virus expressing E6 and E7 from both HPV-16 and HPV-18	E6 and E7 of HPV16 and HPV-18	I	Stage Ib and IIa cervical cancer
		I/II	Advanced cervical cancer
		II	Stage Ib and IIa cervical
PADRE peptide linked to E7 Lipopeptide	HPV-16 E7	I	Cervical cancer
HPV-16 E7 epitopes emulsfied in montanide ISA-51 adjuvant	HPV-16 E7	I/II	Cervical cancer
13 overlapping long peptides covering whole E6 and e7 sequences of HPV 16 plus montanide ISA-51 adjunvant	HPV-16 E6 and E7	I	Advanced cervical can cervical cancer
		II	
DC pulsed with HPV-16 E7	HPV-16 E7	I	Recurrent cervical cancer
pNGVL4a-Sig/E7/Hsp70: DNA plasmid expressing mutated HPV-16 E7 fused to Sig and Hsp70	HPV-16 E7	I	Advanced HNSCC

Fig. 14.1 Clinical trials for cervical cancer immunotherapy

Phase one of immunoediting plays an important role in CC development as this barrier of the immune system against cancer can be overcome by persistent infection with high-risk HPV [3]. Most (90%) cervical HPV infections are cleared within 2 years [3]. In cases that progress to CC, the immune response paradoxically contributes to tumor development rather than to tumor eradication [3]. The type and number of immune cells present in the CC microenvironment are crucial for clinical outcome [4]. T helper 1 (Th1) cells are required to overcome HPV and other oncogenic drivers by inducing a tumor antigen-specific response [4]. Th2 cells protect against extracellular pathogens, and these cells have been shown to support CC progression in immune infiltration studies [4]. Another T cell subtype that has been related to poor survival in several CC studies is Foxp3-positive T regulatory cells (Tregs) [5]. Several CC studies have reported the number and distribution of intraepithelial and stromal T, Treg, Th1, Th2, and Th17 cells, as well as other adaptive and innate immune cells [5, 6]. The infiltration of both adaptive and innate immune cells may predict the prognosis of patients with CC [6]. In particular, adaptive immune cells such as antigen-specific Th1 cells are the most attractive targets for testing which epitopes derived from HPV and non-HPV oncogenic driver proteins are biologically and clinically relevant in the development of effective active antigen-specific immunotherapies for CC [7].

Importantly, although E6 and E7 are the most studied viral proteins and are immunogenic, we do not yet have a clinically available immunotherapy for premalignant cervical lesions or CC based on these proteins [7]. However, it is important to remember that independently of CC is caused by HPV the most attractive targets are viral proteins from the virus, but once malignant transformation occurs, other oncogenic driver proteins are potential targets for the development of active antigen-specific immunotherapies [6, 7]. Such therapies can include both viral and non-viral proteins to improve the cellular and/or humoral immune response and eventually increase the clinical efficacy of immunotherapies for CC [8].

However, CC cells can escape immune system surveillance by promoting an immunosuppressive state in their microenvironment [4, 5]. Many studies have shown that various immunosuppressive cells and molecules are recruited to a primary cervical tumor site [5].

Higher frequencies of CD4+ and CD8+ T cells expressed the immune checkpoint molecules PD-1 and CTLA-4 in positive lymph nodes in patients with CC [9, 10]. Several studies have found high numbers of PD-L1+CD14+ antigen presenting cells (APCs) and T regulatory cells in the microenvironment of positive lymph nodes in CC patients, and the presence of these cell types is correlated [10]. Therefore, a combinatorial active antigen-specific immunotherapy including checkpoint inhibitors and immune modulators might block this immunosuppressive cycle and induce effective anti-tumor immunity to halt metastatic spread in patients with CC (Fig. 14.2).

The main goals of CC immunotherapy using active antigen-specific approaches are to induce an effective Th1 immune response and to overcome some of the

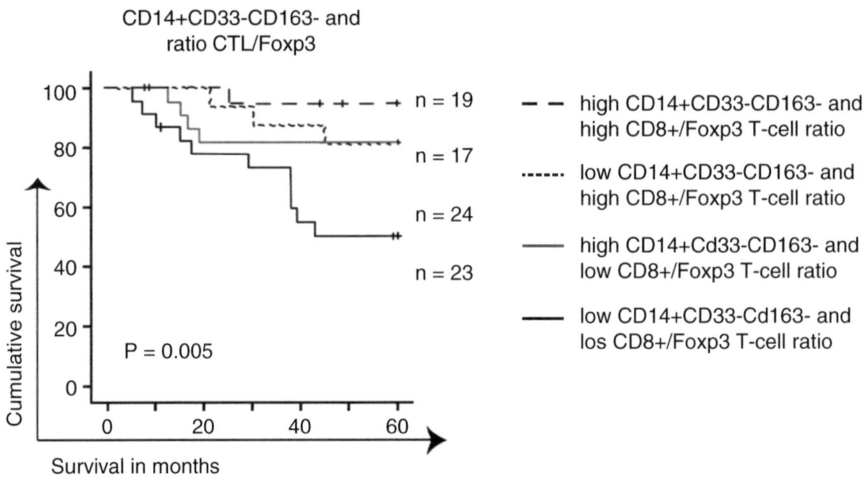

Fig. 14.2 Clinical impact of the ratios of subpopulations of immune infiltrates in cervical cancer

inhibitory mechanisms that impede an effective immune response, as mentioned above. Furthermore, immunotherapy must target the more protected Th1 epitopes on several viral and non-viral proteins to increase the successful induction of an immune response against biologically and clinically relevant oncogenic drivers [11]. Achieving a state of remission does not necessarily imply the elimination of all CC cells and cancer stem cells, as shown by the frequency of CC recurrence after standard-of-care treatment [12]. The administration of active antigen-specific immunotherapy before, during and after standard-of-care regimens to treat CC is an attractive alternative to destroy transformed tumor cells and to provide long-term protection through the generation of memory T cells and antibodies classically induced by active immunotherapy. Despite the limited success in early clinical trials, several new studies using peptides and DNA immunotherapies have shown some success in treating CC and preventing relapse [13].

14.2 Immune Infiltration and Immunogenicity of Cervical Cancer

The role of immune infiltration in opposing tumor growth has only recently been widely appreciated [14]. After years of controversy, it is now established that reactivating the immune system is a potent tool for eradicating some forms of cancer [14]. Recent studies have improved our understanding of the relationship between the innate and adaptive immune systems and cancer development, and there is consistent evidence that lymphocytic infiltration into solid tumors is a beneficial prognostic marker [15] (Fig. 14.3).

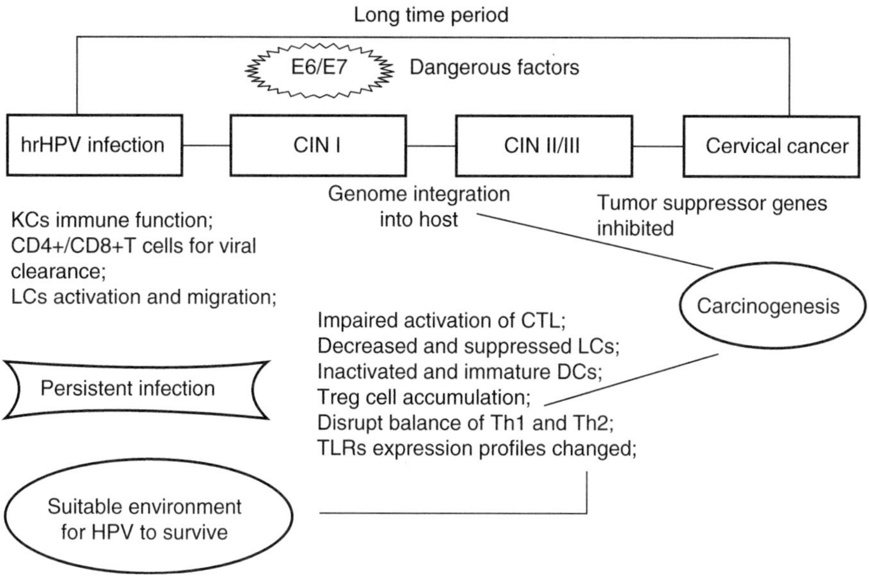

Fig. 14.3 Immune changes during the progression from human papilloma virus infection to cervical cancer

In 2006, Jerome Galon and his colleagues used microarray analysis and immunohistochemistry to document that the presence, type, and location of CD8+ T cell infiltrates in human colon cancer were associated with longer patient survival [14].

Jordanova et al. studied whether the infiltration of T cell subpopulations was correlated with patient survival in cases of cervical adenocarcinoma and squamous cell carcinoma (SCC) ($n = 67$). They analyzed the frequencies of tumor-infiltrating T cells, Tregs, Th17 cells and IL-17+ cells [15] and found that a high total number of Tregs was significantly correlated with improved disease-specific survival (DSS) and disease-free survival (DFS) ($p = 0.010$, $p = 0.007$). Within the tumor epithelium, a high number of T cells was significantly correlated with improved DFS ($p = 0.034$). In particular, a low number of both Tregs and IL-17+ cells was correlated with poor DSS ($p = 0.007$). A low number of Tregs in the presence of Th17 cells was also correlated with poor survival ($p = 0.018$). These data in cervical adenocarcinoma contrast the correlations described in SCC, suggesting a differential contribution of the local immune response to tumor growth in cervical adenocarcinoma versus SCC [15].

In another CC study conducted by Van der Burg et al. ($n = 58$), the infiltration of Tbet+ cells, but not of Foxp3+ cells, was positively associated with DFS and DSS, indicating that the type 1 immune response of the infiltrate, rather than the overall number of immune cells, is an important predictor of the response to subsequent therapy [16].

There are also indications that marked infiltration by Tbet+ cells is associated with better clinical outcome in patients with HPV-induced pre-malignant lesions [16]. Furthermore, tumors from patients without lymph node metastasis had a larger average area occupied by CD45+ immune cells and displayed greater Tbet+ cell infiltration compared to tumors from patients with lymph node metastases [16].

Jordanova et al. investigated the composition of tumor-infiltrating myeloid cells and their relationship to other tumor-infiltrating immune cells, tumor characteristics and the DSS of patients with CC ($n = 86$). Substantial intraepithelial infiltration of CD141 cells, and more specifically, mature M1 macrophages [17], was associated with a large influx of intraepithelial T lymphocytes ($p = 0.008$) and improved DSS ($p = 0.007$) and was identified as an independent prognostic factor for survival ($p = 0.033$). The ratio of intraepithelial CD8 T cells to Tregs was also an independent prognostic factor ($p = 0.010$). Furthermore, the combination of these two prognostic factors revealed a further increased survival benefit in patients whose tumors displayed dense intraepithelial infiltration of mature M1 macrophages and a high CD8 T cell/Treg ratio, indicating that both populations of immune cells simultaneously improve survival [17]. They concluded that the reinforcement and activation of intratumoral M1 macrophages might represent an attractive option for modulating the CC microenvironment [17].

In another study, Yu et al. studied immune infiltration in CC to predict local recurrence [6]. The objective was to establish a predictive model of local recurrence by assessing the prognostic significance of clinicopathologic features and five markers within the tumor microenvironment. The expression of CD3, CD4, CD8, Foxp3, and IL-17 was assessed by immunohistochemistry in tumor tissue ($n = 153$) after radical resection for CC. Local recurrence was observed in 34% of the patients. Independent predictors of tumor recurrence were lymph node status ($p = 0.004$), lymphovascular space invasion ($p = 0.012$), and the number of intratumoral IL-17+ cells ($P = 0.003$). The risk of local recurrence was the highest in patients with few intratumoral IL-17+ cells [6].

14.3 Targets for Immunotherapy in Cervical Carcinoma

Typically, for cancers that are induced by viruses, such as CC, the immunotherapy targets and biomarkers are viral proteins that are important for tumor formation and progression [18]. However, despite the identification of several viral early proteins, such as E2, E5, E6, and E7, as potential targets in CC, no effective active antigen-specific immunotherapy targeting these proteins has been approved for clinical use [18]. Moreover, some viral proteins may not be biologically relevant for tumor survival, but the virus or transformed CC cells may aberrantly express other proteins that could serve as targets for active antigen-specific immunotherapy [19].

Several studies in CC have been conducted to identify and characterize aberrantly expressed proteins that, if immunogenic, could be included in active antigen-specific immunotherapy for CC [20].

For example, NQO1 was studied in uterine cervical lesions, including non-neoplastic cervical tissue (n = 25), CIN (CIN-1 n = 28; CIN-2 n = 38; and CIN-3 n = 27), and squamous CC (n = 177), from patients aged 22–76 years [20].

The investigators found that NQO1 protein was expressed at high levels in several tumors. NQO1 expression in SCC of the uterine cervix and the other above-mentioned clinical conditions was evaluated to ascertain the relationship with clinicopathological parameters and its prognostic value in squamous CC based on survival data [20].

Immunofluorescence staining revealed high NQO1 expression levels in CC (80.23%). The rate of positive NQO1 protein expression was only 12% in non-neoplastic cervical tissues but was significantly higher in CIN lesions (CIN-1 41.38%; CIN-2 52.63%; and CIN-3 55.56%) ($p = 0.01$) [20].

Patients with SCC whose tumors overexpressed NQO1 had lower DFS ($p < 0.01$) and 5-year OS rates ($p < 0.01$) than those whose tumors had low NQO1 expression. In early-stage cervical SCC, patients with high-level NQO1 expression had lower DFS and 5-year OS rates compared with those with low-level NQO1 expression ($p < 0.05$) [20].

Song et al. evaluated astrocyte elevated gene-1 (AEG-1), which plays an important role in the development and progression of certain types of human cancer [21]. In this study, immunohistochemistry was utilized to investigate AEG-1 expression in CIN and CC, and a multivariate analysis was performed. AEG-1 expression increased from CIN-1 to CIN-3, and the high expression in CC (61.1%) was associated with shorter patient survival, as evidenced by univariate and multivariate analyses ($p < 0.05$). This study was the first to show that high AEG-1 expression is significantly associated with CC progression [21] (Table 14.1).

Table 14.1 Potential non-viral targets for active antigen-specific immunotherapy in cervical cancer

Protein	Cervical cancer percent of expression	N
AEG-1	61	90
NQO1	80.23	177
LAPTM4B-35	72.57	113
EZH2	68.3	101
HIF-alpha	94.6	74
API-5	80.3	122
URG4	35.13	167
C14ORF166	39.9	148
FASCIN	67	27
EIF5A2	64	314
B7-H4	69.6	102

14.4 Checkpoint Inhibitors in Cervical Cancer

Checkpoint inhibitors have been barely explored in CC [22].

However, active antigen-specific immunotherapy for CC might be improved by the co-administration of immunomodulatory antibodies that block immunosuppressive signaling, such as that by CTLA-4 or PD-1, to more effectively promote antitumoral T cell responses.

Thus far, limited data suggest that tumor-infiltrating Tregs are present in CC and many types of cancer and usually indicate a poor prognosis [23]. One study found an increased Treg/CD8 ratio in CC, and a similar intratumoral lymphocyte pattern was observed in the TC-1 mouse model of CC [23]. In this animal model of CC, systemic Treg depletion was ineffective at controlling tumor growth. However, when local anti-CTLA-4 antibody production was combined with Treg inhibition, permanent TC-1 tumor regression and immunity were induced. Importantly, no signs of autoimmunity were detected in mice that received local CTLA-4 blockade alone or in combination with Treg depletion [23].

Thus, CC immunotherapy might be combined with immunomodulatory drugs or antibodies that combat local immune suppression in the CC microenvironment.

References

1. Lowy DR. HPV vaccination to prevent cervical cancer and other HPV-associated disease: from basic science to effective interventions. J Clin Invest. 2016;126(1):5–11.
2. Menderes G, Black J, Schwab CL, Santin AD. Immunotherapy and targeted therapy for cervical cancer: an update. Expert Rev Anticancer Ther. 2016;16(1):83–98.
3. Gimenes F, Teixeira JJ, de Abreu AL, Souza RP, Pereira MW, da Silva VR, Bôer CG, Maria-Engler SS, Bonini MG, Borelli SD, Consolaro ME. Human leukocyte antigen (HLA)-G and cervical cancer immunoediting: a candidate molecule for therapeutic intervention and prognostic biomarker? Biochim Biophys Acta. 2014;1846(2):576–89.
4. Adurthi S, Mukherjee G, Krishnamurthy H, Sudhir K, Bafna UD, Umadevi K, Jayshree RS. Functional tumor infiltrating TH1 and TH2 effectors in large early-stage cervical cancer are suppressed by regulatory T cells. Int J Gynecol Cancer. 2012;22(7):1130–7.
5. Shah W, Yan X, Jing L, Zhou Y, Chen H, Wang Y. A reversed CD4/CD8 ratio of tumor-infiltrating lymphocytes and a high percentage of CD4(+)FOXP3(+) regulatory T cells are significantly associated with clinical outcome in squamous cell carcinoma of the cervix. Cell Mol Immunol. 2011;8(1):59–66.
6. Yu Q, Lou XM, He Y. Prediction of local recurrence in cervical cancer by a Cox model comprised of lymph node status, lymph-vascular space invasion, and intratumoral Th17 cell-infiltration. Med Oncol. 2014;31(1):795.
7. Grabowska AK, Kaufmann AM, Riemer AB. Identification of promiscuous HPV16-derived T helper cell epitopes for therapeutic HPV vaccine design. Int J Cancer. 2015;136(1):212–24.
8. Zhang W, Ou J, Lei F, Hou T, Wu S, Niu C, Xu L, Zhang Y. C14ORF166 overexpression is associated with pelvic lymph node metastasis and poor prognosis in uterine cervical cancer. Tumour Biol. 2016;37(1):369–79. doi:10.1007/s13277-015-3806-3. Epub 2015 Jul 29.
9. Howitt BE, Sun HH, Roemer MG, Kelley A, Chapuy B, Aviki E, Pak C, Connelly C, Gjini E, Shi Y, Lee L, Viswanathan A, Horowitz N, Neuberg D, Crum CP, Lindeman NL, Kuo F, Ligon

AH, Freeman GJ, Hodi FS, Shipp MA, Rodig SJ. Genetic basis for PD-L1 Expression in squamous cell carcinomas of the cervix and vulva. JAMA Oncol. 2016;2(4):518–22. doi:10.1001/jamaoncol.2015.6326.
10. Heeren AM, Koster BD, Samuels S, Ferns DM, Chondronasiou D, Kenter GG, Jordanova ES, de Gruijl TD. High and interrelated rates of PD-L1+CD14+ antigen-presenting cells and regulatory T cells mark the microenvironment of metastatic lymph nodes from patients with cervical cancer. Cancer Immunol Res. 2015;3(1):48–58.
11. Yang S, Gao Y, Wang D, Xia B, Liu Y, Qin Y, Ning X, Li G, Hao L, Xiao M, Zhang Y. Overexpression of Eukaryotic initiation factor 5A2 is associated with cancer progression and poor prognosis in patients with early-stage cervical cancer. Histopathology. 2016;69(2):276–87. doi:10.1111/his.12933. Epub 2016 Mar 17.
12. Markman M. Advances in cervical cancer pharmacotherapies. Expert Rev Clin Pharmacol. 2014;7(2):219–23.
13. Melief CJ, van Hall T, Arens R, Ossendorp F, van der Burg SH. Therapeutic cancer vaccines. J Clin Invest. 2015;125(9):3401–12.
14. Galon J, Costes A, Sanchez-Cabo F, Kirilovsky A, Mlecnik B, Lagorce-Pagès C, Tosolini M, Camus M, Berger A, Wind P, Zinzindohoué F, Bruneval P, Cugnenc PH, Trajanoski Z, Fridman WH, Pagès F. Type, density, and location of immune cells within human colorectal tumors predict clinical outcome. Science. 2006;313(5795):1960–4.
15. Heeren AM, de Boer E, Bleeker MC, Musters RJ, Buist MR, Kenter GG, de Gruijl TD, Jordanova ES. Nodal metastasis in cervical cancer occurs in clearly delineated fields of immune suppression in the pelvic lymph catchment area. Oncotarget. 2015;6(32):32484–93.
16. Gorter A, Prins F, van Diepen M, Punt S, van der Burg SH. The tumor area occupied by Tbet+ cells in deeply invading cervical cancer predicts clinical outcome. J Transl Med. 2015;13:295.
17. De Vos van Steenwijk PJ, Ramwadhdoebe TH, Goedemans R, Doorduijn EM, van Ham JJ, Gorter A, van Hall T, Kuijjer ML, van Poelgeest MI, van der Burg SH, Jordanova ES. Tumor-infiltrating CD14-positive myeloid cells and CD8-positive T-cells prolong survival in patients with cervical carcinoma. Int J Cancer. 2013;133(12):2884–94.
18. Albers AE, Kaufmann AM. Therapeutic human papillomavirus vaccination. Public Health Genomics. 2009;12(5–6):331–42.
19. Sagae S, Monk BJ, Pujade-Lauraine E, Gaffney DK, Narayan K, Ryu SY, McCormack M, Plante M, Casado A, Reuss A, Chávez-Blanco A, Kitchener H, Nam BH, Jhingran A, Temkin S, Mileshkin L, Berns E, Scholl S, Doll C, Abu-Rustum NR, Lecuru F, Small Jr W. Advances and concepts in cervical cancer trials: a road map for the future. Int J Gynecol Cancer. 2016;26(1):199–207.
20. Ma Y, Kong J, Yan G, Ren X, Jin D, Jin T, Lin L, Lin Z. NQO1 overexpression is associated with poor prognosis in squamous cell carcinoma of the uterine cervix. BMC Cancer. 2014;14:414.
21. Song E, Yu W, Xiong X, Kuang X, Ai Y, Xiong X. Astrocyte elevated gene-1 promotes progression of cervical squamous cell carcinoma by inducing epithelial-mesenchymal transition via Wnt signaling. Int J Gynecol Cancer. 2015;25(3):345–55.
22. Raval RR, Sharabi AB, Walker AJ, Drake CG, Sharma P. Tumor immunology and cancer immunotherapy: summary of the 2013 SITC primer. J Immunother Cancer. 2014;2:14.
23. Tuve S, Chen BM, Liu Y, Cheng TL, Touré P, Sow PS, Feng Q, Kiviat N, Strauss R, Ni S, Li ZY, Roffler SR, Lieber A. Combination of tumor site-located CTL-associated antigen-4 blockade and systemic regulatory T-cell depletion induces tumor-destructive immune responses. Cancer Res. 2007;67(12):5929–39.

Chapter 15
Palliative Care in Cervical Cancer Patients

Silvia Allende-Pérez, Emma Verástegui-Avilés, Dana A. Pérez-Camargo, Georgina Domínguez-Ocadio, and Frank D. Ferris

Abstract The use of aggressive treatments in patients with advanced cervical cancer at the end of life is frequent. Different studies have suggested no appreciable difference in survival between patients treated aggressively versus those that received palliative care, the term is frequently misconstrued as synonymous with end-of-life. Palliative care is focused on the relief of suffering, in all of its dimensions, throughout the course of a patient's illness. A provisional clinical opinion released by the *American Society of Clinical Oncology* recommends the use of palliative care alongside standard oncologic therapy for patients newly diagnosed with metastatic cancer, according with the patients' needs. The purpose of the chapter is to highlight the importance of palliative care (PC) as an integral part of the care of CaCu patients. A better understanding of PC would help the oncologist to identify potentially eligible patients for PC; researchers to standardize the design for future trials and administrators promote the implementation of PC programs and allocate proper resources.

Keywords Advanced cervical cancer • Palliative care • Symptom management

S. Allende-Pérez, MD • E. Verástegui-Avilés, MD (✉) • D.A. Pérez-Camargo, MSc
G. Domínguez-Ocadio, MD
Palliative Care Service, Instituto Nacional de Cancerología-México,
Av. San Fernando No 22, Mexico City, Mexico, 14080
e-mail: everasteguia@incan.edu.mx

F.D. Ferris, MD
Palliative Medicine Research and Education at OhioHealth in Columbus,
Columbus, OH, USA

J.G. de la Garza-Salazar et al. (eds.), *Cervical Cancer*,
DOI 10.1007/978-3-319-45231-9_15

15.1 Introducción

Non-communicable diseases, including cancer, are becoming the leading health-care threat in middle-income and low-income countries [1]. Latin American and Caribbean countries are struggling to respond to increasing morbidity and death from advanced diseases, such as cancer, even though the overall incidence of cancer is lower in the Region than in Developed countries; the mortality burden is greater, mainly due to presentation at more advanced stages, and partly related to poorer access to cancer care [1–3].

Health-care systems in Latin America are characterized by a lack of health-care coverage for populations with no formal employment; therefore, families are exposed to a high risk of catastrophic expenses, particularly for chronic illnesses [1]. Fragmented health-care systems and poor financing schemes causes diagnostic failures, late referrals and treatment delays that contributes to advanced disease at presentation [1]. Cervical Cancer (CaCu) is a clear example of it, is second most common cause of cancer in Latin America and is a leading cause of cancer mortality among women. Gaps in prevention, screening, diagnostic, and treatment capacities, contribute to poor 5-year survival rates [1, 3]. In consequence, 31,000 women of the close to 70,000 diagnosed with CaCu in Latin America will die of the disease [1–4].

Management of early-stage; locally advanced or metastatic cervical cancer involves multispecialty care, including gynecology oncology, medical oncology, radiology, pathology, radiation oncology, and palliative care [5]. Women with metastatic or recurrent cervical cancer have heterogeneous manifestations and therefore no standard treatment is available at the present time [6–10].

Mexico, promote a major legislative health-care reform leading to universal health coverage through integration of health insurance for poor and uninsured populations, known as Seguro Popular. (SP) [11]. Furthermore, an additional mechanism was also designed to include the coverage of several high cost intervention defined as "Catastrophic health spending" and treatment for CaCu became the first type of adult neoplasm included [12, 13].

The availability SP for the treatment of CaCu has increased the adherence to therapy; however, advanced and recurrent CaCu continues to be a major problem in Mexico, mostly on highly social and economic vulnerable population. In addition to the poor prognosis, patients with advanced CaCu experience several stressful physical symptoms associated tumor location and treatment complications include pain, vaginal bleeding, fatigue, lymphedema, sexual dysfunction, proctitis, cystitis, constipation, diarrhea, foul odor, and recto-vaginal fistulas [14]. They also experience disturbing psychological symptoms depression and anxiety, sleep disturbance, and concentration difficulties, in addition to complex economic and social problems [15].

Despite advances in cancer treatment, a large proportion of CaCu patients still eventually die as a result of their disease. Patients with advanced-stage cancer are receiving increasingly aggressive medical care at the end of life [16]. Indicators of overly "aggressive" end-of-life care includes: (1) repeated hospitalizations or emergency department visits or admission to an intensive care unit within the last month, (2) chemotherapy $\leq$2 weeks before death, and late or absent palliative care referrals [17, 18]. All these practices contributes to poor quality of care, according to the definition provided by the National Cancer Policy Board *"practices of known effectiveness are being underutilized, practices of known ineffectiveness are being overutilized, and when services of equivocal effectiveness are being utilized in accordance with provider rather than patient preferences* [19]". Assessment of these three areas may be useful to identified poor-quality care from the administrative point of view [18].

Several studies have shown that the use of chemotherapy near the end of life may not provide benefit, and suggest that one of the major drivers to recommend it, is physician practice style [20, 21], The discussion about providing symptomatic and supportive care is a difficult, and often is easier to recommend another line of chemotherapy, particularly nontoxic targeted agents [22–24]. From the patient perspective, the request to receive an aggresive treatment right before the end of life, end could be caused because they do not understand their prognosis; therefore, have unrealistic expectations about the benefits of chemotherapy, want to "keep fighting", among several other reasons [25–29].

Aggressive end-of-life care is an indicator of poor quality care; however, if high-quality palliative care is not available, oncologists will continue giving chemotherapy longer than they otherwise would. Uneven access to hospice and palliative care has been documented, particularly in Low and Middle income countries [30, 31].

The purpose of the chapter is to highlight the importance of palliative care (PC) as an integral part of the care CaCu patients. A better understanding of PC would help the oncologist to identify potentially eligible patients for PC; researchers to standardize the design for future trials and administrators promote the implementation of PC programs and allocate proper resources.

15.2 What Is Palliative Care?

The World Health Organization defines Palliative Care *as an approach that improves the quality of life of patients and their families facing the problem associated with life-threatening illness, through the prevention and relief of suffering by means of early identification and impeccable assessment and treatment of pain and other problems, physical, psychosocial and spiritual* [32].

Palliative care:

- *provides relief from pain and other distressing symptoms;*
- *affirms life and regards dying as a normal process;*
- *intends neither to hasten or postpone death;*
- *integrates the psychological and spiritual aspects of patient care;*
- *offers a support system to help patients live as actively as possible until death;*
- *offers a support system to help the family cope during the patients illness and in their own bereavement;*
- *uses a team approach to address the needs of patients and their families, including bereavement counselling, if indicated;*
- *will enhance quality of life, and may also positively influence the course of illness;*
- *is applicable early in the course of illness, in conjunction with other therapies that are intended to prolong life, such as chemotherapy or radiation therapy, and includes those investigations needed to better understand and manage distressing clinical complications.*

According to the *Worldwide Palliative Care Alliance* (WPCA), worldwide, over 6 million people with cancer are estimated to require palliative care at the end of life every year, the majority are adults over 60 years old living in low and middle-income countries [30, 31].

15.2.1 Integrative Model of Palliative Care in Cancer Patients

Palliative care is frequently misconstrued as synonymous with end-of-life care. Palliative care is focused on the relief of suffering, in all of its dimensions, throughout the course of a patient's illness. The use of hospice and other PC services only at the end of life limits the benefit they may gain from these services. Therefore, based on data from several clinical trials, *The American Society of Clinical Oncology* (ASCO) released a provisional clinical opinion (PCO) recommending the use of PC alongside standard oncologic therapy for patients newly diagnosed with metastatic cancer, according with the patients' needs [33]. PC is an all-encompassing approach to cancer care that focuses not only on symptom control, but on other aspects of life important to patients and families in an attempt to prevent and/or alleviate suffering [34].

Despite the support for an early PC referral, at the present time there are not universal criteria for doing so. Most authors agree that the presence of cancer diagnosis, prognosis, physical symptoms, performance status, psychosocial distress, and end-of-life care planning needs, are important issues to be considered. It is important to validate and/or personalize to the local needs the assessment tools, to facilitate and complement clinical judgment for appropriate referrals [35]. An integrative PC model is feasible mainly in tertiary cancer care facilities; however, if not available, the oncologist could manage many PC problems, and could ask for PC consultation for more complex or refractory problems [36, 37]. Basic PC needs should be addressed by the oncologist, including pain and other symptoms, also must have skills to have discussions about prognosis; goals of treatment; suffering and do not resuscitate orders. Referrals to a PC specialist should include the management of refractory symptoms or complex psychosocial issues [36]. When such consultations are initiated, consideration should be given to returning the patient to the oncologist for ongoing PC management, allowing increased access to expert PC consultation and reinforces the patient confidence in his/her care [38].

15.2.2 Palliative Care Assessment Tools

Although there is not a standard format of clinical PC assessment tool, it includes traditional components of medical evaluation (medical and psychosocial history, physical examination), comprehensive palliative assessment involves unique content, focus, and sources of information [39].

A. The content includes six areas examined in a structured manner:
   (a) Pain and other physical symptoms;
   (b) Psychological, psychiatric, and cognitive symptoms;
   (c) Illness understanding and care preferences (ie, personal goals, expectations, understanding of illness trajectory and risks versus benefits of therapies);
   (d) Existential and spiritual concerns;
   (e) Social and economic resources and needs of patients and caregivers, including for care in the home;
   (f) Continuity of and coordination of care across settings.
B. The components of care in palliative are patient-focused and family oriented.
C. Information about the patients not only from the patient, family, medical records. The palliative evaluation utilizes a broad range of sources, each contributing to the final assessment (nursing staff, phycologist, social workers, and nutritionists perform discipline-specific evaluative tasks, together developing the comprehensive palliative assessment).

Effective symptom management requires a good symptom assessment. Different measurement instruments have been created to identify symptoms in oncology practice. Comprehensive reviews of assessment tools and scales are available. For clinical purposes, the Brief Pain Inventory (BPI and its short-form version (BPI-SF)), the revised Edmonton Symptom Assessment Scale (rESAS).

15.2.2.1 Edmonton Symptom Assessment System

In the original version is composed of 10 visual-analogue scales, represented on the left as the least intensity or lack of a symptom and at the right as the worst possible intensity of symptom. The patient marks in her opinion the most appropriate place [40].

15.2.2.2 Quality of Life (QoL)

Is a multidimensional concept regarding self-assessment of patients' situation that to a significant extent is determined by individual needs, beliefs, values, attitudes, which are changing with time.

15.2.2.3 One of the Possibilities of Screening

The psychological state of cancer patients is a distress thermometer that on a scale from 0 to 10 indicates no stress (0) to the strongest psychological distress.

15.2.2.4 The EORTC Quality of Life Questionnaire—Cervical Cancer (QLQ- CX24)

Has been developed and validated to assess the disease- specific and treatment-specific aspects of HRQOL (Health Related) in patients with cervical cancer in a multicultural setting. The QLQ-CX24 consists of 3 multi-item scales and 5 single-item scales [41, 42].

15.2.2.5 Prognostic Scales

Predicting prognosis in advanced cancer aids physicians in clinical decision making and can help patients and their families to prepare for the time ahead. Clinical prediction of survival alone is fairly inaccurate and often presents a bias oriented towards overestimation. Its prognostic capability can potentially be improved by assessing and evaluating a number of clinical symptoms and syndromes. Clinical factors seems to be highly indicative of prognosis in far advanced and palliative phases, (Cancer Anorexia-Cachexia Syndrome), Performance Status Indexes, symptoms such as dyspnea and delirium, and biological parameters, for example, leukocytosis, lymphocytopenia, and C-reactive protein. Several Scales have been validated the most used are the (**A**) Palliative Prognostic Score (PaP Score), (**B**) Delirium-Palliative Prognostic Score (D-PaP Score), Table 15.1 (**C**) Palliative

Table 15.1 Palliative Prognostic Scale (PaP)

Criterion	Assessment	Partial score
Dyspnea	Yes	0
	No	1
Anorexia	Yes	0
	No	1.5
Performance status	>30	0
	10–20	2.5
Clinical prediction (weeks)	>12	0
	11–12	2
	7–10	2.5
	5–6	4.5
	3–4	6
	1–2	8.5
Total WBC	< 8.5	0
	8.6–11	1
	>11	2.5
Lymphocyte percentage	20–40%	0
	12–19.9%	1
	<11	2.5
Risk group	**30 Day survival**	**Total score**
A	>70%	0–5.5
B	30–70%	5.6–11
C	<30%	>11

Table 15.2 Palliative prognostic index

Prognostic domain	Partial score value	
Palliative performance status*		
10–20	4.0	
30–50	2.5	
>60	0	
Clinical symptoms		
Oral intake		
Moderately reduced	1.0	
Severely reduced	2.5	
Normal	0	
Edema	1.0	
Dyspnea at rest	3.5	
Delirium	4.0	
Total score		
Median survival		0–2.0 = 90 days
		2.1–4.0 = 61 days
		>4.0 = 12 day

Modified from: Morita et al. [45]
*The Palliative performance status represents a modified version of the Karnofsky performance scale

Prognostic Index (PPI), Table 15.2 [43–46]. Although there is not consensus, there is a suggestion that the PaP score and especially D-PaP showed slightly better overall accuracy than PPI or PPS [47, 48].

15.3 Palliative Care in Cervical Cancer Patients

Patients with advanced CaCu are a special group of patients to deliver palliative care, they experience a several distressing physical symptoms associated with the anatomic location of their disease, in addition of the physical complications of surgery and/or chemotherapy and radiotherapy. Most of the patients have distressing psychological symptoms related to their frequently low socioeconomic status, complex family issues and the burden of the disease. Common physical symptoms include pain, fatigue, lymphedema, sexual dysfunction, proctitis, cystitis, constipation, diarrhea, foul odor, thrombosis, vaginal bleeding, anorexia, and fistulas. However, despite the appalling impact that the symptoms can have on quality of life, there is no standardized tool for assessing symptoms of gynecologic cancer, and symptom assessment is rarely a part of routine cancer care [49, 50].

15.3.1 Symptoms

15.3.1.1 Pain

Studies conducted by the International Association for the Study of Pain (IASP) have demonstrated that approximately 90% of patients with cancer experience pain [51]. Is one of the most common and devastating symptoms among patients with advanced cancer. It is a multidimensional syndrome that has physical, psychological, and behavioral components, and a multidimensional approach is required for its management.

Pain management is a key element in palliative care and the skills required to provide comfort and relieve other sources of suffering should be acquired by all clinicians involved in the care of populations with life-threatening illnesses. With appropriate use of available pharmacologic agents and other approaches, pain associated with advanced illness in the last weeks of life usually can be controlled.

The pain assessment begins with a detailed characterization of the pain. Specific questions should be directed to pain location; onset, duration, course and daily fluctuation; severity; quality; factors that relieve or provoke the pain; and associated symptoms. The impact of the pain on varied functional domains, including physical activity, mood, interactions in the family and others, should be clarified. Information about the prior evaluation of the pain and the outcomes of prior and existing analgesic therapies should be noted.

(a) Site
(b) Type of pain

- Somatic nociceptive pain involves injury to somatic structures like skin, bone, joints, or muscles. It is usually well localized, and often described by patients as “aching”, “stabbing” or “throbbing”, in quality.
- Visceral nociceptive pain results from distension, injury to, or inflammation of visceral organs. It is usually poorly localized, and characterized as “gnawing” or “crampy” when arising from the obstruction of a hollow viscus (eg, the bowel lumen), or as “aching” or “stabbing” when arising from other somatically innervated visceral structures, such as organ capsules or parietal pleura.
- Neuropathic pain is sustained by abnormal somatosensory processing in the peripheral or central nervous system, or direct damage to nerves. Examples include postchemotherapy neuropathy. Patients may describe unpredictable shooting, burning, numbness, or pruritus.
- Most patients with chronic cancer pain experience periodic flares, often referred to as Breakthrough pain.

(c) Severity and QOL impact. There are a number of simple ways to assess pain severity, including a Faces scale) and Visual Analog Scale.

- Formal instruments have also been developed to rate pain severity in multiple dimensions. The McGill Pain Questionnaire and the BPI have been translated into several languages.

(d) Aggravating and alleviating factors.
(e) Associated symptoms – This includes paresthesias, weakness, nausea.
(f) Temporal patterns – Temporal assessment of the pain may include information about onset, duration, and fluctuation. Both the extent and duration of relief provided by interventions should be determined.

15.3.1.2 Treatment

The WHO analgesic ladder for cancer pain relief is widely accepted as the standard approach in cancer pain control. The foundations for the WHO analgesic ladder were first developed in the early 1980's and the guidelines were published in 1986 [52]. It employs three steps: Step 1: Non-opioid analgesia, e.g. paracetamol/acetaminophen. Step 2: Weak opioid, e.g. codeine. Step 3: Strong opioid, e.g. morphine. Initial studies assessing the efficacy of the WHO ladder showed approximately 80% of patients with cancer pain, will respond to treatment using this. The WHO ladder was quick to be adopted and by 1995, 40 countries had developed policies for the management of cancer pain [53].

Opioids are the standard choice for pharmacologic management of cancer pain, with the goal of analgesic effects with minimum toxicity [54].

A. **Opioids**

Opioids act by binding to specific receptors, the best characterized of which are the mu, kappa, and delta receptors. These receptors are present in tissues throughout the body, including both the peripheral and central nervous systems [55].

Based upon their effects on the mu receptor, opioids are conventionally divided into pure agonists, agonist-antagonists (of which there are two subtypes: partial agonists and mixed agonist-antagonists), and pure antagonists. Mu receptor antagonists have no intrinsic analgesic properties; they are used to prevent or reverse opioid effects.

(a) **Morphine.** Is usually considered to be a standard for comparison across opioid drugs. The morphine is primarily metabolized in the liver and its metabolites are excreted renally. Two active metabolites have been extensively studied, morphine-6-glucuronide (M6G) an opioid, contributes to the analgesia and other opioid effects produced by the administration of morphine and morphine-3-glucuronide (M3G) is not an opioid, binds to other receptors and may be associated with toxic effects.
(b) **Oxycodone.** Have short half-lives similar to morphine and are available in multiple formulations, including an oral formulation and modified release formulations.
(c) **Fentanyl.** Is a synthetic opioid that is available in transdermal, and injectable formulations. Fentanyl may be useful when rotating from one opioid to another and may offer particular advantages for patients who have itching or urticarial in response to opioids, or those with renal insufficiency.

The transdermal formulation, which has duration of effect of 2–3 days, may not be as useful if rapid titration of dose is needed. Furthermore, heat changes the dose delivery rate from the patch. Thus, patients with advanced illness who have recurrent fevers may be at increased risk of unexpected toxicity.

(d) **Methadone.** The use of this drug for pain in populations with advanced illness has steadily increased, driven by its low cost and longstanding clinical benefits. The safe use of methadone requires an understanding of its challenging pharmacokinetic-pharmacodynamic profile [56]. Therefore, uncertainty about how long will take for the patients to reach a steady state after stable dosing begins is always a clinical question. In addition because methadone can prolong the QTc interval, an electrocardiogram (ECG) prior to therapy is recommended. Methadone should be prescribed by a clinician with experience in prescribing and monitoring this drug with complex pharmacokinetics.

(e) **Buprenorphine.** Is a partial agonist. Transdermal buprenorphine, has been licensed in Europe and is commonly prescribed for chronic pain. A 2009 consensus statement from an international panel with expertise in palliative care and pain treatment endorsed the use of transdermal buprenorphine where available.

B. **Opioids Side Effects**

Some patients experience treatment-limiting side effects as the dose of the opioid is increased. Those who initially appear to be poorly responsive to an opioid regimen may have a favorable outcome if the side effects are successfully managed so that the patient can tolerate the dose associated with adequate pain control.

The assessment of opioid side effects in those with advanced illness can be challenging because of the existence of disease complications or comorbidities that may contribute to the problem, change the presentation, or alter the usual approach to therapy. The goals of care may be continually shifting in the context of far advanced illness and the appropriateness of interventions, such as a strategy to reduce somnolence, may change over time. Indeed, near the end of life, somnolence may be viewed as a positive effect of treatment. The most common problems related to pain management in populations with advanced illness are constipation and somnolence or cognitive impairment.

C. **No opioid drugs**

The no opioid analgesics may be used for mild or moderate pain and can provide analgesia that is additive to that produced by the opioids.

Adjuvant analgesics are usually defined as drugs that are indicated for reasons other than pain (eg, depression, epilepsy) but are analgesic in specific circumstances (e.g., gabapentin, pregabalin, and duloxetine).

D. **Neuropathic pain**

Neuropathic pain may be directly related to an illness (eg, nerve compression from tumor) or to a comorbid condition (e.g., chronic back pain with radiculopathy, diabetic peripheral neuropathic pain, or postherpetic neuralgia). When associated with serious illness, opioid therapy usually is tried first. If response is relatively poor, a trial of an adjuvant analgesic often is considered.

15.3.1.3 Special Circumstances for Pain Management

(a) **Chemical Coping.** Opioids are also capable of binding μ receptors in the limbic system to induce reward responses [57]. This double-edged effect of opioids may result in opioid-related problems in patients, including drug-seeking behaviors and a tendency toward dependence. Chemical coping occurs when patients use medications, mainly opioids, in a no prescribed way to cope with the various stressful events associated with the diagnosis and management of cancer, incidence may be as high as 18% of palliative care if diagnosed as by palliative medicine specialists [58].
(b) **Pseudo addiction**. Describes a situation in which a patient's legitimate chronic pain condition is undertreated with pain medication, leading the patient to act in a way that resembles addictive behavior (requesting extra medications and demanding attention); such patients are often labeled as demonstrating "drug seeking behaviors". A careful pain history that emphasizes perceived pain relief will help clarify the issue.

15.3.1.4 Risk Assessment and Management for Patients Receiving Opioids

The public health consequences of opioid abuse drive the imperative that all physicians assume responsibility for risk management; therefore, in some countries the government has taken additional steps to regulate opioids. In the US a Risk Evaluation and Mitigation Strategies (REMS), was designed, one for extended-release and long-acting opioids including transdermal preparations and methadone analgesics, and one for transmucosal immediate release fentanyl formulations (TIRFs) [59]. REMS, prescriber education and patient counseling, are strongly encouraged, but not mandatory. In the US, for transmucosal fentanyl (not available in Mexico) REMS require registration of outpatient prescribers, pharmacies, distributors, and patients in the TIRF REMS access program.

However, clinicians have raised concerns, that the effort to reduce risk could create barriers for cancer pain alleviation. Principles for balancing opioid access with the need to curb misuse and abuse are addressed in a 2016 policy statement on protecting access to opioid treatment for cancer-related pain from the American Society of Clinical Oncology (ASCO) [60].

15.3.2 Total Pain

The perception of discomfort and burden of illness among palliative care patients is highly individualized. To address the complexity of suffering, Dame Cicely Saunders, the foundress of modern hospice and palliative care, introduced the term "total pain." Recalling one of her patient's testimonies, "…The pain began in my

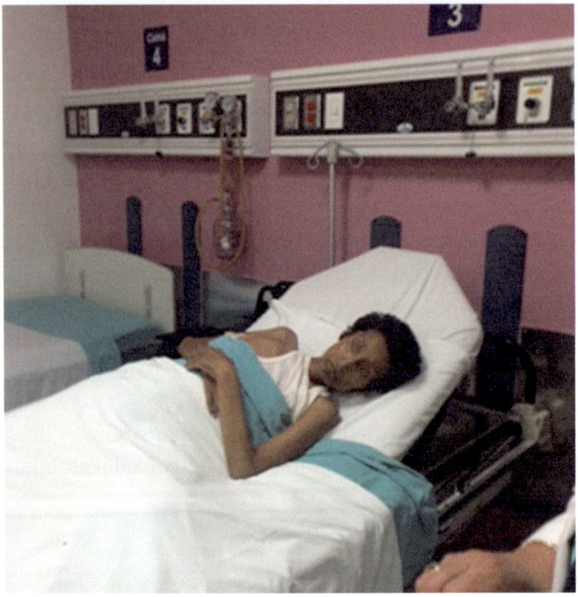

back, but now it seems that all of me is wrong. My husband and my son were marvelous but they were at work and they would have to stay off and lose their money. Everything seemed against me and nobody seemed to understand…" Dr. Saunders observed that her patient's pain included not only physical but also "…emotional and mental suffering, her social problems, and her spiritual need for security and meaning [61–63]". Accordingly, the concept of "total pain," which provides a defining framework for patient assessment in palliative care, refers to the complex mechanisms and manifestations of suffering, including its physical, emotional, socioeconomic, and spiritual components.

15.3.3 Fatigue

Fatigue is a prevalent and poorly understood symptom in patients with advanced serious and/or life-threatening illness. In CaCu patients seen at the palliative Care Service of INCan, up to 99 percent of patients have fatigue.

The assessment of fatigue in palliative care patients can be complex given its subjective and multidimensional nature. Different instruments have been developed for assessment of fatigue in cancer (CRF) patients which assess both severity and functional impact (e.g., the Brief Fatigue Inventory) [64, 65]. Fatigue severity can also be quantified using a 0–10 visual analog scale such as provided in the revised Edmonton Symptom Assessment Scale. The cause of fatigue in palliative care patients is typically multifactorial; therefore, a complete history and physical examination should be undertaken to ascertain the various organ systems affected by the underlying disease and the impact of fatigue on activities of daily living and quality of life, to search for potentially reversible or treatable contributory factors, and to direct the diagnostic work-up. Review of all medications (both prescribed and over the counter, including complementary/alternative therapies) is important.

Potentially treatable causes of fatigue should be sought. These include comorbidities (e.g., anemia, electrolyte abnormalities, alcohol/substance abuse, endocrine dysfunction [e.g., hypothyroidism, hypogonadism, adrenal insufficiency], cardiac, pulmonary, or renal dysfunction), medications, emotional distress, sleep disturbance, pain, nutritional issues (changes in weight/caloric intake), and deconditioning/loss of muscle mass. Symptoms that may contribute to fatigue should be managed appropriately (e.g., pain, dyspnea, nausea, sleep disturbance, depression, anxiety, and anorexia

For patients with cancer-related pain who are receiving opioids, these should be titrated or the schedule/agent modified so as to alleviate pain without causing significant fatigue. If needed, a trial of psychostimulants may help to reverse opioid-related sedation.

Anemia is the most common reversible cause of CRF, particularly among patients receiving chemotherapy. Correction of anemia has been associated with an improvement in health-related quality of life (QOL) and fatigue.

In terminally ill patients who have a high symptom burden that includes fatigue, we suggest a trial of glucocorticoid therapy [66].

15.3.4 Transfusion

Red blood cell (RBC) transfusions are commonly prescribed for palliative care patients. However, RBCs are a limited resource, transfusion is not without risk, and may be of variable benefit in people approaching the end of life [67].

Transfusions of packed red blood cells can improve fatigue due to anemia, although higher-quality studies are needed to determine which patients are most likely to respond, which are not, and the duration of any response [68]. Furthermore, for those patients requiring repeated transfusions, there are potential harms, including blood-borne infection, acute transfusion reaction, transfusion-associated graft-versus-host disease, subtle immune modulation, and iron overload.

15.3.5 Dyspnea

Dyspnea is a common symptom in terminally-ill cancer patients [69]. Is defined only by patient self-report. Objective measures, such as respiratory rate, oxygen saturation, and arterial blood gas determination may not correlate with, nor provide a quantitative measure of the degree of dyspnea, neither physical examination, or pulse oximetry. The prognostic implications of dyspnea, particularly at rest is a prognostic feature.

The most common pharmacologic intervention for dyspnea at the end of life is an opioid analgesic, typically morphine, although other opioids are used successfully. Opioid analgesics function by reducing oxygen demand and dilating pulmonary vessels, which in turn reduce preload to the heart. Other possible interventions include bronchodilators, corticosteroids, sedatives, and tranquilizers. Bronchodilators help open up the airways; corticosteroids help to decrease inflammation and mucous production, benzodiazepines reduce anxiety and, therefore, decrease oxygen demand. Regardless of the cause, severe dyspnea is an emergency and should be treated aggressively. The combination of an opioid and sedative can markedly relieve patients who have end-stage disease.

15.3.6 Gastrointestinal Symptoms

15.3.6.1 Anorexia

Is frequently seen in patients in palliative care and is often a foremost concern of patients and their families. Can be a consequence of chronic fatigue or associated with barely noticeable nausea; depression, pain, xerostomia, or constipation [70].

15.3.6.2 Cachexia

Is a hypercatabolic state that is characterized by an accelerated loss of skeletal muscle in the context of a chronic inflammatory response, and should be distinguished from sarcopenia, loss of muscle. The profound weight loss suffered by patients with cachexia cannot be entirely attributed to poor caloric intake. Insufficient oral intake is superimposed upon complex metabolic aberrations that lead to an increase in basal energy expenditure and culminate in a loss of lean body mass from skeletal muscle wasting. The anorexia-cachexia syndrome often results in psychosocial distress for both patients and family and is associated with a poor prognosis [71].

There are no formal validated cachexia assessment instruments based upon these domains, and malnutrition assessment tools are generally in use to assess cachexia. Patients with anorexia-cachexia syndrome who are able to eat should be recommended to have small, frequent meals that are dense in calories. While some patients may benefit from nutritional supplementation, patients and families should be counseled that increasing caloric intake does not reverse the underlying process and that anorexia/cachexia is not an uncommon symptom, it is different from starvation, and it is a natural process that occurs at the end of life. For patients with persistent anorexia, pharmacologic treatments are available that predominantly stimulate appetite; however, they will not reverse cachexia in most patients [72].

15.3.6.3 Nausea and Vomit

Are a frequent symptoms in palliative care and cause of physical and psychological distress for patients and their families, and significantly impact quality of life (QOL). The etiology is often multifactorial: in addition to cancer treatment, hypercalcemia, malignant bowel obstruction, gastroparesis, or drug-induced constipation. Emesis is not merely a more severe degree of nausea, since the neural circuits responsible for nausea appear to be anatomically distinct from those that generate emesis, the mechanisms underlying the symptom of nausea are not well understood; however, unlike vomiting, nausea requires conscious awareness and cerebral function. An effort should be made to identify and correct reversible underlying causes [73]. Metoclopramide 5 to 10 mg four times daily intravenously, orally, or subcutaneously.

15.3.6.4 Malignant Bowel Obstruction (MBO)

A well-recognized complication in patients with advanced CaCu. Most of these patients are inoperable, and their survival is generally short. Clinical management of MBO requires a specific and individualized approach that is based on disease prognosis and the objectives of care. In most cases, there are few or no data addressing the relative value of palliative surgery versus medical management, and a decision to proceed to surgical intervention requires careful weighing of risks and benefits, including an assessment of the estimated life expectancy and patient goals and preferences [74].

For patients with inoperable MBO, management with IV fluids and temporary nasogastric suctioning to decrease a large amount of secretions before the start of specific pharmacologic management can reduce nausea, vomiting, and pain. Medical management of inoperable patients has focused on adequate control of pain, distention, and vomiting using hydration, opioids, and pharmacologic agents that may reduce symptoms by lessening peritumoral edema (glucocorticoids) and or diminishing intraluminal secretions and peristaltic movements (octreotide reduce propulsive as well as nonpropulsive gut motility, and decrease intraluminal secretions). Prokinetic agents are contraindicated in patients with a complete bowel obstruction. IV haloperidol is considered a first choice antiemetic for patients with malignant bowel obstruction in conjunction with dexamethasone.

Olanzapine is an antipsychotic medication that has affinity for multiple neurotransmitters that may play a role in modulating nausea and vomiting, including dopamine, serotonin, adrenergic, muscarinic, and histamine receptors.

15.3.6.5 Constipation

Constipation has been defined as a stool frequency of less than three per week based upon epidemiological studies in the United States and the United Kingdom; however, this definition is not universally applicable, and for some, it may mean that stools are too hard or too small, or that defecation is too difficult or infrequent. Risk includes advanced disease, decreased physical activity, low fiber diet, depression, and cognitive impairment. Medications include opioids, calcium channel blockers, diuretics, anticholinergic drugs, iron, and serotonin antagonists. The choice of laxative therapy is empiric [75].

15.3.6.6 Xerostomia

Is a highly prevalent symptom in palliative care, can alter taste and make it difficult for patients to eat and swallow, mouth pain and difficulty with speaking Risk factors include medications, mouth breathing, advanced age, and in cancer patients.

15.3.7 Obstructive Nephropathy

Treatment of advanced cancer is always challenging, in advanced stage CaCu is difficult to offer definitive treatment as they present in uremia due to associated obstructive uropathy. There are no clear-cut guidelines for performing to implement invasive palliative procedures such as percutaneous nephrostomy which in some cases may compromise quality of life to offer additional non- curative therapy. Thus interventions should prioritize the patient's quality of life, pain relief, assurance of hygiene and psychological care [76].

15.3.8 Palliative Interventions to Control Vaginal Bleeding in Advanced Cervical Cancer

Bleeding is the immediate cause of death in 6% of women with cervical cancer and its management often poses a challenge; thus, vaginal bleeding remains a common consequence of advanced cervical cancer. A pragmatic approach would be to try simple local measures such as vaginal packing and the commonly available oral hemostatic agents e.g. tranexamic acid before considering more interventional approaches such as radiotherapy. The more unorthodox and unevaluated suggestions should be considered only once the more familiar measures have been exhausted [77].

According to a Cochrane Systematic review there is an absence of evidence that tranexamic acid, vaginal packing (with or without formalin-soaked packs), interventional radiology techniques or other interventions are as effective or safe as radiotherapy for palliative control of bleeding from the vagina in advanced cervical cancer [78]. For those whose bleeding cannot be controlled successfully, use of a benzodiazepine in doses adequate to sedate patients can ease fears and minimize awareness of the circumstances.

Bleeding is visually impactant and the use of red towels to absorb bleeding can ease the anguish for families who want to remain close to a patient. It is impossible, however, to completely disguise and disregard. Patients and families should be reassured that it will be handled as sensitively and effectively as possible and that the goal of care continues to be maximization of quality of life.

15.3.9 Lower Extremity Deep Vein Thrombosis (DVT)

Reports of the incidence of DVT in patients with cervical cancer vary widely, ranging from 0% to 34%. Concerns have been raised that substantial under-reporting of DVT in cervical cancer might be occurring. The pathogenic mechanisms of thrombosis involve a complex interaction between tumor cells, the hemostatic system, and characteristics of the patient. CaCu patients have additional risk factors for thromboembolism, long-term immobilization, especially in hospital, surgery, chemotherapy, the presence of chronic renal disease, liver disease, some patients are obese, may have a central venous lines. Classic symptoms of DVT include swelling, pain, and erythema of the involved extremity. There is not necessarily a correlation between the location of symptoms and the site of thrombosis [79].

Initial treatment for most patients is subcutaneous injections of therapeutic doses (adjusted to body weight) of low molecular weight heparines (LMWH) once or twice daily. The main issues for a clinician managing a Palliative CaCu patient who has an episode of venous thrombosis are the most appropriate duration and intensity of anticoagulation, the risk of extension or recurrence of venous thromboembolism during anticoagulation, and the potential for an increased risk of bleeding during anticoagulant therapy [80].

15.3.10 Lymphedema

Lymphedema is defined as the abnormal accumulation of interstitial fluid and fibro adipose tissues resulting from different causes, is a chronic, incurable condition, the effects of which include limb swelling and feelings of heaviness, tightness, and pain. Lymphedema can take a psychological toll and adversely affect their quality of life [81].

Symptoms of peripheral lymphedema include extremity swelling, skin changes, limb pain and discomfort, restricted range of motion, and nonpitting edema. The differential diagnosis of lymphedema includes acute deep venous thrombosis, post-thrombotic syndrome, limb hypertrophy, lipedema, peripheral edema due to other systemic illness, drug-induced edema (AINES, pregabalin, bisphosphonates and taxotere), hypoalbuminemia.

The diagnosis of lymphedema can be made by history, physical exam, and extremity measurements comparing the affected with the unaffected limb. While imaging of the lymphatic system is usually not necessary to confirm the diagnosis of lymphedema, imaging can be helpful to distinguish lymphedema from no lymphatic causes of edema. Lymphedema cannot be cured but it requires complex and individualized, palliative patients with lymphedema can benefit from pain reduction, infection minimization, skin protection and the psychological support that lymphedema treatment provides. Cancer patients with lymphedema are more likely to experience greater disability, poorer quality of life, and greater psychological distress as compared to cancer patients without lymphedema. Among patients with refractory lymphedema in the palliative care setting, there are few data to guide optimal management.

15.3.11 Psychological, Psychiatric, and Cognitive Symptoms

Patients with CaCu have complex socioeconomic environments and terminal disease add additional distress. Clinicians should screen for the multiple factors that increase the prevalence and/or severity of psychological distress.

15.3.11.1 Delirium

In advanced serious or life-threatening illness, delirium is common, but it is reversible in up to 50 percent of cases, underscoring the importance of early recognition and aggressive evaluation and management. A mnemonic FACT recalls the diagnostic criteria of delirium: Fluctuating cognitive deficit(s) with acute onset; Attention deficits and either; consciousness level disturbance, or thought disorganization.

Several tools are available to screen for delirium including the Confusion Assessment Method (CAM), the bedside confusion scale (ability to recite the months backwards and assessment of consciousness state [82], use of serial-sevens, and spelling a word such as "farm" or "world" backward (or language proper words).

Haloperidol is the drug of choice 0.5–1.0 mg haloperidol (PO, intravenous [IV], intramuscular [IM], or subcutaneous [SC]) is administered, with repeat doses every 45–60 min titrated against symptoms. Older patients may require lower doses in order to avoid side effects including extrapyramidal symptoms. Symptomatic treatment should be considered a palliative measure while other strategies, such as a change in the type of opioid, hydration, or the management of metabolic or infectious complications, are introduced. Hyperactive symptoms improve within 3–5 days in most patients if the underlying etiology is corrected. If no response is observed within 24–48 h of administering full doses of haloperidol, other more sedating neuroleptics such as olanzapine or chlorpromazine are potential alternatives in patients with persistent signs and symptoms of delirium refractory to treatment with haloperidol.

15.3.11.2 Depression

The spectrum of mood disorders and conditions seen in palliative care patients includes normal grief reaction (including anticipatory grief), pathologic grief, adjustment disorder with depressed features, and minor as well as major depression.

15.3.11.3 Mood disorders

The mood disorders are frequent in patients with a serious and/or life-threatening illness. In general, a single-item inquiry, "Have you been depressed most of the time for the past 2 weeks?", appear to be as effective as longer instruments to screen for depression, and the Distress and Impact Thermometer.

15.3.11.4 Anxiety

Anxiety may also be the result of a pre-existing anxiety disorder, substance abuse, delirium, or undertreated symptoms, most commonly pain. Significant factors that may exacerbate anxiety include concerns about future symptom control, the course of the disease, and other components of total pain. A screening item, "Are you bothered by feeling nervous, anxious, or unable to stop worrying? ", can be utilized.

15.3.11.5 Coping

Coping refers to a patient's adjustment and psychological rebalancing to manage a life-threatening illness. Adaptive processing of stressors may utilize a variety of factors and styles, including humor, anticipation (planning, active management), disclosure and sharing with others/seeking support, positive reframing, sublimation, and suppression (distraction, compartmentalization).

15.3.12 Wound Care

Wound care is an important palliative care issue as untreated wounds can lead to physical discomfort and impair quality of life. The focus of wound care in palliative settings is the management of related symptoms, such as odor, exudate, bleeding, pain, and infection.

Patients at the end of life are at risk for skin breakdown because of fragile skin, excess pressure and friction, lack of proper nutrition, compromised mobility, dehydration, incontinence, advanced age, surgical wounds, fistulas, stomas, fungating tumors, peripheral edema, and lymphedema [83, 84]. Often as death approaches the skin begins to fail because of increased pressure and altered perfusion, which put patients at risk for further breakdown. It is important to inform patients and families that the wounds have limited chance of healing. Topical anesthetics can be used in the wound bed to manage lower levels of pain. Crushed metronidazole also can be sprinkled into the wound bed to help decrease odor and the amount of exudate from the wound. Dressings should be selected carefully with the intention of minimizing trauma with dressing changes and preventing further deterioration of the wound or surrounding should be on what can be done.

15.4 Last Days of Life

15.4.1 Place of Death

The place where the patients receive end of life care influences the type of management of symptoms. Death in a hospital is associated with more physical and emotional distress, worse quality of life at the end of life, and more prolonged grief disorder among caregivers [85, 86]. Some CaCu patients included in the SP in Mexico often chose the hospital environment to receive treatment.

Cervical cancer patients in the last days/hours of life have unrelieved physical suffering, but most significantly, emotional, spiritual, and social distress. Recognizing that a patient is dying or terminal phase of their illness is very important to shift standard medical care to comfort care.

15.4.2 Physiologic Changes and Symptoms

There are multiple physiologic changes that occur in the last hours and days of life, and these are generally accompanied by functional decline and a variety of symptoms [87–89].

(a) **Weakness, fatigue, and functional decline**, Increasing weakness and fatigue and eventually the patient is Bed-bound
(b) **Decreased oral intake**, as part of profound generalized weakness the inability to take in food and fluids parallels the overall physiologic decline. It may develop in the final days, or be due to potentially reversible sedation due to medications, or metabolic disturbances such as hypercalcemia.

   - Although it's a major cause of distress in family members, neither parenteral nutrition nor tube feeding is recommended for nutritional support of patients in the dying phase of an advanced terminal illness. Family education and counseling on the normal dying process is of paramount importance.
   - The possibility that dehydration may contribute to suffering and accelerate death at the end of life is a subject of debate with arguments for and against parenteral fluid administration.

(c) **Inability to close eyes,** the cachexia leads to loss of the retroorbital fat pad, causing the eyelids may not fully appose. Avoidance of dry eyes can be aided by the use of ophthalmic lubricants.
(d) **Reduction in the cardiac output** and intravascular volume leads to decreased perfusion, Tachycardia, hypotension, peripheral cooling, peripheral and central cyanosis, mottling of the skin and loss of peripheral pulses are common.
(e) **Neurologic changes** associated with the dying process may manifest themselves in two different ways: decreasing levels of consciousness leading to coma and death, or a terminal delirium, presenting as confusion, restlessness, agitation.

(f) **Periods of apnea or a Cheyne-Stoke**s pattern of respirations may develop. This may be perceived by family members as breathlessness, or impending suffocation. Therefore, similar to other anticipated changes at the end of life, this should be discussed with the family early on.
(g) **Accumulation of upper airway secretions**, loss of the ability to swallow may result from weakness and decreased neurologic function. The gag reflex and reflexive clearing of the oropharynx decline, and secretions from the tracheobronchial tree accumulate. The buildup of saliva and oropharyngeal secretions may lead to gurgling, crackling, or rattling sounds with each breath, which some refer to as the "death rattle".
(h) **Loss of sphincter control** in the last hours of life may lead to incontinence of urine and/or stool, both of which are distressing to patients and family members.

15.4.3 End of Life Care

15.4.3.1 Reviewing Medication Orders

Polypharmacy is common in patients at the end of life, and presents a burden for many [90, 91].

(a) Nonessential drugs that are no longer consistent with the overall care plan should be discontinued. Anticonvulsants are generally maintained;
(b) Drugs for common symptoms (including pain, dyspnea, nausea, delirium, anxiety, and noisy respiratory secretions) should be prescribed according to an agreed upon protocol. This ensures that needed medications are available for comfort care at any time, without delay in obtaining an order.
(c) Route of medication administration. We prefer the subcutaneous route for most patients as it is safe, broadly feasible, and fairly no burdensome.

- Transdermal systems might not be helpful in the dying phase as absorption might be reduced when circulation is centralized or patients are very cachectic. In addition, the use of a transdermal administration approach may not be optimal if dose changes are needed quickly.
- Medications whose injectable formulations can be absorbed by the buccal, sublingual, and nasal routes include the opioids fentanyl, midazolam, lorazepam, ketamine, and methadone [92–97].
- Given that bioavailability will never exceed the IV route of administration, a general guideline for buccal, sublingual, or nasal dosing is to start with the recommended IV dose, and titrate to response.
- Rectal – With the increasing numbers of medications that can be given by SC injection, transmucosally (buccal, sublingual, or nasal) and transdermally, the rectal route is used less often.

15.4.3.2 Pain and Dyspnea

Opioids are the mainstay of treating pain and dyspnea. We recommend a short acting oral, usually morphine. Sustained release opioids, including morphine, oxycodone, and fentanyl may accumulate excessively.

15.4.3.3 Routine Administration of Oxygen

To patients who are near death is not supported by clinical evidence [98]. The use of supplemental oxygen should ideally be restricted to dyspneic patients who are hypoxemic. In this setting, oxygen masks are not generally recommended because they are uncomfortable and interfere with patient communication and are more restrictive.

15.4.3.4 Airway Secretions

Occur late in the dying process. Discontinuing non-essential IV fluids or enteral feedings combined with positioning the patient on his or her side helps move the secretions out of the airway [99].

15.4.4 Palliative Sedation

Palliative Sedation (PS) is an important and necessary tool in the management of a small number of patients in whom the intentional reduction of a state of consciousness is required to relieve one or more refractory symptoms or spiritual distress at the end of life [100, 101] Patients with CaCu after a careful evaluation of a multidisciplinary team may require palliative sedation in cases of malignant obstruction, terminal agitation, massive hemorrhage, or other refractory symptom.

15.4.5 Use of Antimicrobials at the End of Life

Infections and febrile episodes are among the most common acute complications experienced by terminally ill patients, and they may represent a terminal event. Antimicrobials are commonly prescribed to dying patients in the absence of clinical symptoms to support bacterial infection [102]. The decision to treat infections at the end of life must be individualized, and the approach taken should align with the patient's stated goals of care. Even if the decision is made not to pursue antibiotics, around the clock acetaminophen may be beneficial if the patient has rigors or chills.

15.4.6 Preparing the Family for the Dying Process

Patients and families are usually unaware of the changes that typically occur during the last hours of life and the actual moment of death. Health care professionals should explain the expected changes in cognition and physical function before they occur in order to alleviate distress and prevent panic. This is particularly useful for families planning a home death, or for those closely involved in institutional care.

15.4.7 When Death Occurs

In Mexico, regulations require that a physician pronounce death and complete a death certificate. Different procedures are used in other countries. For patients who die in the hospital, the death certificate is provided by the physician.

15.5 Conclusions

The use of aggressive treatments in patients with advanced CaCu at the endo of life is frequent. Different studies have suggested no appreciable difference in survival between patients treated aggressively versus those that received palliative care. Similarly, patients without palliative care may have had more uncontrolled symptoms and possibly are more likely to have regular clinic visits and visits to the emergency departments.

Increased awareness of palliative care services with referral for these services may have an economic impact as a large amount medical spending is used for end-of-life care, and of paramount importance an improvement in quality of life and death in these patients.

References

1. Goss PE, Lee BL, Badovinac-Crnjevic T, Strasser-Weippl K, Chavarri-Guerra Y, St Louis J, et al. La planificación del control del cáncer en América Latina y el Caribe. Lancet Oncol. 2013;14:391–436.
2. Ferlay J, Steliarova-Foucher E, Lortet-Tieulent J, Rosso S, Coebergh JW, Comber H, et al. Cancer incidence and mortality patterns in Europe: estimates for 40 countries in 2012. Eur J Cancer. 2013;49:1374–403.
3. Bychkovsky BL, Ferreyra ME, Strasser-Weippl K, Herold CI, de Lima Lopes Jr G, Dizon DS, et al. Cervical cancer control in Latin America: a call to action. Cancer. 2016;122: 502–14.
4. Palacio-Mejia L, Rangel-Gomez G, Hernandez-Avila M, et al. Cervical cancer, a disease of poverty: mortality differences between urban and rural areas in Mexico. Salud pública Méx. 2008;48:315–25.Availablefrom:http://scielo.unam.mx/scielo.php?script=sci_arttext&pid=S0036-

5. van Meir H, Kenter GG, Burggraaf J, Kroep JR, Welters MJ, Melief CJ, et al. The need for improvement of the treatment of advanced and metastatic cervical cancer, the rationale for combined chemo-immunotherapy. Anticancer Agents Med Chem. 2014;14:190–203.
6. Ramondetta L. What is the appropriate approach to treating women with incurable cervical cancer? J Natl Compr Canc Netw. 2013;11(3):348–55.
7. Coronel-Martínez* J, Rivera-Rubí LM, Azuara-Forcelledo H, Floriano-Sánchez E. Tratamiento en cáncer cervicouterino localmente avanzado. Gaceta Mexicana de Oncología. 2014;13(Supl 4):67–70.
8. Candelaria M, Arias-Bonfill D, Chávez-Blanco A, et al. Lack inefficacy for imatinib mesylate as second line treatment of recurrent or metastatic cervical cancer expressing platelet-derivedgrowth factor receptor alpha. Int J Gynecol Cancer. 2009;19:1632–7.
9. Coronel J, Cetina L, Candelaria M, et al. Weekly topotecan assecond- and third-line treatment in patients with recurrent ormetastatic cervical cancer. Med Oncol. 2009;26:210–4.
10. Kim HS, Kim T, Lee ES, Kim HJ, Chung HH, Kim JW, et al. Impact of chemoradiation on prognosis in stage IVB cervical cancer with distant lymphatic metastasis. Cancer Res Treat. 2013;45:193–201.
11. Frenk J, de Ferranti D. Universal health coverage: good health, good economics. Lancet. 2012;380:862–4.
12. Frenk J. Bridging the divide: global lessons from evidence-based health policy in Mexico. The Lancet. 2006;368:954–61.
13. Knaul FM, Gonzalez-Pier E, Gomez-Dantes O, et al. The quest foruniversal health coverage: achieving social protection for all in Mexico. Lancet. 2012;380:1259–79.
14. Wenzel L, DeAlba I, Habbal R, et al. Quality of life in long-term cervical cancer survivors. Gynecol Oncol. 2005;97(2):310–7.
15. Distefano M, Riccardi S, Capelli G, et al. Quality of life and psychological distress in locally advanced cervical cancer patients administered pre-operative chemoradiotherapy. Gynecol Oncol. 2008;111(1):144–50.
16. Wright AA, Keating NL, Ayanian JZ, Chrischilles EA, Kahn KL, Ritchie CS, et al. Family perspectives on aggressive cancer care near the end of life. JAMA. 2016;315(3):284–92. http://doi.org/10.1001/jama.2015.18604.
17. Earle CC, Park ER, Lai B, Weeks JC, Ayanian JZ, Block S. Identifying potential indicators of the quality of end-of-life cancer care from administrative data. J Clin Oncol. 2003;21(6): 1133–8.
18. Earle CC, Landrum MB, Souza JM, Neville BA, Weeks JC, Ayanian JZ. Aggressiveness of cancer care near the end of life: is it a quality-of-care issue? J Clin Oncol. 2008;26(23):3860–6. http://doi.org/10.1200/JCO.2007.15.8253
19. National Cancer Policy Board. Ensuring quality cancer care. Washington, DC: National Academy Press; 1999.
20. Murillo Jr JR, Koeller J. Chemotherapy given near the end of life by community oncologists for advanced non-small cell lung cancer. Oncologist. 2006;11:1095–9.
21. Emanuel EJ, Young-Xu Y, Levinsky NG, et al. Chemotherapy use among medicare beneficiaries at the end of life. Ann Intern Med. 2003;138(639–643):10.
22. von Gunten CF. Discussing hospice care. J Clin Oncol. 2003;21:31s–6s.
23. Glare P, Virik K, Jones M, Hudson M, Eychmuller S, Simes J, Christakis N. A systematic review of physician's survival predictions in terminally ill cancer patients. BMJ. 2003;327:195–8.
24. Martoni AA, Tanneberger S, Mutri V. Cancer chemotherapy near the end of life: the time has come to set guidelines for its appropriate use. Tumori. 2007;93:417–22.
25. Weeks JC, Cook EF, O'Day SJ, et al. Relationship between cancer patients' predictions of prognosis and their treatment preferences. JAMA. 1998;279:1709–14.
26. Matsuyama R, Reddy S, Smith TJ. Why do patients choose chemotherapy near the end of life? A review of the perspective of those facing death from cancer. J Clin Oncol. 2006;24:3490–6.
27. Slevin ML, Stubbs L, Plant HJ, et al. Attitudes to chemotherapy: comparing views of patients with cancer with those of doctors, nurses, and general public. BMJ. 1990;300:1458–60.

28. Mack JW, Wolfe J, Cook EF, et al. Hope and prognostic disclosure. J Clin Oncol. 2007;25:5636–42.
29. Hui D, Bruera E, Li Z, Palmer JL, de la Cruz M, Elsayem A. Utilization of antineoplastic therapy in advanced cancer patients admitted to an acute palliative care unit at a comprehensive cancer center. J Clin Oncol. 2009;27:505s. abst n.9590.
30. Jackson K. Global atlas of palliative care at the end of life worldwide palliative care Alliance. In: Connore R, editor. Sepulveda Bermedo, World Health Organization 2014. Consultado en línea el 9 de diciembre de 2015 en. http://www.who.int/nmh/Global_Atlas_of_Palliative_Care.pdf.
31. Sepulveda CM, Yoshida A, Ullrich T. Palliative care: the world health organization's global perspective. J Pain Symptom Manage. 2002;24:91–6.
32. WHO definition of palliative care. 2015. Available from: http://www.who.int/cancer/palliative/definition/en/.
33. Smith TJ, Temin S, Alesi ER, Abernethy AP, et al. American society of clinical oncology provisional clinical opinion: the integration of palliative care in to standard oncology care. J Clin Oncol. 2012;30:880–7.
34. Ferris FD, Bruera E, Cherny N, Cummings C, Currow D, Dudgeon D, et al. Palliative cancer care a decade later: accomplishments, the need, next steps—from the American society of clinical oncology. J Clin Oncol. 2009;27(18):3052–8.
35. Hui D, Meng Y-Ch, Bruera S, Geng Y, Hutchins R, Mori M et.al. Referral criteria for outpatient palliative cancer care: a systematic review. Oncologist. 2016;21:895–901; first published on May 16, 2016. doi:10.1634/theoncologist.2016-0006.
36. Quill TE, Abernethy AP. Generalist plus specialist palliative care—creating a more sustainable model. N Engl J Med. 2013;368:1173–5.
37. Center to Advance Palliative Care. National palliative care registry annual survey summary: results of the 2012 national palliative care registry survey, as of July 2014. Accessed at https://registry.capc.org/cms/portals/1/Reports/National_Palliative_Care%20Registry_Annual_Survey_Summary_9.2.2014.pdf on 24 July 2015.
38. Kamal AH, Currow DC, Ritchie CS, Bull J, Abernethy AP. Community-based palliative care: the natural evolution for palliative care delivery in the U.S. J Pain Symptom Manage. 2012;46:254–64. (Epub ahead of print)
39. Lorenz KA, Lynn J, Dy SM, Shugarman LR, Wilkinson A, Mularski RA, et al. Evidence for improving palliative care at the end of life: a systematic review. Ann Intern Med. 2008;148(2):147.
40. Bruera E, Kuehn N, Miller MJ, Selmser P, Macmillan K. The Edmonton Symptom Assessment System (ESAS): a simple method for the assessment of pallative care patient. J Palliat Care. 1991;7:6–9.
41. Jayasekara H, Rajapaksa L, Greimel ER. The EORTC QLQ-CX24 cervical cancer- specific quality of life questionnaire: psychometric properties in a South Asian sample of cervical cancer patients. Psychooncology. 2008;17(10):1053–7.
42. Greimel ER, Kuljanic Vlasic K, Waldenstrom AC, Duric VM, Jensen PT, Singer S, et al. The European Organization for Research and Treatment of Cancer (EORTC) Quality of Life Questionnaire Cervical Cancer Module: EORTC QLQ-CX24. Cancer. 2006;107(8):1812–22.
43. Rirovano M, Maltoni M, Nanni O, et al. A new Palliative Prognostic Score: a first step for the staging of terminally ill cancer patients. Italian multicenter study group on palliative care. J Pain Symptom Manage. 1999;17:231–9.
44. Maltoni M, Nanni O, Pirovano M, et al. Successful validation of the Palliative Prognostic Score in terminally ill cancer patients. Italian multicenter study group on palliative care. J Pain Symptom Manage. 1999;17:240–7.
45. Morita T, Tsunoda J, Inoue S, et al. The Palliative Prognostic Index: a scoring system for survival prediction of terminally ill cancer patients. Support Care Cancer. 1999;7:128–33. [PubMed]
46. Anderson F, Downing GM, Hill J, et al. Palliative Performance Scale (PPS): a new tool. J Palliat Care. 1996;12:5–11.

47. Maltoni M, Scarpi E, Pittureri C, Martini F, Montanari L, Amaducci E. Prospective comparison of prognostic scores in palliative care cancer populations. Oncologist. 2012;17(3):446–54. doi:10.1634/theoncologist.2011-0397.
48. Hui D. Prognostication of survival in patients with advanced cancer: predicting the unpredictable? Cancer Control. 2015 Oct;22(4):489–97.
49. Allende PS et al. Cuidados Paliativos en Cáncer Cervicouterino Avanzado. Rev Inst Nal Cancerol (Mex). 2000;46(1):11.
50. Kim YJ, Munsell MF, Park JC, Meyer LA, Sun CC, Brown AJ, et al. Retrospective review of symptoms and palliative care intervension in women with advanced cervical cancer. Gynecol Oncol. 2015 Dec;139(3):553–8. doi:10.1016/j.ygyno.2015.09.079.
51. Caraceni A, Portenoy RK. An international survey of cancer pain characteristics and syndromes. IASP Task Force on Cancer Pain. International Association fo r the Study of Pain. Pain. 1999 Sep;82(3):263–74.
52. World Health Organization. Cancer pain relief. Geneva: World Health Organization; 1986. ISBN 9241561009 © World Health Organization.
53. Ventafridda V, Tamburini M, Caraceni A, De Conno F, Naldi F. A validation study of the WHO method for cancer pain relief. Cancer. 1987;59(4):850–6.
54. Foley K. The treatment of cancer pain. N Engl J Med. 1984;313:84–95.
55. Cancer pain management with opioids: optimizing analgesia. Upto date. Disponible en Línea en http://www.uptodate.com/contents/cancer-pain-management-with-opioids-optimizing-analgesia?source=see_link&sectionName=Management+of+breakthrough+pain&anchor=H20#H20 Consultado 21–2-2016.
56. Plummer JL, Gourlay GK, Cherry DA, Cousins MJ. Estimation of methadone clearance: application in the management of cancer pain. Pain. 1988;33(3):313.
57. Koob GF. Dynamics of neuronal circuits in addiction: Reward, antireward, and emotional memory. Pharmacopsychiatry. 2009;42(suppl 1):S32–41.
58. Kwon JH, Tanco K, Park JC, Wong A, Seo L, Liu D, et al. Frequency, predictors, and medical record documentation of chemical coping among advanced cancer patients. Oncologist. 2015;20(6):692–7. http://doi.org/10.1634/theoncologist.2015-0012.
59. Califf RM, Woodcock J, Ostroff S. A proactive response to prescription opioid abuse. N Engl J Med. 2016;374:1480.
60. ASCO Policy Stattement on Opioid Therapy: Protecting access to treatment for cancewr-related pain. Policy statement available online at http://www.asco.org/sites/new-www.asco.org/files/content-files/advocacy-and-policy/documents/2016_ASCO%20Policy%20Statement%20on%20Opioid%20Therapy.pdf. Accessed on 20 July 2016.
61. Saunders C. The depths and the possible heights. Med News. 1964;10:16.
62. Wilson KG, Chochinov HM, McPherson CJ, et al. Suffering with advanced cancer. J Clin Oncol. 2007;25:1691.
63. Cassell EJ. Recognizing suffering. Hastings Cent Rep. 1991;21:24.
64. Radbruch L, Strasser F, Elsner F, et al. Fatigue in palliative care patients -- an EAPC approach. Palliat Med. 2008;22:13.
65. Mendoza TR, Wang XS, Cleeland CS, et al. The rapid assessment of fatigue severity in cancer patients: use of the Brief Fatigue Inventory. Cancer. 1999;85:1186.
66. Escalante CP. Cancer-related fatigue: treatment. UpToDate. Available at: http://www.uptodate.com/contents/cancer-related-fatigue-treatment?source=related_link. Consulted 15 May 2016.
67. Timothy HM, Luen Bik T, Currow David C. Can we detect transfusion benefits in palliative care patients? J Palliat Med. 2016. Ahead of print. doi:10.1089/jpm.2016.0073.
68. Preston NJ, Hurlow A, Brine J, Bennett MI. Blood transfusions for anaemia in patients with advanced cancer. Cochrane Database Syst Rev. 2012;15:CD009007.
69. Reuben DB, Mor V. Dyspnea in terminally ill cancer patients. Chest. 1986;89:234.
70. Bruera E. ABC of palliative care. Anorexia, cachexia, and nutrition. BMJ. 1997;315:1219.
71. Kotler DP. Cachexia. Ann Intern Med. 2000;133:622.

72. Vigano A, Del Fabbro E, Bruera E, Borod M. The cachexia clinic: from staging to managing nutritional and functional problems in advanced cancer patients. Crit Rev Oncog. 2012; 17:293.
73. Davis MP, Walsh D. Treatment of nausea and vomiting in advanced cancer. Support Care Cancer. 2000;8:444.
74. Ripamonti C, Twycross R, Baines M, Bozzetti F, Capri S, De Conno F. Working group of the European Association for Palliative Care Clinical-practice recommendations for the management of bowel obstruction in patients with end-stage cancer. Support Care Cancer. 2001;9(4):223.
75. Candy B, Jones L, Larkin PJ, Vickerstaff V, Tookman A, Stone P. Laxatives for the management of constipation in people receiving palliative care. Cochrane Database Syst Rev. 2015;13:CD003448.
76. Paula de Souza AC, Souza AN, Rubens K, Kirsztajn GM. Cervical cancer: renal complications and survival after percutaneous nephrostomy. Rev Assoc Med Bras. 2016;62(3): 255–61. Available from: http://www.scielo.br/scielo.php?script=sci_arttext&pid=S0104-42302016000300255&lng=en. http://dx.doi.org/10.1590/1806-9282.62.03.255.
77. Tranexamic acid as a vaginal pessary. In: Bulletin Board. Palliativedrugs.com Ltd. Available from www.palliativedrugs.com.
78. Eleje GU, Eke AC, Igberase GO, Igwegbe AO, Eleje LI. Palliative interventions for controlling vaginal bleeding in advanced cervical cancer. Cochrane Database of Systematic Reviews 2015, Issue 5. Art. No.: CD011000. doi:10.1002/14651858.CD011000.pub2.
79. Lip GY, Chin BS, Blann AD. Cancer and the prothrombotic state. Lancet Oncol. 2002;3:27.
80. Akl EA, Kahale L, Neumann I, et al. Anticoagulation for the initial treatment of venous thromboembolism in patients with cancer. Cochrane Database Syst Rev. 2014;19:CD006649.
81. Todd M. Understanding lymphoedema in advanced disease in a palliative care setting. Int J Palliat Nurs. 2009;15:474–6.
82. O'Regan NA, Ryan DJ, Boland E, Connolly W, McGlade C, Leonard M, Clare J, Eustace JA, Meagher D, Timmons S. Attention! A good bedside test for delirium? J Neurol Neurosurg Psychiatry. 2014;85(10):1122–31. Epub 2014 Feb 25.
83. Hughes R, Bakos A, O'Mara A, et al. Palliative wound care at the end of life. Home Health Care Manage Pract. 2005;17(3):196–202.
84. Tice M. Wound care in the face of life-limiting illness. Home Healthc Nurse. 2006;24(2):115–8.
85. Wright AA, Keating NL, Balboni TA, et al. Place of death: correlations with quality of life of patients with cancer and predictors of bereaved caregivers' mental health. J Clin Oncol. 2010;28:4457.
86. Zhang B, Nilsson ME, Prigerson HG. Factors important to patients' quality of life at the end of life. Arch Intern Med. 2012;172:1133.
87. Ferris FD, von Gunten CF, Emanuel LL. Competency in end-of-life care: last hours of life. J Palliat Med. 2003;6:605.
88. Tang ST, Mccorkle R. Determinants of congruence between the preferred and actual place of death for terminally ill cancer patients. J Palliat Care. 2003;19:230.
89. Hui D, Dos Santos R, Chisholm G, et al. Bedside clinical signs associated with impending death in patients with advanced cancer: preliminary findings of a prospective, longitudinal cohort study. Cancer. 2015;121:960.
90. McNeil MJ, Kamal AH, Kutner JS, et al. The burden of polypharmacy in patients near the end of life. J Pain Symptom Manage. 2016;51:178.
91. LeBlanc TW, McNeil MJ, Kamal AH, et al. Polypharmacy in patients with advanced cancer and the role of medication discontinuation. Lancet Oncol. 2015;16:e333.
92. Anderson SL, Shreve ST. Continuous subcutaneous infusion of opiates at end-of-life. Ann Pharmacother. 2004;38:1015.
93. Herndon CM, Fike DS. Continuous subcutaneous infusion practices of United States hospices. J Pain Symptom Manage. 2001;22:1027.

94. Justad M. Continuous subcutaneous infusion: an efficacious, cost-effective analgesia alternative at the end of life. Home Healthc Nurse. 2009;27:140.
95. Gardner-Nix J. Oral transmucosal fentanyl and sufentanil for incident pain. J Pain Symptom Manage. 2001;22:627.
96. McDonough JH, Van Shura KE, LaMont JC, et al. Comparison of the intramuscular, intranasal or sublingual routes of midazolam administration for the control of soman-induced seizures. Basic Clin Pharmacol Toxicol. 2009;104:27.
97. Spaner D. Effectiveness of the buccal mucosa route for methadone administration at the end of life. J Palliat Med. 2014;17:1262.
98. Campbell ML, Yarandi H, Dove-Medows E. Oxygen is nonbeneficial for most patients who are near death. J Pain Symptom Manage. 2013;45:517.
99. Lokker ME, van Zuylen L, van der Rijt CC, van der Heide A. Prevalence, impact, and treatment of death rattle: a systematic review. J Pain Symptom Manage. 2014;47:105.
100. Cherny N. Editorial. The use of sedation to relieve cancer patients' suffering at the end of life: addressing critical issues. Ann Oncol. 2009;20:1153–5. doi:10.1093/annonc/mdp302. Consulted on line: http://annonc.oxfordjournals.org/, 3 May 2016
101. Palliative Sedation Position Statement Approved by the AAHPM Board of Directors on 5 Dec 2014. Consulted on line at: http://aahpm.org/positions/palliative-sedation, Jan 2016.
102. Thompson AJ, Silveira MJ, Vitale CA, Malani PN. Antimicrobial use at the end of life among hospitalized patients with advanced cancer. Am J Hosp Palliat Care. 2012;29:599.

Chapter 16
Special Conditions and Follow-Up in Cervical Cancer

Flavia Morales-Vásquez, Claudia Cano-Blanco, Jaime Alberto Coronel-Martínez, Lucely Cetina-Pérez, Julio César Velasco-Rodríguez, Horacio N. López-Basave, and Jaime G. de la Garza-Salazar

Abstract The present chapter reviews cervical cancer (CC) management in conditions of various co-morbidities and provides general guidelines for the proper follow-up of patients. We address the most common special management conditions: renal insufficiency, senility, fragility, AIDS, and pregnancy.

Renal insufficiency and obstruction require patient management to be further adjusted compared to cases with a neoplasia only. The general population is living longer, thus producing a considerable increase in the prevalence of chronic degenerative diseases, such as diabetes, hypertension, and metabolic syndrome. Therefore, we are facing more cases with co-morbidities, which necessitates rethinking therapeutic options.

Both geriatric and non-geriatric patients with CC present with morbidities and conditions that limit the use of cisplatin chemotherapy, which is the standard treatment.

F. Morales-Vásquez, MD, MSc (✉) • C. Cano-Blanco, MD
Department of Medical Oncology, Instituto Nacional de Cancerología-México, Av. San Fernando No 22, Col. Toriello Guerra, Tlalpan, Mexico City, Mexico 14070
e-mail: dra.morales.oncomed@gmail.com

J.A. Coronel-Martínez, MSc • L. Cetina-Pérez, MSc
Clinical Research Department, Instituto Nacional de Cancerología-México, Mexico City, Mexico

J.C. Velasco-Rodríguez, MD
Department of Medical Oncology, Hospital Español de México, Mexico City, Mexico

H.N. López-Basave, MD, MSc
Department Surgical Oncology, Instituto Nacional de Cancerología-México, Mexico City, Mexico

J.G. de la Garza-Salazar, MD
Department of Clinical Investigation, Instituto Nacional de Cancerología-México, Mexico City, Mexico

J.G. de la Garza-Salazar et al. (eds.), *Cervical Cancer*,
DOI 10.1007/978-3-319-45231-9_16

Other equally relevant challenges in treating patients with CC include AIDS and pregnancy; here, we aim to elucidate general principles that can orient patient management in these unique situations.

Finally, we focus on describing the ideal time of and requirements for adequate follow-up and reincorporation into daily life.

Keywords Cervical cancer (CC) • Renal insufficiency • Fragility-CC • AIDS-CC • Pregnancy-CC • Follow-up in CC

16.1 Cervical Cancer in Special Situations

16.1.1 Cervical Cancer in Patients with Renoureteral Obstruction

Patients with bilateral ureteral obstruction and uremia secondary to CC metastasis pose a considerable challenge for specialists. For the sake of therapeutic purposes, patients are divided in two subgroups: (1) those that have not received radiotherapy; and (2) those that present with recurrent disease after pelvic radiotherapy [1].

In the second group, a small percentage of patients present with bilateral renoureteral obstruction as a sequela of radiotherapy without evidence of tumoral disease; identifying these patients is of vital importance because they are potentially curable.

In patients who present with a bilateral ureteral obstruction due to untreated CC or those with recurrent pelvic involvement after surgical intervention, a urinary diversion must be seriously considered and then followed by radiotherapy. Few patients fall into this category of complications, but it is a real issue that must be addressed.

A ureteral obstruction is a sudden block in one or both ureters; pressure increases inside the urinary system upstream of the obstruction and is transmitted to renal tubules until it nears the filtration pressure values. Glomerular filtration does not decrease to zero because some of the tubular liquid is reabsorbed, and this allows the tubule to admit a volume equal to the glomerular filtrate. In advanced disease, functional and anatomical changes occur that eventually lead to total destruction of functional renal mass. Finally, infections can increase renal damage under conditions of any obstruction and can cause pyonephrosis, which is dilation of the pelvis and calyces that is usually caused by ureteropelvic or ureterovesical obstructions (hydronephrosis); such infection-related complications are associated with the formation of purulent liquid and total destruction of functional renal mass. Immediately after a ureteral obstruction occurs, vasodilation promotes an increase in renal blood flux that persists for 3–4 h. Then, the blood flux gradually decreases over 5–6 h to the level prior to the obstruction; at this point, renal vasoconstriction occurs and progressively reduces blood flux during the subsequent 24–48 h to 20–30% of the control values. This vasoconstriction seems to be related to intrarenal prostaglandin (PGN) production; blocking PGN synthesis with indomethacin prevents the vasodilation that follows a ureteral obstruction. In summary, during the initial few hours of the obstruction, the raise in intratubular pressure determines the drop in glomerular filtration in spite of vasodilation and increased plasmatic flux secondary to the PGN increase. When the obstruction persists for more than 24–48 h, intratubular pressure decreases to normal, but glomerular filtration remains low; at this stage, hydrostatic pressure in the glomerular capillary is lower than normal, indicating an increase in resistance caused by vasoconstriction of the afferent arteriole. Finally, ureteral obstructions also decrease glomerular filtration by destroying the renal parenchyma, which suppresses nephron function. This mechanism becomes more important for prolonged obstructions but is present after the first 24 or 48 hours.

16.1.1.1 Tubular Alteration

For partial urinary obstructions, the inability to concentrate urine is manifested as nephrogenic insipidus diabetes because it does not respond to vasopressin. These findings suggest that the tubular defect is reversible. The inability to acidify urine is another tubular alteration.

In such situations, bicarbonate reabsorption is increased in the proximal tubule but is incomplete in the distal tubule. This leads to an abnormal increase in urinary pH, which prevents the excretion of titratable acidity and drastically decreases ammonium excretion. These changes necessarily limit net acid excretion and promote a positive hydrogen ion balance. After releasing the obstruction, abundant diuresis can lead to massive loss of sodium, potassium, chlorine, and other solutes; the magnitude of the post-obstructive diuresis is the extracellular volume immediately before the obstruction release. Usually, these patients have some degree of renal insufficiency and sodium and water retention that cause variable expansion of the extracellular volume. This extracellular expansion activates natriuretic factors that increase when the blockage is released, and glomerular filtration intensifies.

16.1.1.2 Vasopressin Suppression and Consequential Tubular Resistance

The excretion of retained water and electrolytes enables the pre-existing extracellular expansion to be corrected and undoubtedly constitutes the most important post-obstructive polyuria mechanism. However, an increase in tubular phosphate reabsorption in the affected kidney during the post-obstructive period after unilateral occlusions has been observed in humans. The signs and symptoms of obstructive nephropathy are often limited or nonspecific. Clinical anomalies can manifest as impaired renal function or symptoms related to an associated urinary infection, and some appear as extrarenal manifestations of other pathologic processes, local metastases, or distant metastases [2].

16.1.1.3 Hypertension and Urinary Obstruction

The presence of acute or chronic unilateral or bilateral hydronephrosis is often accompanied with a significant rise in arterial pressure. Hypertension can be coincidental or caused by renal damage due to the inability of the kidney to excrete sodium through abnormal renin release. Treatment of an obstructive uropathy complicated by infection and generalized sepsis involves antibiotics and immediate release of the obstruction.

A total urinary tract obstruction causes irreversible damage to the kidney. There is only modest excretion at 6 weeks after the obstruction, and kidney function is completely lost after 8 weeks.

Relieving the obstruction is undoubtedly the first step that must be taken; initially, the placement of anterograde ureteral devices is preferred (J stent) before initiating radiotherapy.

The obstruction can also be resolved through nephrostomy (surgical or percutaneous), but the associated complications and morbidities are higher than those for the Double J stent, and there is a decrease in patient quality of life [3].

For Double J stents, the prevalence of complications, such as infection, the formation of kidney stones, or recurrent obstruction, increases with time. Stent replacement is mandatory for these reasons; the ideal replacement interval is between 2 and 4 months. Different techniques, including cystoscope- and fluoroscope-based strategies, have been described for performing this task [4].

The treatment of patients with bilateral renal obstructions who have received ideal-dose radiotherapy is more complicated. Less than 5% of these patients present with obstructions due to radiotherapy-induced fibrosis; nevertheless, one should try to resolve obstructions because these patients can potentially be cured. It is important to detect this pathological condition as soon as possible, before renal damage becomes irreversible [1].

In cases of recurrent obstructions, the decision process for releasing one urinary tract becomes complex and, in some occasions, even philosophical because many studies have suggested that a urinary diversion does not provide a substantial increase in survival and, unfortunately, increases the incidence of complications that hinder quality of life. Hence, in each disease scenario, patients who are candidates for urinary diversion must be carefully selected after considering the wishes of the patient and her family, as there is a risk of dying with each option: uremic syndrome versus increased bleeding, pain, infection, fistulae and a higher number of hospitalizations [5].

16.1.2 Cervical Cancer in Geriatric Patients

There are two emerging problems in health care: an increase in the geriatric population and an increase in the frequency of diseases such as diabetes mellitus and systemic arterial hypertension. These issues add an extra variable to the management of patients with CC; there are populations of geriatric CC patients with or without co-morbidities and of non-geriatric patients who present with co-morbidities; in both conditions, the use of standard cisplatin chemotherapy is limited. Such demographic changes will necessitate modifying the therapeutic approach.

16.1.2.1 The Geriatric Patient

Geriatric patients are 65 years or older; senescence-related biological changes start to become evident between 65 and 70 years of age. Geriatric fragile patients meet one of the following criteria: older than 80 years, lives alone, recently lost her partner, chronic pathology (cerebrovascular disease, ischemic cardiopathy, Parkinson's disease, arthrosis or advanced osteoarticular disease, important auditory or visual deficits, falls, polypharmacy, hospitalization during the last year, dementia, depression or other cognitive hindrance, and economic deficiency), or an insufficient support network [6]. These situations create a challenge for the already-complex process of CC treatment; patients with CC that meet the fragility criteria are not candidates for standard treatment [7, 8]. This problem is not properly addressed, and there is a tendency to minimize it. Demographic transition caused by an increase in life expectancy (fueled by sanitary improvement) is a global phenomenon. In the USA, the geriatric population increased from 25 million in 1980 to 35 million in 2000, and it is estimated to reach 72 million in 2030 [9]. In Latin America and the Caribbean, the population of people older than 60 years grew three-fold, from 9,260,300 in 1950 to 41,290,200 in 2000; the UN estimates indicate that in 2050, there will be 181,218,000 persons older than 60 years, and 18% of these persons will be older than 80 [10]. Cancer is generally considered a disease of ageing. Ershler used experimental systems to show that the same number of Lewis carcinoma or B16 melanoma cells produced more metastases and shorter survival in young compared to elderly mice [8]. These data may indicate that tumors are less aggressive in older organisms, although it is important to underscore that in humans, cancer prognosis can either improve or worsen based on patient age [8]. In the case of geriatric patients, additional prognoses represent another important factor because they can affect systems such as hepatic and renal physiology; these changes have a general impact on pharmacokinetics and pharmacodynamics, which could lead to increased toxicity from chemotherapy.

16.1.3 Cervical Cancer in Fragile Patients

The fragile patient concept (not to be confused with the geriatric fragile patient) is emerging, and the definition that we propose is a non-geriatric patient with an associated co-morbidity that prevents the use of standard anti-tumor therapy. Diabetes mellitus and systemic arterial hypertension are the main causes of general organ or renal functional deterioration. Between 20% and 30% of diabetic patients develop nephropathy 7–10 years after initial diagnosis [11]. Both diabetic and hypertensive nephropathies have a considerable impact on decreased glomerular function, which leads to renal failure [12]. Hence, there is a need to focus on decreasing factors that accelerate renal damage. In fact, locally advanced CC can produce obstructive nephropathy.

Few studies have been performed in geriatric and fragile patients, and these populations are automatically excluded from large clinical trials. However, they are often encountered in everyday clinical practice. At the National Cancer Institute of Mexico, there has been an effort to develop a systemic and orderly approach for the management of these patients, including those with locally advanced CC or metastatic disease. One of the first such studies was published in 2004; this study included new patients with stage IIIB and IVA CC with obstructive nephropathy that placed them in the fragile condition category. These patients were treated with radiotherapy and gemcitabine as a radiosensitizer [13]. Radiotherapy-associated carboplatin was also evaluated. Fifty-nine patients with stage IB2-IIIB disease, including geriatric patients and those with co-morbidities, were included. The treatment regimen was well tolerated, with minimal toxicity (grades 3–4); nonetheless, although responses were observed, the gemcitabine and carboplatin patient groups were not compared to a control group, and thus, the results are inconclusive [14]. Another recently published study compared cisplatin with oral vinorelbine [15] in a cohort that included geriatric patients and those with co-morbidities. In total, 40 patients with locally advanced uterine CC were included. Oral vinorelbine was well tolerated, and cisplatin can also be safely administered to this patient population. Although there was less toxicity in the vinorelbine group, a larger cohort is required to confirm these results [15].

We can conclude that geriatric, fragile geriatric, and fragile patients with CC must not be excluded from receiving the benefits of chemoradiotherapy for the treatment of locally advanced disease or of systemic chemotherapy for the treatment of metastatic disease. Here, we have described some treatment alternatives that, when supported by exploratory studies, have proven feasible and applicable.

16.1.4 Cervical Cancer in Patients with Aids

Cervical Cancer was identified as an AIDS-associated disease in 1993 [16]. Fortunately, the incidence of this disease is low among women infected with HIV: although the prevalence of intraepithelial lesions (IEL) and intraepithelial cervical neoplasia (ICN) is low, the prevalence of HIV infection in cancer patients is 1.2%, which is higher than the 0.1% prevalence among cancer-free patients. Thus, the USA guidelines recommend routine HIV testing in patients with cancer [17].

CC is an important AIDS-related disease, and it is possible that the malignant processes related to CC are upregulated or aberrantly activated in this patient population, especially in areas with a high prevalence of human papilloma virus (HPV) infection [18].

HPV infection progresses to advanced stage ICN in 14% of cases, and chronic infections can lead to CC [19]. Currently, studies in women with HIV/AIDS have revealed that cytology is not sensitive enough to diagnose CC because of the high rate of false negatives. Thus, some authors concluded that this test is not sufficiently useful and proposed that colposcopy is a more accurate procedure [18, 20].

HIV-positive women are more prone to suffer from certain conditions, including bacterial vaginosis caused by *Gardnerella vaginalis*, *Mobiluncus*, *Bacteroides*, *Mycoplasma hominis*, *Ureaplasma parvum*, or *Ureaplasma urealyticum*. Women diagnosed with bacterial vaginosis by either Nugent's or Amsel's criteria must undergo further diagnostic microbiological exams to enable adequate treatment, which will help prevent future genital tract diseases [21].

Currently, we have a theory that links bacterial vaginosis to the development of cervical dysplasia and, ultimately, to CC. Many anaerobic bacterial species (which constitute one of the factors that cause infection) produce nitrosamines, which are potent human carcinogens that cause cervical damage. In one of three patients, an intermediate vaginal flora is observed according to Nugent's criteria, with evidence of a decrease in lactobacilli, which play a fundamental role in vaginal flora maintenance. This condition renders patients more susceptible to bacterial vaginosis or vaginitis caused by fungi, parasites, or other types of bacteria. The multidisciplinary team that evaluates these patients must perform complete gynecological exams that include vaginal exudate, cytology, and colposcopy in order to prevent CC or to detect it in the earliest possible stages.

Among the main treatment recommendations are the following:

- For all HIV-infected women, cervical surveillance must be performed in close collaboration with the team monitoring and controlling the HIV infection (level of evidence 1B). An initial colposcopy and annual cytology should be performed if resources permit (level of evidence 2C).
- We recommend subsequent colposcopy for cytological abnormalities, and the age range recommended for screening should be the same as that for HIV-negative women (level of evidence 1B).
- We suggest that CIN 2/3 (HSIL) should be managed with standard treatment. Lesions less advanced than CIN 2 should most likely not be treated according to the CIN 2/3 recommendations, as these low-grade lesions represent persistent HPV infection of the cervix rather than a pre-malignant state (level of evidence 2B). Women with HIV and CIN 2/3 who are treated by excisional procedures have a significantly higher treatment failure rate than HIV-negative women. Numerous studies have shown that such relapses are less frequent in the presence of HAART or higher CD4 cell counts or in cases with an undetectable viral load. Multidisciplinary management of such women is thus recommended.
- We recommend that women with HIV and invasive CC be managed in the same way as HIV-negative women according to international guidelines, again within a multidisciplinary team framework (level of evidence 1B) [22].

16.1.5 Pregnant Patients with Cervical Cancer

CC is one of the most common tumors in women of fertile age. Therefore, it is not surprising to find an association between this neoplasia and pregnancy. The coexistence of both conditions does not worsen the tumor prognosis; however, a multidisciplinary, specialized team is required to ensure the best oncologic result and safety of the fetus. The therapeutic strategy depends on clinical stage, tumor size, nodal status, histologic subtype, and the desire and potential to preserve the pregnancy. Radiotherapy is prohibited throughout the entire pregnancy.

Abnormal cervical cytology is reported in approximately 5% of pregnancies. CC and pregnancy co-occur at an incidence of 1 in 10,000 women. According to the literature, more than 70% of the cases reported in developed countries are stage I. Conversely, in developing countries, most patients have advanced stage disease at initial diagnosis. Treatment is challenging because it requires the participation of a multidisciplinary team that must consider clinical stage, tumor size, nodal status, gestational age, and the will to preserve the pregnancy as fundamental elements in therapeutic decisions, while striving for the best results for both mother (in terms of oncology) and fetus. Treatment options are usually divided according to gestational age (before or after 20 weeks gestation) [23–25].

16.1.5.1 Screening During Pregnancy

Cervical cytology screening is a routine part of prenatal management. Most cases are detected after 20 weeks gestation. When a high-grade intraepithelial lesion (ICN 2–3) or an invasive cancer is detected, a confirmation biopsy must be taken. A cervical cone can be performed if the biopsy is insufficient. It is recommended that this procedure be performed between 14 and 20 weeks gestation, taking into consideration the main complications: hemorrhage (10%), infection (5%), fetal death (5%), and preterm birth (15%) [26].

Staging FIGO staging is based on clinical findings. Conclusions from imaging studies must account for the secondary effects of radiation and contrast medium. Thorax postero-anterior teleradiography is recommended beginning with stage IB1, with universal safety measures, such as abdominal protection. In cases of advanced disease (even suspected cases), an abdominal MRI can be performed, which has 88% sensitivity and 91% specificity. The use of tomography and PET/CT is contraindicated. When CC is diagnosed near the end of pregnancy or in women harboring tumors larger than 4 cm or with positive pelvic nodes, cesarean delivery is recommended, along with surgical sampling of the pelvic and para-aortic nodes. In the most aggressive histologic subtypes, such as small cell CC, pregnancy preservation is generally not recommended [27].

Stage IA1 Diagnosis is performed through cervical conization. The use of a cold knife cone is preferred, and this procedure should be performed in the second trimester of pregnancy; under such conditions, less than 10% fetal loss is expected. If the margins are negative, clinical surveillance and colposcopy during each trimester are recommended. If the margin is positive, clinical surveillance must be strictly performed along with colposcopy each trimester; additional excisions or hysterectomy will be considered 6–8 weeks after pregnancy resolution [24].

Stages IA2 and IB1 The therapeutic decision is based on nodal status, gestational age, patient preference, and the skills of the treating team. MRI and laparoscopic lymphadenectomy may be performed between 18 and 22 weeks gestation. If the presence of nodal disease is not demonstrated, the pregnancy can continue, and treatment can be postponed under close surveillance. Trachelectomy is an option for women who want to preserve fertility; however, this process must be performed in highly specialized centers because it has been associated with fetal loss. Pregnancy termination can be considered if CC is diagnosed in the first trimester or if there is nodal involvement. Paclitaxel based induction therapies are an option, in case of the pregnancy is in first two trimesters, and the tumors are not larger than 4 cm, carboplatin or cisplatin they are not approved [28, 29].

Stages IB2 through IV It is convenient to determine the para-aortic nodal status by MRI. As with the other scenarios, the treatment plan must be individualized. Paclitaxel and cisplatin/carboplatin neoadjuvant chemotherapy is recommended after second trimesters, when there is desire to preserve the pregnancy, and concurrent chemoradiotherapy can be administered 6–8 weeks after pregnancy resolution. Carboplatin is preferred based on a better toxicity profile: it has a higher upper safety limit of 800 mg. Neoadjuvant chemotherapy helps reduce tumor size and control micrometastases. The gestational period that is the most vulnerable to chemotherapy and radiotherapy is organogenesis, from 10 days to 8 weeks gestation; the risks include major malformations, spontaneous abortion, and embryonic death in up to 20% of cases. During the second trimester, malformations such as growth retardation, preterm birth, and transitory myelosuppression are less severe. During the first trimester, the risk of fetal malformation after in utero exposure is 5–15% for combination treatments and 10% for monotherapy; the rate drops to 1.3% in the second trimester, which is similar to the rate of 3% in the general population. There are reports of spontaneous abortions after 40 Gy of treatment, or 3 weeks from the beginning of radiotherapy, in patients at less than 12 weeks gestation who were treated with chemoradiotherapy. Targeted therapy is not recommended during pregnancy because there is no previous experience [30, 31].

Supportive therapy Usually, supportive therapy can be provided according to general recommendations. Regarding steroids, methylprednisolone and hydrocortisone are preferred because they are metabolized in the placenta. In animal models, repeated use of dexamethasone/betamethasone resulted in decreased body and brain weight, growth retardation, and hormonal anomalies; in utero exposure to these drugs is thought to be related to cerebral palsy and attention problems. Colony-stimulating and erythropoiesis-stimulating factors have been used without complications in pregnant women. Table 16.1 shows the fetal safety profile of the most frequently used supportive drugs [32, 33].

Table 16.1 Supportive drugs and their fetal safety profile

Drug	Fetal safety
Antiemetics	
Metoclopramide	Can be used throughout the entire pregnancy
4HT antagonists	Do not avoid. Animal models suggest low risk. Has been used to effectively control nausea without adverse effects
NK1 antagonists	Do not avoid. Animal models suggest low risk
Steroids	Can be used during the first trimester. Prednisolone and hydrocortisone are preferred
Growth factors	
Filgrastim	Do not avoid. Crosses placenta into the fetus
Erythropoietin	Do not avoid. Most likely does not cross the placenta into the fetus
Analgesics	
Paracetamol	Preferably dosed at no more than 4 g/day
NSAIDs	Can be used from gestational weeks 12 through 32

Pregnancy resolution Vaginal birth has been associated with a higher risk of CC recurrence; therefore, delivery by cesarean section is recommended. One of seven (14%) women with CC who had a cesarean section experienced disease recurrence, while ten of seventeen (59%) who gave birth vaginally had distant metastasis [34].

CC in reproductive-age patients Up to 15% of women diagnosed with CC are less than 40 years old. Some are diagnosed during pregnancy prior to bearing the desired number of children. Patients diagnosed with stage IA1 disease without lymphovascular invasion but with negative margins can be treated with conization. Radical vaginal trachelectomy with laparoscopic lymphadenectomy is the most accepted procedure when attempting to preserve fertility, with 700 case reports of 250 pregnancies and 100 live births [35, 36].

16.2 Follow-Up

Historically, the main objective of follow-up for cancer patients has been to detect recurrence at an early stage; nevertheless, after a cancer diagnosis, patients face a series of challenges in different aspects of their life, including physical, psychosocial, spiritual, and existential issues. Furthermore, patients must cope with loss of economic income, inability to continue schooling or a job, hindrances in personal development, and lifestyle changes regarding societal, familial, and partner relationships. Some of the changes related to the disease or its treatment are transitory (e.g., loss of hair, nausea, and fatigue), while others are irreversible, such as infertility and late secondary effects, including cardiac toxicity, neuropathy and cognitive deterioration [37].

These patients frequently face the challenge of restarting their sexual life and rebuilding their life as a partner. For these reasons, CC patients, as well as all other cancer survivors, face different degrees of transitory or permanent anxiety and stress. For most patients, their biggest fear is related to the risk of recurrence [38].

Symptoms related to the treatment are also common once the treatment period ends. During this phase, anguish, insomnia, or depression often occur; patients suffering from these syndromes may need special psychological support. Most surgical treatments for CC do not affect sexual function. However, patients consciously or unconsciously perceive changes in their femininity because of treatment consequences or emotional conditions, causing meaningful changes in sexual performance. Radiotherapy can weaken the lining of the bladder, rectum or vagina, thus causing consequential, yet usually reversible, problems with urination, defecation, and sexual intercourse. Nonetheless, lack of open-mindedness on the part of the patient and the physician because of sociocultural issues leaves these problems unresolved.

Other typical effects of chemotherapy, such as memory disorders, difficulty concentrating, and fatigue, disappear within months.

16.2.1 Medical Follow-Up

After treatment is concluded, specialists propose a follow-up plan consisting of periodic consultations as detailed below.

The detection of possible tumor recurrence: The frequency and methodology of tumor surveillance is dependent on the initial clinical stage and the adequacy of the treatment provided for the patient's clinical condition. Other relevant aspects include histology and histological grade.

In general terms, for a previously treated clinical stage 0 patient with 3 sequential tests that yielded normal results within 2 years, the risk of CC recurrence is the same as the risk of primary CC in a healthy woman. After 2 years, these women can follow the regular surveillance scheme for healthy women (Papanicolaou test every 3 years).

In patients with more advanced stage disease, the recommendation is to perform clinical and gynecological exams (including Papanicolaou tests) at a 3-month periodicity during the first 2 years, a 6-month periodicity during the next 3 years, and yearly thereafter.

In previously treated patients with advanced stage disease, medical history should be periodically reviewed along with symptomatic consultations and physical examinations, and further exams should be performed whenever an anomaly is found. Moreover, the adverse effects of the treatment must be evaluated and addressed, and psychological support should be provided to help the patient return to her normal daily life.

Recurrences can be local, regional or distant. Based on our current knowledge, there are no specific recommendations for reducing the risk of recurrence after concluding treatment. Both the disease itself and the adverse effects of treatment can make it difficult to return to normal daily life.

16.2.2 Recurrent CC

The risk of recurrence is 70% in the first 2–3 years after diagnosis for cases of locally advanced disease; this probability decreases continuously thereafter, but it never reaches zero. Recurrences have been reported 13, and even 30, years after initial diagnosis.

16.3 General Recommendations

16.3.1 Proper Follow-Up After the End of Treatment

The main objective of follow-up in patients who have already completed or are still receiving adjuvant therapy is to detect recurrences early in order to initiate adequate and timely treatment. Table 16.2 describes the internationally accepted recommendations for these patients and their periodicity: orientation and education about the signs and symptoms of recurrence. Self-examinations, physical examinations by an oncologist, cytology, imaging, and pertinent laboratory tests. There are numerous diagnostic resources, but not all have demonstrated value.

An oncologist cannot see metastases and current imaging and laboratory tests are unable to diagnose a recurrence, according to international consensus. Tumor markers, thorax radiography, tomography, nuclear medicine studies and PET/CT are not recommended as a first option but are indicated in specific circumstances and as secondary options.

Table 16.2 Recommendations for patient follow-up

Procedure	Frequency
Patient orientation about signs and symptoms of recurrence	At the end of the initial treatment
Physical examination by an oncologist or a gynecologic oncologist	Every 3 months during the first 2 years
	Every 6 months from years 3–5
	Annually beginning in year 5
Tomography, bone scintigraphy, PET, PET/CT or MRI	Only when symptoms are present
Laboratory tests: complete blood count, blood chemistry, creatinine, blood urea nitrogen and LFT	Only when recurrence is suspected
Tumor markers	Not recommended
Scrutiny for other neoplasias, such as endometrial, ovarian or colon cancer	Annually
Patient education regarding symptoms of potential recurrence, lifestyle, obesity, exercise, smoking cessation and nutrition counseling	After treatment and every 3 or 4 months as necessary
Patient education regarding sexual health, vaginal dilator use, and vaginal lubricants/moisturizers (e.g., estrogen creams)	After treatment and every 3 or 4 months as necessary

Signs and symptoms of recurrent cervical cancer are described in Table 16.3.

In the case of a documented recurrence with a confirmatory biopsy, meticulous physical examinations and restaging are necessary based on the laboratory and imaging findings and the symptoms.

Classifying the disease as local or disseminated will enable the clinical to establish the scope of the treatment.

In CC, the treatment objectives are as follows:

- Prolong progression-free survival and overall survival;
- Palliate the symptoms;
- Maintain a proper quality of life and a good functional state.

To achieve such objectives, the best therapeutic strategy must be chosen after considering the tumor biology and clinical factors and the unique characteristics of each patient, such as the following:

- Patient age
- Symptoms
- Functional state
- Concomitant diseases
- Disease-free interval
- Disease aggressiveness
- Number, localization, and volume of metastases
- Previous treatment and associated response
- Patient preferences

In cases of recurrent disease, other additional factors must be evaluated, such as the patient's support network, her family, economic resources, and medical services. Clinicians rely on these important factors to orient the patient and her relatives and friends to ensure the best possible care while taking into account the emotional, spiritual and social support structures. It is important to remember that children in the family may be extremely worried about their mother's disease and may require additional attention to help them cope with the situation.

Table 16.3 Signs and symptoms of recurrent cervical cancer

Weight loss
Leg edema
Pelvic and/or thigh-buttock pain
Serosanguineous vaginal discharge
Progressive ureteral obstruction
Supraclavicular lymph node enlargement
Cough
Hemoptysis
Chest pain
Lumbar pain

16.4 Conclusions

Considering the unique circumstances of each woman with CC, it is fundamental to provide established treatment based on clinical stage, but with specific adjustments, to best influence symptomatic improvement and overall survival. The oncologists who attend to patients suffering from this pathology know that the cancer, co-morbidity factors, and sociocultural limitations continuously faced by these patients must be addressed in unison.

Medical follow-up must be continuously reinforced with educational, psychological, emotional and sexual support in order to enable a patient to recover her regular sexual, familial, social, and professional life.

CC is detectable in the early phase and is currently preventable through the application of vaccines and a non-promiscuous sexual code of conduct. Thus, efforts must be tireless in eradicating this pathology during the premalignant phases.

References

1. DiSaia PJ, Creasman WT. Invasive cervical cancer. In: Clinical gynecologic oncology. 5th ed. ST Louis: Mosby; 1997.
2. Horan G, McArdle O, Martin J, Collins CD, Faul C. Pelvic radiotherapy in patients with hydronephrosis in stage IIIB cancer of the cervix: renal effects and the optimal timing for urinary diversion? Gynecol Oncol. 2006;101(3):441–4.
3. Hausegger KA, Portugaller HR. Percutaneous nephrostomy and antegrade ureteral stenting: technique-indications-complications. Eur Radiol. 2006;16(9):2016–30.
4. Kose O, Gorgel SN, Ozbir S, Yenigurbuz S, Kara C. Manual replacement of double j stent without fluoroscopy (Double j stent replacement). Int Surg. 2015;100(2):381–5. doi:10.9738/INTSURG-D-13-00248.1.
5. Kouba E, Wallen EM, Pruthi RS. Management of ureteral obstruction due to advanced malignancy: optimizing therapeutic and palliative outcomes. J Urol. 2008;180(2):444–50. doi:10.1016/j.juro.2008.04.008. Epub 2008 Jun 11. Review.
6. Hogan DB, Ebly EM, Fung TS. Disease, disability, and age in cognitively intact seniors: results from the Canadian Study of health and aging. J Gerontol A Biol Sci Med Sci. 1999;54(2):M77–82.
7. Erhsler WB. A gerontologist's perspective on cancer biology and treatment. Cancer Control, J Moffitt Cancer Center. 1994;1:103–8.
8. Erhsler WB. Tumor-host interaction in the experimental system. In: Balducci L, Lyman GH, Ershler WB, editors. Comprehensive geriatric oncology. London: Harwood Academic Publishers; 1998. p. 201–2.
9. Antoni S, Soerjomataram I, Møller B, Bray F, Ferlay J. An assessment of GLOBOCAN methods for deriving national estimates of cancer incidence. Bull World Health Organ. 2016;94(3):174–84. doi:10.2471/BLT.15.164384. Epub 2016 Jan 28.
10. Department of Economic and Social Affairs. Population division. World population aging: 1950–2050. New York: Naciones Unidas ; 2001.ISBN 92-1- 051092-5.
11. Gross JL, de Azevedo MJ, Silveiro SP, Canani LH, Caramori ML, Zelmanovitz T. Diabetic nephropathy: diagnosis, prevention, and treatment. Diabetes Care. 2005;28(1):164–76. Review.
12. Cerasola G, Mule' G, Cottone S, Nardi E, Cusimano P. Hypertension, microalbuminuria and renal dysfunction: the Renal Dysfunction in Hypertension (REDHY) study. J Nephrol. 2008;21(3):368–73.

13. Cetina L, Rivera L, Candelaria M, de la Garza J, Dueñas-González A. Chemoradiation with gemcitabine for cervical cancer in patients with renal failure. Anticancer Drugs. 2004;15(8):761–6.
14. Cetina L, Garcia-Arias A, Uribe MJ, Candelaria M, Rivera L, Oñate-Ocaña L, Coronel J, Dueñas-Gonzalez A. Concurrent chemoradiation with carboplatin for elderly, diabetic and hypertensive patients with locally advanced cervical cancer. Eur J Gynaecol Oncol. 2008;29(6):608–12.
15. Coronel JA, Cetina Ldel C, Cantú D, Cerezo O, Hernández CS, Rivera L, Chacón AP, Duenas-Gonzalez A. A randomized comparison of cisplatin and oral vinorelbine as radiosensitizers in aged or comorbid locally advanced cervical cancer patients. Int J Gynecol Cancer. 2013;23(5):884–9. doi:10.1097/IGC.0b013e3182915c69.
16. Autran R, Figueredo MK, Leite A, Souza CR, Chaorro J, Chada E. Association of cervical intraepitelial neoplasia with CD 4 T cell counts and viral loadin HIV- infected women. RBGO. 2004;26(2):56–67.
17. Hwang JP, Granwehr BP, Torres HA, Suarez-Almazor ME, Giordano TP, Barbo AG, Lin HY, Fisch MJ, Chiao EY. HIV testing in patients with cancer at the initiation of therapy at a large US Comprehensive Cancer Center. J Oncol Pract. 2015;11(5):384–90. doi:10.1200/JOP.2015.005116. Epub 2015 Aug 4.
18. Russomano F, Reis A, Camargo MJ, Grinszteja B, Tristao MA. Recurrence of cervical intraepitelial neoplasia grades 2 or 3 in HIV- infected women treated by large loop escisión of the transformation zone(LLETZ). Sao Paulo Med. 2008;26(1):17–22.
19. Massad LS, Xie X, Burk RD, D'Souza G, Darragh TM, Minkoff H, Colie C, Burian P, Palefsky J, Atrio J, Strickler HD. Association of cervical precancer with human papillomavirus types other than 16 among HIV co-infected women. Am J Obstet Gynecol. 2016;214(3):354.e1–6. doi:10.1016/j.ajog.2015.09.086. Epub 2015 Nov 14.
20. Mamprim R, Giri AA, Cavatorta AL. Nature of the papillomavirus infection in human inmunodeficiency virus- infected women. Actual. SIDA. 2009;17(64):44–51.
21. Denslow SA, Westreich DJ, Firnhaber C, Michelow P, Williams S, Smith JS. Bacterial vaginosis as a risk factor for high-grade cervical lesions and cancer in HIV-seropositive women. Int J Gynaecol Obstet. 2011;114(3):273–7. doi:10.1016/j.ijgo.2011.03.011. Epub 2011 Jun 16.
22. Bower M, Palfreeman A, Alfa-Wali M, Bunker C, Burns F, Churchill D, Collins S, Cwynarski K, Edwards S, Fields P, Fife K, Gallop-Evans E, Kassam S, Kulasegaram R, Lacey C, Marcus R, Montoto S, Nelson M, Newsom-Davis T, Orkin C, Shaw K, Tenant-Flowers M, Webb A, Westwell S, Williams M, British HIV Association. British HIV Association guidelines for HIV-associated malignancies 2014. HIV Med. 2014;15(Suppl 2):1–92. doi:10.1111/hiv.12136.
23. Cardonick E, Iacobucci A. Use of chemotherapy during pregnancy. Lancet Oncol. 2004;5:283–91.
24. Gustafsson L, Ponten J, Zack M, et al. International incidence rates of invasive cervical cancer after introduction of cylogical screening. Cancer Causes Control. 1997;8:755–63.
25. Pavlidis NA. Coexistence of pregnancy and malignancy. Oncologist. 2002;7:279–87.
26. Mcintyre SK, Lesnock JL. Cervical cancer, screening in pregnancy. Obstet Clin N Am. 2008;35:645–58.
27. Morice P, Uzam C, Gouy S, Verschraegen C, Haie-Meder C. Gynaecological cancers in pregnancy. Lancet. 2012;379(9815):558–69.
28. Alouini S, Rida K, Mathevet P. Cervical cancer complicating pregancy: implicatons of laparoscopic lymphadenectomy. Gynecol Oncol. 2008;108(3):472–7.
29. Ishioka S, Endo T, Hayashi T, Baba T, Umemura K, Saito T. Pregnancy-related complicatons after vaginal radical trachelectomy for early-stage-invasive uterine cervical cancer. Int J Clin Oncol. 2007;12:350–5.
30. Caluwaerts S, VAN Calsteren K, Mertens L, Lagae L, Moerman P, Hanssens M, Wuyts K, Vergote I, Amant F. Neoadyuvant chemotherapy followed by radical hysterectomy for invasive cervical cancer diagnosed duringe pregnancy: report of a case and review of literatura. Int J Gynecol Cancer. 2006;16(2):905–8.
31. du Bois A, Quinn M, Thigpen T, et al. 2004 consensus statements on the management of ovarian cancer: final document of the 3rd International Gynecologic Cancer Intergroup Ovarian Cancer Consensus Conference (GCIG OCCC). Ann Oncol. 2005;16:viii7–12.

32. Blanford AT, Murphy BE. In vitro metabolism of prednisolone, dexamethasone, betamethasone and cortisol by the human placenta. Am J Obstet Gynecol. 1977;127:264–7.
33. Gralla RJ, Osoba D, Kris MG, Kirkbride P, Hesketh PJ, Chinnery LW, Clark-Snow R, Gill DP, Groshen S, Grunberg S, Koeller JM, Morrow GR, Perez EA, Silber JH, Pfister DG. Recommendations for the use of antiemetics: evidence-based, clinical practice guidelines. American Society of Clinical Oncology. J Clin Oncol. 1999;17:2971–94. Erratum in: J Clin Oncol 2000 Aug;18(16):3064. J Clin Oncol 1999 Dec;17(12):3860.
34. Sood AK, Sorosky JI, Mayr N, Anderson B, Buller RE, Niebyl J. Cervical cancer diagnosed shortly after pregnancy: pronostic variables and delivery routes. Obstet Gynecol. 2000;95:832–8.
35. Nishio H, Fujii T, Sugiyama J, Kuji N, Tanaka M, Hamatani T, Miyakoshi K, Minegishi K, Tsuda H, Iwata T, Tanaka K, Fukuchi T, Takehara Y, Yoshimura Y, Aoki D. Reproductive and obstetric outcomes after radical abdominal trachelectomy for esarly-stage cervical cancer in a series of 31 pregnancies. Hum Reprod. 2013;28(7):1793–8. doi:10.1093/humrep/det118. Epub 2013 Apr 26.
36. Gien LT, Convens A. Fertility-sparing options for early stage cervical cancer. Gynecol Oncol. 2010;117:350–7.
37. Ness KK, Krull KR, Jones KE, Mulrooney DA, Armstrong GT, Green DM, Chemaitilly W, Smith WA, Wilson CL, Sklar CA, Shelton K, Srivastava DK, Ali S, Robison LL, Hudson MM. Physiologic frailty as a sign of accelerated aging among adult survivors of childhood cancer: a report from the St Jude Lifetime cohort study. J Clin Oncol. 2013;31(36):4496–503. doi:10.1200/JCO.2013.52.2268. Epub 2013 Nov 18.
38. Jefford M, Karahalios E, Pollard A, Baravelli C, Carey M, Franklin J, Aranda S, Schofield P. Survivorship issues following treatment completion-results from focus groups with Australian cancer survivors and health professionals. J Cancer Surviv. 2008;2(1):20–32. doi:10.1007/s11764-008-0043-4. Epub 2008 Jan 25.

Index

J.G. de la Garza-Salazar et al. (eds.), *Cervical Cancer*,
DOI 10.1007/978-3-319-45231-9

MIX
Papier aus verantwortungsvollen Quellen
Paper from responsible sources
FSC® C105338

If you have any concerns about our products,
you can contact us on
ProductSafety@springernature.com

In case Publisher is established outside the EU,
the EU authorized representative is:
Springer Nature Customer Service Center GmbH
Europaplatz 3, 69115 Heidelberg, Germany

Printed by Libri Plureos GmbH
in Hamburg, Germany